Gastrointestinal Bleeding

Gastrointestinal Bleeding

Edited by

Neville Krasner

Consultant Gastroenterologist
Fazakerley Hospital, Liverpool, UK

BMJ
Publishing
Group

© BMJ Publishing Group 1996

First published 1996
by the BMJ Publishing Group, BMA House, Tavistock Square,
London WC1H 9JR

British Library Cataloguing in Publication Data

A catalogue record for this book is available from the
British Library

ISBN 0-7279-1008-6

Typeset by Latimer Trend & Company Ltd, Plymouth
Printed by Craft Print, Singapore

Contents

Part IV   Bleeding from varices

Part V   Lower gastrointestinal haemorrhage

Part VI Diagnosis and management of lower intestinal haemorrhage

Part VII Paediatric gastrointestinal bleeding

Part VIII Conclusions

Contributors

David J Allison
Professor and Director
Department of Imaging Radiology, Royal Postgraduate Medical School,
Hammersmith Hospital, London, UK

J N Baxter
Professor of Surgery and Consultant Surgeon
Morriston Hospital, Swansea, UK

Ian W Booth
Professor of Paediatric Gastroenterology and Nutrition
Institute of Child Health, Birmingham, UK

Michael J Bourke
Fellow in Therapeutic Endoscopy and Endoscopic Oncology
Division of Gastroenterology, The Wellesley Hospital, Toronto, Canada

A K Burroughs
Consultant Physician and Hepatologist
Department of Liver Transplantation and Hepatobiliary Medicine, Royal
Free Hospital, London, UK

John D Cunningham
Assistant Professor of Surgery
Department of Surgery, Mount Sinai Medical Center, New York, USA

R Dick
Consultant Radiologist
Department of Radiology, Royal Free Hampstead NHS Trust, London,
UK

Grant M Fullarton
Consultant Gastrointestinal Surgeon
West Glasgow Hospitals University NHS Trust, Department of Surgical
Gastroenterology, Gartnavel General Hospital, Glasgow, UK

David J Galloway
Consultant Colorectal Surgeon
West Glasgow Hospitals University NHS Trust, Department of Surgical
Gastroenterology, Gartnavel General Hospital, Glasgow, UK

A E S Gimson
Consultant Physician and Hepatologist
Cambridge Hepatobiliary and Liver Transplant Unit, Addenbrooke's
Hospital, Cambridge, UK

Adrian J Greenstein
Professor of Surgery
Department of Surgery, Mount Sinai Medical Center, New York, USA

C J Hawkey
Professor
Division of Gastroenterology, University Hospital, Nottingham, UK

James E Jackson
Senior Lecturer and Honorary Consultant
Department of Imaging Radiology, Royal Postgraduate Medical School,
Hammersmith Hospital, London, UK

A K Kubba
Research Registrar
Gastrointestinal Unit, Western General Hospital, Edinburgh, UK

Neville Krasner
Consultant Gastroenterologist
Fazakerley Hospital, Liverpool, UK

John G Lee
Assistant Professor of Medicine
Oregon Health Sciences University, Gastroenterology Section, Portland
Veterans Administration Medical Center, Portland, USA
Division of Gastroenterology, University of California Davis Medical
Center, Sacramento, California, US

Joseph W Leung
Professor of Medicine and Chief of Gastroenterology
University of California Davis Medical Center, Sacramento, California,
US

G R Lipscomb
Senior Registrar
Department of Gastroenterology, Manchester Royal Infirmary,
Manchester, UK

Norman E Marcon
Chief
Division of Gastroenterology, The Wellesley Hospital, Toronto, Canada

A I Morris
Consultant Physician and Gastroenterologist
Royal Liverpool University Hospital, Liverpool, UK

M Stephen Murphy
Senior Lecturer in Paediatrics and Child Health and Honorary
Consultant in Paediatric Gastroenterology
Institute of Child Health, Birmingham, UK

K R Palmer
Consultant Physician
Gastrointestinal Unit, Western General Hospital, Edinburgh, UK

D Patch
Department of Liver Transplantation and Hepatobiliary Medicine, Royal
Free Hospital, London, UK

W D W Rees
Consultant Physician/Gastroenterologist
Salford Royal Hospitals NHS Trust, Salford, UK

Paul Swain
Reader in Medicine/Consultant Gastroenterologist
The Royal London Hospital, London, UK

J Tibbals
Department of Radiology, Royal Free Hampstead NHS Trust, London,
UK

J M T Willoughby
Consultant Physician and Gastroenterologist
Lister Hospital, Stevenage, Hertfordshire, UK

Andrew Wu
Consultant Surgeon
Fazakerley Hospital, Liverpool, UK

Preface

Overall mortality rates from upper gastrointestinal bleeding remain unacceptably high at 8–10%, when perhaps a realistic and more acceptable figure would be half of that. The initial diagnosis and management of upper gastrointestinal bleeding is traditionally the province of physicians, whereas bleeding from the lower gastrointestinal tract tends to be referred to surgeons. However, individual units will handle such cases in their own way, with or without adherence to a defined protocol, and herein lies the problem.

Endoscopy undoubtedly allows more accurate diagnosis of bleeding lesions throughout the gastrointestinal tract, but the timing of the procedure and the necessity for emergency endoscopy is open to debate in the individual case. Can any competent clinician assume responsibility for an "acute bleeder", or should the patient be admitted to a high dependency "bleeding unit"? Should a management care plan be implemented or can the same results be achieved by a committed team with a less formal protocol? Whatever system a unit adopts, regular audit of the management of upper and lower gastrointestinal bleeding is essential and should assess the use of endoscopic and radiological facilities.

Physicians and surgeons will find a comprehensive review of gastrointestinal bleeding, from the scope of the problem and its background aetiology, through the clinical recognition and investigation of the condition, to current and new approaches to its management. I have been fortunate in assembling a distinguished international team of contributors, and it is a pleasure to acknowledge and thank them for their involvement.

Neville Krasner
Liverpool
1996

Part I
Upper gastrointestinal haemorrhage: the nature of the problem

1: Epidemiology and aetiology of upper gastrointestinal bleeding

C J HAWKEY

Upper gastrointestinal bleeding remains the most common gastrointestinal emergency. In western countries it is the cause of 50–100 hospital admissions per 100 000 of the population each year,[1–13] and in the UK causes about 5000 deaths per annum.[1–3] A recent audit by the British Society of Gastroenterology (BSG) found an overall incidence of 100 per 100 000 adults per annum, confirming earlier impressions that the rate of presentation with upper gastrointesinal bleeding has not changed appreciably over the past 30–40 years.[13] Mortality also remains obstinately irreducible.[1–6 8 9] The BSG audit found an overall mortality of 14%,[13] suggesting that outcome, like incidence, has changed little in recent years.

Changing Epidemiology

These statistics conceal more than they reveal. Upper gastrointestinal bleeding in general and peptic ulcer bleeding in particular have become diseases of the elderly to a much greater extent than they were previously.[1 3 6–9 11 12–18] Because mortality from upper gastrointestinal bleeding is more common in elderly people[3 19–21] the stability or even slight decline of the death rate probably reflects an improvement in age related outcomes (Figure 1.1). Peptic ulcer remains the commonest cause of gastrointestinal bleeding in nearly all series (Table 1.1), but there is considerable variation in the proportion of patients with variceal bleeding, which tends to be low in United Kingdom series and high in those from the US.[2 7 16 17 22–30] The age of the patient and the nature of the underlying lesion strongly affect outcome, so it is difficult to know whether wide differences in mortality—which ranges in different series from 4 to 15% and in the BSG

3

audit from 0 to 28% in different hospitals—reflect differences in case mix or management.[13]

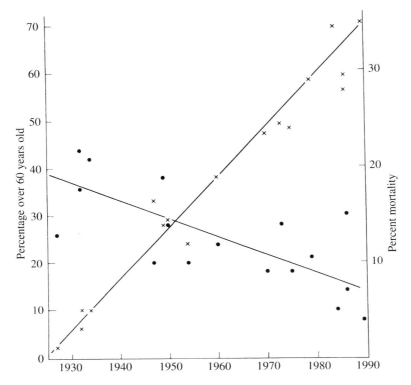

FIGURE 1.1—*Trends in mortality (•) and age distribution (x) for upper gastrointestinal bleeding (reproduced with permission from Dronfield MW. Upper gastrointestinal bleeding.* In: Misiewicz JJ, Pounder RE, Venables CW, eds. *Diseases of the gut and pancreas,* Blackwell Scientific, 1994, p. 368).

Causes of Upper Gastrointestinal Bleeding

The commonest causes of upper gastrointestinal bleeding reported from major trials are listed in Table 1.1, and some less common causes in Box 1.1.

Box 1.1 Rarer causes of upper gastrointestinal bleeding

Ulcers
- Stomal ulcer
- Stress ulcer

Vascular causes
Osler–Weber–Rendu syndrome
Pseudoxanthoma elasticum
continued

Neoplasms	Ehlers–Danlos syndrome
• Carcinoma	Blue rubber bleb naevus syndrome
• Leiomyoma	Other arteriovenous malformations
• Lymphoma	Vasculitis
• Polyps	
• Other malignancies	

Peptic ulceration

Peptic ulcer accounts for 30–60% of all episodes of upper gastrointestinal bleeding, while bleeding is the commonest complication of peptic ulceration and occurs relatively often. It used to be said that 15–20% of patients with ulcers experience haemorrhage, the annual risk being 4%.[31-35] More recent information suggests that the prevalence of peptic ulcer, which is often silent, may be higher than previously recognised, at around 20% for patients not taking non-steroidal anti-inflammatory drugs (NSAIDs) and similar values for patients taking NSAIDs;[37] both figures are compatible with a complication rate close to 1% per annum.

Causes of ulcer bleeding

Most peptic ulcers are caused by *Helicobacter pylori* infection or NSAID usage.[20 21 37-51] Several series have suggested that NSAID usage accounts for 22–31% of all ulcer bleeds in elderly patients.[38 44 46 47] When ulcer bleeds associated with (sometimes surreptitious[52]) aspirin usage are also included, about half of peptic ulcer bleeds can be attributed to aspirin and nonaspirin NSAIDs. The presumption has been that the rest are attributable to *H. pylori* infection, but in two recent trials a significant number of patients with bleeding peptic ulcer were neither infected by *H. pylori* nor taking NSAIDs;[50 51] whether this finding reflects occult or undetected NSAID usage is not clear.[52] Provisional data also suggest that *H. pylori* and NSAIDs act as relatively independent risk factors for ulcer bleeding, with the risk of NSAID associated ulcer bleeding being similar whether or not patients are infected with *H. pylori*.[51]

Risk factors for presentation

The main factors that increase the risk of a patient with a peptic ulcer developing upper gastrointestinal bleeding are past history, age, and NSAID usage.[20 21 37 46 47 53 54] The epidemiology of peptic ulcer complications (mainly bleeding) was investigated using data from the VAMP computer system (Figure 1.2). VAMP is the computer system used by the largest number of GPs. It was found that patients over 60 are about three times more likely than patients under 60 to present with ulcer bleeding,[20] while NSAID users are overall about three times more likely than nonusers to present with ulcer bleeding. Age and NSAID usage show a positive interaction

TABLE 1.1—*Common causes (%) of upper gastrointestinal bleeding reported from major trials.*

Country	US	England	England	Australia	Scotland	Wales	Denmark	Several	England	US	England
Year of report	1981	1983	1985	1985	1986	1986	1986	1986	1990	1991	1991
Reference	22	23	27	24	26	16	25	28	17	30	29
No. of patients	100	775		201	326	330	539	443	430	445	1147
Peptic ulcer	40	50		43	52	48	53	37	50	40	40
Gastric ulcer	18	24			16	19			25	13	15
Duodenal ulcer	22	26			30	29			25	27	75
Erosions	6	7		12	6	14	12	7	22	3	9
Gastric										3	7
Duodenal											2
Oesophageal varices	20	3		8	2	3	11	13	4	31	2
Oesophageal ulcer			7		15	7	13	4	12	2	15
Mallory–Weiss tear			5	4	2	5	3	3	4	13	3
Malignancy		2	2		1	3	2	3	1	1	1
Vascular lesions										1	0·1
Other cause	16	11·8		17	23	20	5	34	7	9	21·7

that may be additive or multiplicative. Patients with a past history of known peptic ulcer or ulcer bleeding have increased risk that interacts positively with NSAID usage.

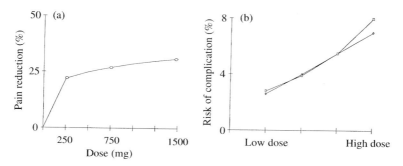

FIGURE 1.2—*Interaction of non-steroidal anti-inflammatory drugs (NSAIDs) with patient's age and past history in determining increased risk of upper gastrointestinal bleeding.*[20]

Risk factors among NSAID users

Established risk factors specific to NSAID users are dose, individual drug, and steroid usage.[20 21 37 46 47 53 54] Many studies (but not all[20]) suggest that about one half of patients will present with ulcer bleeding within 3 months of starting an NSAID.[38 42 47]

Several studies (Figure 1.3) have shown a linear relationship between the risk of NSAID associated ulcer bleeding and the dose of the NSAID used.[20 21 42 45–47] More than 12 have included data on individual NSAIDs. A meta analysis of these suggests strongly that the level of risk associated with ibuprofen is significantly lower than the average NSAID related risk,[20 21 49 54] and this conclusion is supported by two large studies that have investigated individual NSAIDs.[20 21 49] NSAIDs associated with an increased risk of peptic ulcer bleeding seem to be azapropazone, piroxicam and indomethacin. Differences in toxocity may, for many of these drugs, relate to differences in potency. The particularly high risks associated with azapropazone have not been explained, and might reflect the type of patient receiving the drug or the pattern of usage.

The absolute risk of peptic complications in NSAID users (who are usually elderly) has been estimated in several studies to be in a range between 1 in 20 and 1 in 200 patient years.[37 42 44 46 53 55] A prospective trial has shown a rate of one complication per 45 patient years in a cohort of patients over the age of 52 (mean age 68). On the basis that half of these complications involve ulcer bleeding, the risk is about 1 in 100 patient years.[55]

Most NSAID associated ulcer bleeds occur early,[38 42 47] about half in the first 3 months of usage; risk thereafter declines, probably by a process of

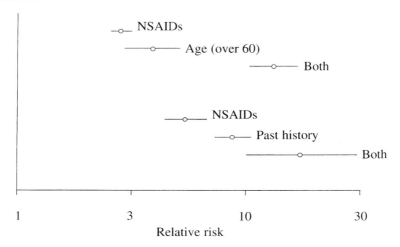

FIGURE 1.3—*Finding a balance in therapy with non-steroidal anti-inflammatory drugs: dose dependence of (a) benefit and (b) risk of ulcer bleeding complications.*

attrition, but remains elevated. The most likely reason for early presentation is provocation of bleeding in a pre-existing silent ulcer by the antihaemo-static effects of NSAIDs.[56]

Duodenal versus gastric ulceration

Duodenal ulcers predominate in most series of bleeding ulcers, but the ratio of duodenal to gastric ulcers (whether NSAID related or not) is usually less than two;[7 16 17 22–30] this ratio is lower than that of uncomplicated ulcers, and suggests that gastric ulcers are relatively more prone to bleed than duodenal ulcers.

Uncertain risk factors

Patients with congenital coagulation defects, those receiving warfarin, and those with abnormal platelet function or thrombocytopenia are more likely to present with ulcer bleeding.[2 25 26 57] Men are slightly more likely that women to present with ulcer bleeding,[20] reflecting the underlying prevalence of ulcer disease; women are slightly more likely than men to present with NSAID associated ulcer bleeding because they are more likely to receive the drugs. Older texts[31 32] mentioned renal failure, arthritis, portal hypertension, rheumatoid arthritis, alcohol and cirrhosis as risk factors for ulcer bleeding but there are no systematic data to suggest that they are.

Protective factors

Informal evidence and two clinical trials suggest that use of H_2 receptor antagonists not only reduces ulcer recurrence rate but also is disproportionately effective in reducing bleeding from ulcers that do recur.[9 58–60] One possible reason is that elevation of intragastric pH improves haemostasis.[61] Another is that ulcers that recur in patients taking H_2 antagonists may be less deep than those in patients not taking these drugs. Data also suggest that, for patients with bleeding ulcers unrelated to NSAID usage, eradication of *H. pylori* protects them from further ulcer bleeding.[62] NSAID users who take the cytoprotectant misoprostol appear to have a lower incidence of ulcer bleeding than do NSAID users not taking this drug.[55]

Gastric and duodenal erosions

Gastric and duodenal erosions (sometimes misleadingly described as gastritis and duodenitis, respectively) are often listed as the second commonest cause of upper gastrointestinal bleeding. This ranking is at variance with my own experience (and that of others[2]) and grossly over-estimates the importance of true erosions. The misconception probably arises for several reasons. Patients with erosions may vomit 'coffee grounds' or small amounts of blood, but erosions are seldom the cause of life threatening bleeding or large transfusion requirements.[30 65] Erosions may also be over-estimated as a cause of upper gastrointestinal bleeding by diagnostic inaccuracy, where a superficial ulcer may be reported as an erosion, or a bleeding ulcer missed but the often accompanying erosions reported. It seems likely also that some lesions diagnosed as erosions by one endoscopist would be diagnosed as ulcers by another.[66] The commonest causes of gastric erosions detected in patients with haematemesis and melaena are NSAIDs (where bleeding may be from an associated ulcer), and physical stress in patients being ventilated (in whom minor bleeding is common but major bleeding often results from an associated Cushing/Curling's ulcer.[67] Erosions can also occur because of acute alcohol ingestion,[30] but bleeding then is often trivial or confused with regurgitated Guinness!

Oesophagitis/oesophageal ulcer

Bleeding from oesophageal lesions is relatively common, and when from ulcers can be quite significant.[7 16 17 22–30]

Mallory–Weiss syndrome

A traumatic mucosal tear at the gastro-oesophageal junction[68–70] caused mechanically by prior retching or vomiting accounts for 1–16% of cases of upper gastrointestinal bleeding.[7 16 17 22–30] The classical history of vomiting without blood, followed by (often fresh) blood, may be absent. Mallory–Weiss tears appear to run a relatively benign course. Rarely they may cause a large, submucosal haematoma that results in dysphagia; this usually settles spontaneously.[71]

Oesophageal varices

The proportion of patients with upper gastrointestinal bleeding who have oesophageal varices ranges from 2–33% in different series.[7 13 16 17 22–30] Varices accounted for 4% of admissions in the BSG audit,[13] while in a previous survey by the American Society for Gastrointestinal Endoscopy, about 10% of patients were bleeding from oesophageal varices.[7 60] Bleeding from varices tends to be severe, and is associated with more complications, blood transfusions, interventions and deaths than are other causes of upper gastrointestinal bleeding.[30 72 73]

Patients with oesophageal varices account for about half of the patients classified as having severe or persistent haemorrhage (that is, requiring five or more units of blood to be transfused).[30 60 67 72]

Risk factors for variceal bleeding

Between 12% and 77% of patients with cirrhosis have oesophageal varices[73 74] and about 30% of patients with varices bleed from them.[73–78] Patients with cirrhosis therefore have a risk of variceal bleeding of about 15–20%. The risk appears to be lower in those with noncirrhotic portal hypertension.[79 80] Patients who have had one bleed from oesophageal varices are at increased risk compared with those who have not yet bled.[81] The main endoscopic determinant of risk is variceal size,[75] reflecting portal pressure.[76 82] Reflux of acid does not appear to be important.[83] Red markings detected on oesophageal varices may be associated with a higher risk of subsequent bleeding.[84–86]

Malignancy

Tumours, commonly cancer of the stomach, account for between 2–4% of cases of gastrointestinal bleeding.[7 13 16 17 22–30] Lymphoma, sarcoma and ulcerated leiomyomas may occasionally present with bleeding.

Portal hypertensive gastropathy

The congested gastropathy associated with portal hypertension results in endoscopic appearances that include pink speckling, a red mosaic pattern and red spots caused by vascular dilation and ectasia, which may be confused with intramuscosal petechiae and erosions.[86 88] Portal hypertensive gastropathy seems relatively uncommon, accounting for 20%, at most, of upper gastrointestinal bleeding in patients with portal hypertension, and less than 5% overall.

Aortoduodenal fistula

A fistula developing between an abdominal aortic aneurysm and the gastrointestinal tract is an uncommon but important cause of gastrointestinal bleeding. The haemorrhage can be severe and life threatening and diagnostically cryptic, because about three-quarters of aortoenteric fistulas communicate with the duodenum (usually the third part).[89–92] They occur in patients with abdominal aortic aneurysms and are more common in those who have had reconstructive surgery, where they develop in 0·5–2·4% of patients.[89 92] An aortoduodenal fistula is the classic cause of significant melaena without haematemesis followed by a normal bloodless endoscopy and should always be suspected, because an exsanguinating bleed usually ultimately occurs from an unrecognised fistula.

Vascular anomalies

A wide variety of vascular anomalies can rarely cause upper gastrointestinal bleeding. These include hereditary haemorrhagic telangiectases (Osler–Weber–Rendu syndrome),[93] pseudoxanthoma elasticum,[94] Ehlers–Danlos syndrome[95] and the blue rubber bleb naevus syndrome.[96 97] Patients with chronic renal failure appear to bleed relatively often from vascular ectasias.[98] Brisk bleeding can also occur from larger arteries, known as Dieulafoy's lesions or calibre persistent arteries,[99–101] which are mucosal end arteries that remain as large as their feeding submucosal arteries; they are most commonly found in the proximal stomach and can bleed without any ulceration of the overlying mucosa. Bleeding can be substantial and the diagnosis is difficult to make unless the lesion is actively bleeding at the time of endoscopy. Dieulafoy's lesions therefore account for a significant number of cases of recurrent upper gastrointestinal bleeding where a cause proves difficult to find.

Prognosis: Immediate Mortality

The risk of immediate death from gastrointestinal bleeding depends mainly on the nature of the underlying lesion and the age of the patient.[104–107] Older patients, those with ulcer bleeding, and those with varices are at a higher risk. Prior NSAID usage is probably not associated with increased in-hospital mortality.[108] Most deaths result not from exsanguination but from a complication provoked by the bleed, such as renal failure or stroke, or as a result of surgery for the bleed.[7 13 16 17 22–30 106–108]

Peptic ulcer

Gastric ulcers cause more deaths than do duodenal ulcers but this may reflect the age of the patients. Patients at particularly high risk can be identified at presentation and endoscopy. Factors associated with increased mortality are older age, comorbidity, shock, low haemoglobin, rebleeding, the underlying diagnosis and stigmata of recent haemorrhage.[13 30 110–112] These factors have been used to devise prognostic indices.[13] Some, but not all, series have associated ulcer bleeding with cardiovascular disease.[55 113–116]

Oesophageal varices

The acute mortality of variceal bleeding is in the range of 15–40%.[78–81][117–120] Variceal size, severity of liver disease and red markings on the varices are the most important predictive factors.[75][76][84][85][121][122] At least one-third of patients with oesophageal varices rebleed during the same hospital admission.[73][74][118–120]

Prognosis: Late Mortality

For some causes of upper gastrointestinal bleeding, such as gastric cancer or varices with cirrhosis, the underlying lesion that caused the bleeding is the main determinant of late morbidity and mortality; for others, such as peptic ulcer, this may not be so.

Peptic ulcer

The previously high rate of ulcer rebleeding after survival of a first episode[123][125] may have declined. A recent study found that the risk of death in elderly patients who had presented with ulcer bleeding was increased compared with that in controls. However, the cause of death was seldom recurrent ulcer pathology, most commonly being cardiovascular disease, respiratory disease including bronchopneumonia, or cancer.[116] The reason for these associations is not clear, but in some series cardiovascular disease has been a risk factor for initial or subsequent ulcer bleeding,[55][113–116] supporting the notion that local vascular disease may determine the likelihood of bleeding from an ulcer.

Oesophageal varices

As many as 60–80% of patients who present with bleeding oesophageal varices may be dead within 1–4 years.[126–128] Further variceal bleeding and liver failure are the main causes of death in advanced cirrhosis. Long term mortality increases with severe underlying liver disease particularly if the latter deteriorates rapidly.[78–81] Alcohol use, high bilirubin concentrations and low prothrombin time are also predictive of further rebleeding and death.[118–120][126–128]

Future Trends

It is hard to predict whether upper gastrointestinal bleeding will become more or less common. The influence of *H. pylori* may decline, either as a cohort of infected patients die or because of mass eradication, or it may increase if the prevalence of infection continues to increase in the currently middle aged as they grow older. The growing population of elderly patients may yield more ulcer bleeds associated with NSAID use, and current epidemiology identifies these as possibly more important than *H. pylori* infection in respect of ulcer complications. Alternatively, if non-gastrotoxic NSAIDs are well accepted and effective prophylaxis widely used, the NSAID associated ulcer bleed may become a rarity.

Key points

- Upper gastrointestinal bleeding is the commonest gastrointestinal emergency

- Incidence and mortality remain steady; the increasing proportion of elderly patients who present with bleeding and have a higher mortality probably masks improvements in age-related outcome

- Peptic ulcer is the commonest cause of upper gastrointestinal bleeding

- Most peptic ulcers are caused by infection with *Helicobacter pylori* or use of non-steroidal anti-inflammatory drugs

---

References

1 Dronfield MW. Upper gastrointestinal bleeding. In: Misiewicz JJ, Pounder RE, Venables CW, eds. *Diseases of the gut and pancreas.* Oxford: Blackwell Scientific, 19xx;367–80.
2 Laine L. Rolling review: upper gastrointestinal bleeding. *Aliment Pharmacol Ther* 1993;7: 207–32.
3 Allan R, Dykes P. A study of the factors influencing mortality rates from gastrointestinal haemorrhage. *Q J Med* 1976;45:533–50.
4 Elashoff JD, Grossman MI. Trends in hospital admission and death rates from peptic ulcer in the United States from 1970 to 1978. *Gastroenterology* 1980;78:280–5.
5 National Center for Health Statistics. *Annual summary for the United States, 1979.* Hyattsville, Maryland: National Center for Health Statistics 1980; DHSS Publication 28: 13.
6 Coggon D, Lambert P, Langman MJS. 20 years of hospital admissions for peptic ulcer in England and Wales. *Lancet* 1981;i:1302–4.
7 Gilbert DA, Silverstein FE, Tedesco FJ. National ASGE survey on upper gastrointestinal bleeding; complications of endoscopy. *Dig Dis Sci* 1981;26:55–9.
8 Kurata JH, Honda GD, Frankl H. Hospitalisation and mortality rates for peptic ulcers: a comparison of a large health maintenance organisation and United States data. *Gastroenterology* 1982;83:1008–16.
9 Kurata JH, Elashoff J, Haile BM, Honda GD. A re-appraisal of time trends in ulcer disease: factors related to changes in ulcer hospitalisation and mortality rates. *Am J Public Health* 1983;73:1066–72.
10 Scheerer DE, DeKryger LL, Dean RE. Surgical treatment of peptic ulcer disease before and after introduction of H$_2$ blockers. *Am J Surg* 1987;53:392–5.
11 Bardhan KD, Cust G, Hinchcliffe RFC, Williamson FM, Lyon C, Bose K. Changing pattern of admissions and operations for duodenal ulcer. *Br J Surg* 1989;76:230–6.
12 Henry D, Robertson J. Nonsteroidal anti-inflammatory drugs and peptic ulcer hospitalization rates in New South Wales. *Gastroenterology* 1993;104:1083–91.
13 Rockall TA, Logan RFA, Devlin HB, Northfield TC. Incidence and mortality of acute upper gastrointestinal bleeding (UGIB) in the UK. *Gut* 1994;33:Suppl 5:S47.
14 Dronfield MW. Medical or surgical treatment for haematemesis and melaena. *J R Coll Physicians Lond* 1979;13:84–6.
15 Hunt PS, Francis JK, Hansky J, *et al.* Reduction in mortality from upper gastrointestinal haemorrhage. *Med J Aust* 1983;2:552–5.
16 Madden MV, Griffith GH. Management of upper gastrointestinal bleeding in a district general hospital. *J R Coll Physicians* 1986;20:212–5.
17 Holman RAE, Davis M, Gough KR, Cartell P, Britton DC, Smith RB. Value of centralized approach in the management of haematemesis and melaena: experience in a district general hospital. *Gut* 1990;31:504–8.

18 Ohmann C, Thon K, Hengels J, Imhof M. Incidence and pattern of peptic ulcer bleeding in a defined geographical area. *Scand J Gastroenterol* 1992;**27**:571–81.

19 Langman MJS. Ulcer complications and nonsteroidal anti-inflammatory drugs. *Am J Med* 1988;**84**:15–19.

20 Garcia-Rodriguez LA, Jick H. Risk of upper gastrointestinal bleeding and perforation associated with individual non-steroidal anti-inflammatory drugs. *Lancet* 1994;**343**:769–72.

21 Langman MJS, Weil J, Wainwright P, *et al.* Risks of bleeding peptic ulcer associated with individual non-steroidal anti-inflammatory drugs. *Lancet* 1994;**343**:1075–8.

22 Peterson WL, Barnett CC, Smith HJ, Allen MH, Corbett DB. Routine early endoscopy in upper gastrointestinal tract bleeding. A randomized controlled trial. *N Engl J Med* 1981;**304**:925–9.

23 Barer D, Ogilvie A, Henry D, *et al.* Cimetidine and tranexamic acid in the treatment of acute upper gastrointestinal tract bleeding. *N Engl J Med* 1983;**26**:1571–5.

24 Rofe SB, Duggan JM, Smith ER, Thursby CJ. Conservative treatment of gastrointestinal haemorrhage. *Gut* 1985;**26**:481–4.

25 Wara P, Stodkilde H. Bleeding pattern before admission as guideline for emergency endoscopy. *Scand J Gastroenterol* 1985;**20**:72–8.

26 Clason AE, Macleod DAD, Elton RA. Clinical factors in the prediction of further haemorrhage or mortality in acute upper gastrointestinal haemorrhage. *Br J Surg* 1986;**73**:985–7.

27 Somerville KW, Henry DA, Davies JG, Hine KR, Hawkey CJ, Langman MJS. Somatostatin in treatment of haematemesis and melaena. *Lancet* 1985;**i**:130–2.

28 Morgan AG, Clamp SE. OMGE international gastrointestinal bleeding survey, 1978–1986. *Scand J Gastroenterol* 1988;**144(Suppl)**:51–8.

29 Daneshmend TK, Hawkey CJ, Langman MJS, Logan RFA, Long RG, Walt RP. Omeprazole versus placebo for acute upper gastrointestinal bleeding: randomised double blind controlled trial. *Br Med J* 1992;**304**:143–7.

30 Laine L. Upper gastrointestinal hemorrhage. *West J Med* 1991;**155**:274–9.

31 Lewin DC, Truelove S. Haematemesis. *Br Med J* 1949;**i**:383–6.

32 Ihamaki T, Varis K, Siurala M. Morphological, functional and immunological state of the gastric mucosa in gastric carcinoma families. *Scand J Gastroenterol* 1979;**14**:801–12.

33 Araki S, Goto Y. Peptic ulcer in male factory workers: survey of prevalence, incidence, and etiological factors. *J Epidemiol Comm Health* 1985;**39**:82–5.

34 Schoon IM, Mellstrom D, Oden A, Ytterberg BO. Incidence of peptic ulcer disease in Gothenburg 1985. *Br Med J* 1989;**299**:1131–4.

35 Bonnevie O. Survival in peptic ulcer. *Gastroenterology* 1978;**75**:1055–64.

36 Vaira D, Migloli M, Mule P, Holton J, Menegatti M, Vergura M, *et al.* Prevalence of peptic ulcer in *Helicobacter pylori* positive blood donors. *Gut* 1994;**35**:309–12.

37 Hawkey CJ, Hudson N. Mucosal injury induced by drugs, chemicals and stress. In: Haubrich W, Snaffer F, eds. *Bochu's gastroenterology*. 5th edn. London: Saunders, 1994.

38 Somerville K, Faulkner G, Langman M. Non steroidal anti-inflammatory drugs and bleeding peptic ulcer. *Lancet* 1986;**i**:462–4.

39 Committee on Safety of Medicines. Non-steroidal anti-inflammatory drugs and serious gastrointestinal adverse reactions. *BMJ* 1987;**292**:1190–1.

40 Armstrong CP, Blower AL. Non steroidal anti-inflammatory drugs and life threatening complications of peptic ulceration. *Gut* 1987;**28**:527–32.

41 Beard K, Walker AM, Perera DR, Jick H. Non steroidal anti-inflammatory drugs and hospitalization for gastroesophageal bleeding in the elderly. *Arch Intern Med* 1987;**147**:1621–3.

42 Carson JL, Strom BL, Soper KA, West SL, Morse L. The association of nonsteroidal anti-inflammatory drugs with upper gastrointestinal tract bleeding. *Arch Intern Med* 1987;**147**:85–8.

43 Levy M, Miller DR, Kaufman DW, *et al.* Major upper gastrointestinal tract bleeding. Relation to the use of aspirin and other nonarcotic analgesics. *Arch Intern Med* 1988;**148**:281–5.

44 Hawkey CJ. Non steroidal anti inflammatory drugs and ulcer: facts and figures multiply, but do they add up? *BMJ* 1990;**300**:278–84.

45 Laporte JR, Carne X, Vidal X, Moreno V, Juan J. Catalan countries study on upper gastrointestinal bleeding in relation to previous use of analgesics and non-steroidal anti-inflammatory drugs. *Lancet* 1991;**337**:85–9.

46 Griffin MR, Piper JM, Daughtery J, Snowden M, Ray WA. Nonsteroidal anti-inflammatory drug use and increased risk for peptic ulcer disease in elderly persons. *Ann Intern Med* 1991;**114**:257–63.
47 Gabriel SE, Jaakkimainen L, Bombardier C. Risk for serious gastrointestinal complications related to use of nonsteroidal anti-inflammatory drugs. A meta-analysis. *Ann Intern Med* 1991;**115**:787–96.
49 Bateman DN. NSAIDs: time to re-evaluate gut toxicity. *Lancet* 1994;**343**:1051–2.
50 Jensen DM, Cheng S, Kovacs TOG, *et al.* A controlled trial of ranitidine for the prevention of recurrent haemorrhage from duodenal ulcer. *N Engl J Med* 1994;**330**:382–6.
51 Cullen DJE, Hawkey GM, Humphries H, *et al.* Role of non steroidal anti inflammatory drugs and *Helicobacter pylori* in bleeding peptic ulcers [abstract]. *Gastroenterology* 1994; **106**:A66.
52 Lanas L, Sekar MC, Hirscowitz BI. Objective evidence of aspirin use in both ulcer and non-ulcer upper and lower gastrointestinal bleeding. *Gastroenterology* 1992;**103**:862–9.
53 Henry D, Dobson A, Turner C. Variability in the risk of major gastrointestinal complications from non aspirin nonsteroidal anti-inflammatory drugs. *Gastroenterology* 1993;**105**: 1078–88.
54 Henry DA. Meta analysis of the gastroduodenal risks of individual NSAIDs. International Conference in Pharmacoepidemiology, Stockholm 1994. *Pharmacoepidemiology and Drug Safety* 1995;
55 Silverstein FE, Geis GS, Struthers BJ, and the MUCOSA study group. NSAIDs and gastrointestinal injury: Clinical outcome, the mucosa trial. *Gastroenterology* 1994;**106**: A180.
56 Hawkey CJ, Hawthorne AB, Hudson N, Cole AT, Mahida YR, Daneshmend. Separation of the impairment of haemostasis by aspirin from mucosal injury in the human stomach. *Clin Sci* 1991;**81**:565–73.
57 Mittal R, Spero JA, Lewis JH, *et al.* Patterns of gastrointestinal haemorrhage in haemophilia. *Gastroenterology* 1985;**88**:515–22.
58 Gustavsson S, Kelly KA, Melton JL, Zinsmeister A. Trends in peptic ulcer surgery. *Gastroenterology* 1988;**94**:688–94.
59 Penston J, Wormsley KG. Efficacy and safety of long-term maintenance therapy of duodenal ulcers. *Scand J Gastroenterol* 1989;**24**:1145–52.
60 Jensen DM, Cheng S, Kovacs TOG, *et al.* Controlled study of ranitidine for the prevention of recurrent hemorrhage from duodenal ulcer. *N Engl J Med* 1994;**330**:382–6.
61 Cole AT, Brundell S, Hudson N, Hawthorne AB, Mahida YR, Hawkey CJ. Ranitidine-differential-effects on gastric bleeding and mucosal damage induced by aspirin. *Aliment Pharm Therap* 1992;**6**:707–15.
62 Graham DY, Hepps KS, Ramirez FC, Lew GM, Saeed ZA. Treatment of *Helicobacter pylori* reduces the rate of rebleeding in peptic ulcer disease. *Scand J Gastroenterol* 1993; **28**:939–42.
63 Labenz J, Borsch G. Evidence for the essential role of *Helicobacter pylori* in gastric ulcer disease. *Gut* 1994;**35**:19–22.
64 Santander C, Perez-Miranda M, Cedenilla AG, Carpintero P, Gravalos RG, Pajares JM. *Helicobacter pylori* eradication *vs* maintenance therapy for the prevention of recurrent bleeding from duodenal ulcer [abstract]. *Gut* 1994;**35**Suppl 5:W67.
65 Silverstein FE, Gilbert DA, Tedesco FJ, *et al.* The national ASGE survey on upper gastrointestinal bleeding. II. Clinical prognostic factors. *Gastrointest Endosc* 1981;**27**:80–93.
66 Hudson N, Everitt S, Hawkey CJ. Inter observer variability in assessment of nonsteroidal anti-inflammatory drug associated gastric lesions by video endoscopy. *Gut* 1994;**35**:1665–7.
67 O'Niell JA Jr, Pruitt BA Jr, Moncrief JA. Surgical treatment of Curling's ulcer. *Surg Gynecol Obstet* 1968;**126**:40–4.
68 Mallory GK, Weiss S. Haemorrhages from lacerations of the cardiac orific of the stomach due to vomiting. *Am J Med Sci* 1929;**178**:506–15.
69 Foster DN, Miloszewski KJA, Losowsky MS. Diagnosis of Mallory–Weiss lesions. A common cause of upper gastrointestinal bleeding. *Lancet* 1976;**ii**:483–5.
70 Knauer CM. Mallory–Weiss syndrome. Characterization of 75 intestinal haemorrhages. *Gastroenterology* 1976;**71**:5–8.
71 McIntyre AS. Spiller RC. Dissecting intramural haematoma of the oesophagus (DIHO): description of 4 cases and videoendoscopic appearances. *Gut* 1992;**33 Suppl 12**:S34.
72 Fleischer D. Etiology and prevalence of severe persistent upper gastrointestinal bleeding. *Gastroenterology* 1983;**84**:538–43.

73 Baker LA, Smith C, Liberman G. The natural history of oesophageal varices: a study of 115 cirrhotic patients in whom varices were diagnosed prior to bleeding. *Am J Med* 1959; **26**:228–37.

74 Dagradi AE. The natural history of oesophageal varices in patients with alcoholic liver cirrhosis. An endoscopic and clinical study. *Am J Gastroenterol* 1972;**57**:520–40.

75 Lebrec D, de Fleury P, Rueff B, Nahum H, Benhamou JP. Portal hypertension, size of oesophageal varices, and risk of gastrointestinal bleeding in alcoholic cirrhosis. *Gastroenterology* 1980;**79**:1139–44.

76 Tsao-Garcia G, Groszmann RJ, Fisher RL, Conn HO, Atterbury CE, Glickman M. Portal pressure, presence of gastroesophageal varices and variceal bleeding. *Hepatology* 1985;**3**: 419.

77 Sarin SK, Lahoti D, Saxena SPJ, *et al.* Prevalence, classification and natural history of gastric varices. A long term follow-up study in 568 portal hypertension patients. *Hepatology* 1992;**16**:1343–9.

78 Steigmann GV, Goff JS, Michaletz-Onody PA, *et al.* Endoscopic sclerotherapy as compared with endoscopic ligation for bleeding oesophageal varices. *N Engl J Med* 1992;**326**: 1527–32.

79 Merkel C, Bolognesi M, Bellon S, *et al.* Long term follow-up study of adult patients with non-cirrhotic obstruction of the portal system. Comparison with cirrhotic patients. *J Hepatol* 1992;**15**:299–303.

80 Okuda K, Konon K, Ohnishi K, *et al.* Clinical study of eighty-six cases of idiopathic portal hypertension and comparison with cirrhosis with splenomegaly. *Gastroenterology* 1984;**86**:600–10.

81 Burroughs AK, D'Heygere F, McIntyre N. Pitfalls in studies of prophylactic therapy for variceal bleeding in cirrhotics. *Hepatology* 1986;**6**:1407–13.

82 Polio J, Groszmann RJ. Hemodynamic factors involved in the development and rupture of esophageal varices. A pathophysiologic approach to treatment. *Semin Liver Dis* 1986; **6**:318–31.

83 Grace ND. The misuse of cimetidine in patients with cirrhosis. *Hepatology* 1983;**3**:124–5.

84 Beppu K, Inokuchi K, Koyanagi N, *et al.* Prediction of variceal haemorrhage by esophageal endoscopy. *Gastrointest Endosc* 1981;**27**:213.

85 North Italian Endoscopic Club for the Study and Treatment of Oesophageal Varices. Prediction of the first variceal haemorrhage in patients with cirrhosis of the liver and oesophageal varices. A prospective multicentre study. *N Engl J Med* 1988; **319**:918–21.

86 Poynard T, Cales P, Pasta L, *et al.* Beta-adrenergic-antagonist drugs in the prevention of gastrointestinal bleeding in patients with cirrhosis and esophageal varices: an analysis of data and prognostic factors in 589 patients from four randomized clinical trials. *N Engl J Med* 1991;**324**:1532–8.

87 McCromack TT, Sims J, Eyre-Brook I, *et al.* Gastric lesions in portal hypertension: inflammatory gastritis or congestive gastropathy? *Gut* 1985;**26**:1226–32.

88 Inokuchi K. Cooperative Study Group of Portal Hypertension of Japan. Improved survival after prophylatic portal nondecompression surgery for esophageal varices a randomized clinical trial. *Hepatology* 1990;**12**:1–6.

89 Elliot JP Jr, Smith RF, Szilagyi DE. Aortoenteric and paraprosthetic-enteric fistulas. *Arch Surg* 1974;**108**:479–88.

90 Moulton S, Adams M, Hohansen K. Aorotoenteric fistulas: a 7-year urban experience. *Am J Surg* 1986;**151**:607–11.

91 Goldstone J, Cunningham CC. Diagnosis, treatment and prevention of aortoenteric fistulas. *Acta Chir Scand* 1990;**555 Suppl**:165–72.

92 Low RN, Wall SD, Jeffery RB, Solitto RA, Reilly LM, Tierney LM. Aortoenteric fistula and perigraft infection: evaluation with CT radiology. 1990;**175**:157–62.

93 Vase P, Grove O. Gastrointestinal lesions in hereditary haemorrhagic telangiectasia. *Gastroenterology* 1986;**91**:1079–83.

94 McCreedy A, Zimmerman TJ, Webster SF. Management of upper gastrointestinal haemorrhage in patients with pseudoxanthoma elasticum. *Surgery* 1989;**105**:170–4.

95 Scully RE, Galdabini JJ, McNeely BU. Weekly Clinicopathological Exercises. Case records of the Massachusetts General Hospital. *N Engl J Med* 1979;**300**:129–35.

96 Sandhu KS, Cohen H, Radin R, Buck FS. Blue rubber bleb nevus syndrome presenting with recurrence. *Dig Dis Sci* 1987;**32**:214–19.

97 Jennings M, Ward P, Maddocks JL. Blue rubber bleb naevus disease: an uncommon cause of gastrointestinal tract bleeding. *Gut* 1988;**29**:1408–12.

98 Zuckerman GR, Cornette GL, Clouse RE, Harter HR. Upper gastrointestinal bleeding in patients with chronic renal failure. *Ann Int Med* 1985;**102**:588–92.

99 Gallard T. Aneurysms miliaires de l'estomac, donnant lieu a des hematemeses mortelles. *Bull Soc Med Hop Paris* 1884;**1**:84–91.

100 Dieulafoy G. Exulceratio simplex. L'intervention chirurgicale dans les hematemeses foudroyantes consecutives a l'exulceration simple de l'estomac. *Bull Acad Med* 1898;**49**: 49–84.

101 Van Zanten SJOV, Bartelsman JFWM, Schipper MEI, Tytgat GNJ. Recurrent massive haematemesis from Dieulafoy vascular malformations—a review of 101 cases. *Gut* 1986; **27**:213–22.

102 Boron B, Morbarhan S. Endoscopic treatment of Dieulafoy haemorrhage. *J Clin Gastroenterol* 1987;**9**:518–20.

103 Jaspersen D. Dieulafoy's disease controlled by Doppler ultrasound endoscopic treatment. *Gut* 1993;**34**:857–8.

104 Larson G, Schmidt T, Gott J, Bond S, O'Connor CA, Richardson JD. Upper gastrointestinal bleeding: predictors of outcome. *Surgery* 1986;**100**:765–72.

105 NIH Consensus Conference. Therapeutic endoscopy and bleeding ulcers. *JAMA* 1989; **262**:1369–72.

106 Branicki FJ, Coleman SY, Fok PJ, *et al.* Bleeding peptic ulcer: a prospective evaluation of risk factors for rebleeding and mortality. *World J Surg* 1990;**14**:262–70.

107 Turner IB, Jones M, Piper DW. Factors influencing mortality from bleeding peptic ulcers. *Scand J Gastroenterol* 1991;**26**:661–6.

108 Henry DA, Johnston A, Dobson A, Duggan J. Fatal peptic ulcer complications and the use of non-steroidal anti-inflammatory drugs, aspirin, and corticosteroids. *BMJ* 1987; **295**:1227–9.

109 Laine L, Cohen H, Brodhead J, Cantor D, Garcia F, Mosquera M. Prospective evaluation of immediate versus delayed refeeding and prognostic value of endoscopic findings in patients with upper gastrointestinal hemorrhage. *Gastroenterology* 1992;**102**:314–6.

110 Coghill NF, Wilcox RG. Factors in the prognosis in bleeding gastric and duodenal ulcer. *Q J Med* 1960;**29**:575–96.

111 Griffiths WJ, Neumann DA, Welsh JD. The visible vessel is an indicator of uncontrolled or recurrent gastrointestinal haemorrhage. *N Engl J Med* 1979;**300**:1411–3.

112 Northfield TC. Endoscopic prediction of recurrent bleeding in peptic ulcers. *N Engl J Med* 1981;**305**:915–6.

113 Morrison LM, Gonzales WF. The relationship of chronic peptic ulcer to coronary thrombosis. *Am J Med Sci* 1952;**224**:314–7.

114 Douglas D, Melrose AG. The relationship of coronary atherosclerosis and chronic peptic ulcer: a postmortem study. *Glasgow Med J* 1955;**36**:147–53.

115 Duggan JM. Ten year follow-up of gastrointestinal haemorrhage patients. *Aust NZ J Med* 1986;**16**:33–8.

116 Hudson N, Faulkner G, Smith SJ, Langman MJS, Hawkey CJ, Logan RFA. Late mortality in elderly patients surviving acute peptic ulcer bleeding. *Gut* 1995;**37**:177–81.

117 Westaby D, Hayes PC, Gimson AE, *et al.* Controlled clinical trial of infection sclerotherapy for active variceal bleeding. *Hepatology* 1989;**9**:274–7.

118 Graham DY, Smith JL. The course of patients after variceal haemorrhage. *Gastroenterology* 1981;**80**:800–9.

119 The Copenhagen Oesophageal Varices Sclerotherapy Project: sclerotherapy after first variceal haemorrhage in cirrhosis. *N Engl J Med* 1984;**311**:1594–1600.

120 Paquet KJ, Feussner H. Endoscopic sclerosis and oesophageal balloon tamponade in acute haemorrhage from oesophageal gastric varices: A prospective controlled randomized trial. *Hepatology* 1985;**5**:580.

121 Burroughs AK, D'Heygere F, Philips A, McIntyre N. Predictive model for early failure to control variceal bleeding [abstract]. *Hepatoloygy* 1986;**6**:1153.

122 De Franchis R, Primignani M. Why do varices bleed? *Gastroenterol Clin North Am* 1992; **21**:85–101.

123 Harvey RF, Langman MJS. The late results of medical and surgical treatment for bleeding duodenal ulcer. *Q J Med* 1970;**39**:539–47.

124 Smart HL, Langman MJS. Late outcome of bleeding gastric ulcers. *Gut* 1986;**27**:926–8.

125 Krag E. Acute haemorrhage in peptic ulcer. A clinical radiographic and statistical follow-up study. *Acta Med Scand* 1986;**180**:339–48.

126 Christensen E, Fauerholdt L, Schlichting P, *et al*. Aspects of the natural history of gastrointestinal bleeding in cirrhosis and the effect of prednisone. *Gastroenterology* 1981; **81**:944–52.

127 Westaby D, MacDougall BRD, Williams R. Improved survival following injection sclerotherapy for oesophageal varices: final analysis of a controlled trial. *Heptaology* 1985; **5**:827–30.

128 Cello JP. Endoscopic sclerotherapy versus portacaval shunt in patients with severe cirrhosis and acute variceal haemorrhage: long term follow up. *N Engl J Med* 1987;**316**: 11–15.

Part II
Diagnosis and gastrointestinal bleeding

2: Pathophysiology of bleeding lesions in the upper gastrointestinal tract

GRANT M FULLARTON

We understand little of the pathophysiological changes that accompany upper gastrointestinal bleeding, and treatment regimens have often been based on long-standing, widely held, but often unsubstantiated beliefs. A better understanding of the pathophysiological events underlying non-variceal and variceal gastrointestinal bleeding may provide new and more rational approaches to therapy.

Local Physiological Factors that Inhibit Haemostasis

Bleeding lesions in the upper gastrointestinal tract are in an adverse environment for haemostasis, to which several local factors, both luminal and mural, contribute.

Luminal factors

Luminal factors influencing haemostasis in the stomach and duodenum are:

- Gastric acid
- Pepsin
- Fibrinolysis.

Gastric acid

Gastric acid may start upper gastrointestinal haemorrhage by its erosive effect on vessels, and is a potent inhibitor of normal blood coagulation and platelet aggregation.[1] Gastric mucosal haemostasis, unlike that in the skin or vascular system, depends primarily on processes involving the coagulation system rather than platelet aggregation,[2] but both pathways are particularly sensitive to alterations in free hydrogen ion activity or pH.

Inhibition of platelet aggregation at low pH occurs in rabbits[3] and man,[4] and was thought to be caused by either a change in platelet shape or a reduction in the plasma factors required for aggregation. However, an in vitro study, showed

21

that coagulation and platelet aggregation were extremely sensitive to relatively minor increases in hydrogen ion concentration, being abnormal at pH 6·8 and virtually abolished by pH 5·4.[5] Previously formed platelet aggregates also disaggregated at the only slightly acid pH of 6·8. Similar studies have shown that elevation of pH from acidosis to pH 7·0 induces platelets to aggregate and release calcium and serotonin, and increases the availability of platelet factor VIII.[6]

The fasting pH in the stomach lies between 1 and 2 and that in the proximal duodenum between 2·2 and 7·0, in both normal volunteers[7 8] and in patients with duodenal ulcer[9]. It is surprising that haemostasis occurs at all in such an adverse acidic environment.

Pepsin

Pepsin is a potent proteolytic enzyme found in the stomach. It can start bleeding by eroding an exposed vessel wall at the base of an ulcer, and promote rebleeding by actively digesting the clot that forms over a bleeding lesion.[10]

Human gastric juice contains at least seven different pepsins (I–VII) and one non-pepsin proteinase.[11] The gastric juice from patients with chronic gastric or duodenal ulcers contains an increased concentration of pepsin I.[12] Pepsin I is secreted by the fundic glands in the stomach,[13] and has a powerful collagenolytic action up to five times greater than that of pepsin III, which is the major constituent of normal gastric juice.[14]

The mucus/bicarbonate barrier is an important part of the protection provided by the gastroduodenal mucosa.[15] In a bleeding peptic ulcer, adherent mucus and clot would probably be the initial defence against acid/peptic attack and reduce the risk of continuing bleeding. Pepsins I to III function at their maximum rates in the pH range of 1·0–3·5,[16] but pepsin I may remain active against gastric glycoprotein up to pH 5.[17] Addition of pepsin in vitro also increases the rate of platelet disaggregation when pH is lowered only modestly to 4·7–7·8.[5] Pepsin may, therefore, retain its ability to break down the mucus barrier and disaggregate platelets at pH values up to 5·0. In relation to upper gastrointestinal bleeding, it seems that acid/pepsin attack may continue until gastroduodenal pH is above 5 and will be abolished only at pH values approaching 6.

Fibrinolysis

The intermittent nature of upper gastrointestinal haemorrhage may reflect a cycle in which temporary haemostasis with clot formation is followed by fibrinolysis, clot disruption and rebleeding. This alternation between clot formation and lysis depends on the presence in the upper gastrointestinal tract of both potent activators and inhibitors of proteolysis. The gastrointestinal mucosa is rich in plasminogen activator[18] and local release of this activator may induce fibrinolysis and rebleeding.[19 20] Gastric pepsin and pancreatic proteases may also induce fibrinolysis and clot digestion.[21]

An in-vitro study of the fibrinolytic activity of human gastroduodenal juice showed that pepsin was approximately 100 times more active against fibrin than were pancreatic trypsin, chymotrypsin or elastase.[21] Gastric juice also had 50 times more fibrinolytic activity than did the same volume of duodenal juice. Gastroduodenal secretion amounts to 2–3 l per day under normal conditions, so there is a large reservoir of potential fibrinolytic activity in the upper gastrointestinal tract.

Limited studies suggest that antifibrinolytic agents may be of therapeutic benefit in upper gastrointestinal haemorrhage.[22–24] Haemostasis in the upper gastrointestinal tract may therefore depend on the balance between lytic activity (plasminogen activators, peptic activity, pancreatic enzyme activity) and clot formation. Preliminary studies have suggested enhanced fibrinolytic activity in the gastric juice of patients with upper gastrointestinal bleeding compared with that in the juice of non-bleeding patients.[20 25 26] It is not known whether this enhanced fibrinolytic activity accounts for the small proportion of patients who rebleed.

Mural factors

Mural factors influencing haemostasis in the stomach and duodenum are:

- Vascularity
- Motility.

Vascularity

The upper gastrointestinal tract is highly vascular. It receives up to one-fifth of the total cardiac output, and the mucosa receives about 70% of this visceral blood supply through an extensive anastomotic circulation within the bowel wall.[27 28] The mucosal circulation usually has a close functional link with gastric secretion,[29 30] and the gastroduodenal mucosal circulation may be capable of considerable autoregulation in response to varying physiological events.[31] Such autoregulation may be mediated by arteriovenous shunts in the submucosa, which could allow rapid shifting of large amounts of blood from one region of the stomach to another.

The outcome of ulcer bleeding depends on both the size of the bleeding vessel and the ability of local mechanisms to produce haemostasis. Although the vessels involved in an ulcer haemorrhage are usually diseased and incapable of normal haemostatic responses, up to 68% of ulcer bleeds stop spontaneously.[32] This may reflect alterations in mucosal blood flow, as the latter is capable of considerable autoregulation under other physiological conditions. Such alterations in mucosal blood flow may be accompanied by changes in gastric secretion, as these parameters usually change in parallel.[33]

Motility

The stomach and duodenum are highly motile during normal physiological fasting. They participate in the migrating motor complex, which is a cyclic sequence of alternating motor activity and quiescence.[34] Such motility is likely to be detrimental to haemostasis in two ways.

Increased vascular stress. Continuing active peristalsis may dislodge fresh clot from the bleeding site and increase intramural and intravascular pressure.[35] Such added stresses on already breached vessels in an ulcer base may cause persistent bleeding or rebleeding. Powerful smooth muscle contractions may also overstretch undamaged mucosal or submucosal vessels, leading to vessel wall disruption and bleeding.[36]

Enhanced acid/pepsin digestion. The physical mixing effect of gastroduodenal peristalsis may increase the rate of acid/peptic clot digestion[35] and promote rebleeding. Continuing gastric motility allows the emptying of an acid/pepsin load directly onto a duodenal bleeding site, which may interfere with haemostasis as well as induce clot and vessel digestion. Reduction of gastroduodenal motility during upper gastrointestinal bleeding therefore seems desirable, and therapeutic regimens with early feeding have been introduced as a means of inhibiting gastric peristalsis.[38 39]

The effect of gastrointestinal haemorrhage on the motility of the upper gastrointestinal tract is unknown. The propensity of upper gastrointestinal bleeds to stop spontaneously, however, suggests the presence of some inhibitory effect to facilitate haemostasis.

The paradox that 80% of all upper gastrointestinal bleeds stop spontaneously, despite the multiplicity of aggressive local physiological factors, strongly suggests the presence of specialised defence mechanisms to promote haemostasis.

Protective Physiological Responses

Two possible local protective responses to upper gastrointestinal bleeding are a temporary inhibition of acid secretion[39] and inhibition of gastric motility, the latter being suggested by the decreased gastric emptying observed after a simulated intragastric bleed.[40] There may also be a response that promotes haemostasis.

Gastric mucosal bleeding time was shorter in patients with upper gastrointestinal haemorrhage than in a control group of ulcer patients without haemorrhage (Figure 2.1).[41] This effect occurred without a change in systemic haemostasis, as measured by skin bleeding time, suggesting a local protective response. In addition to local changes in mucosal haemostasis a recent study demonstrated that upper gastrointestinal haemorrhage induces a hypercoagulable state that may act in a protective manner to promote haemostasis and thereby reduce rebleeding.[42]

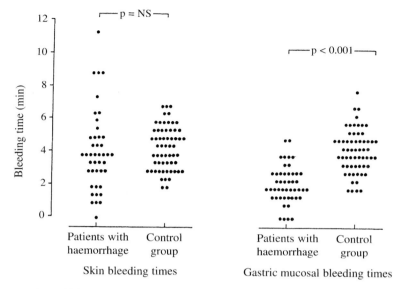

FIGURE 2.1—*Skin and gastric mucosal bleeding times in 47 patients with upper gastrointestinal haemorrhage and 61 control patients.*

Pathophysiology of Non-variceal Haemorrhage

Most non-variceal upper gastrointestinal haemorrhage arises from peptic ulcers, the precursors of which are gastric erosions.

Gastric erosions

A gastric erosion is a breach of the epithelial surface that does not extend beyond the muscularis mucosa. Such erosions are common in patients taking non-steroidal anti-inflammatory drugs (NSAIDs), in whom there is often a progression of gastric mucosal damage from tiny erosions to an ulcer, which is an epithelial defect that penetrates through the muscularis mucosa into the submucosa.[43 44] NSAIDs induce gastric damage both by local irritant action and by inhibition of prostaglandin synthesis. Increased mucosal permeability subsequent to gastric injury leads to further attack by acid and pepsin and hence even greater mucosal injury.

Peptic ulcers

The pathological characteristics of a bleeding, chronic gastric ulcer were first clearly described by the French pathologist Jean Cruveilhier in 1829.[45]

He reported a postmortem study of a young carpenter who died after several upper gastrointestinal bleeds.[45]

> At the level of the lesser curve there is a deep ulceration. The edge and floor of the ulcer are cicatrised excepting at a point where there is a clot of blood elevated like a nipple: a stylet introduced into the coronary (left gastric) artery of the stomach and directed toward the end of the vessel, pushes the clot out and enters the cavity of the stomach; but on withdrawing the stylet a little and pushing it in the same direction it can be made to re-enter the vessel which was not completely severed but only cut about three-quarters of its circumference.

Since Cruveilhier's time, several authors have noted the association between major peptic ulcer haemorrhage and exposed vessels in the ulcer base.[46–48] The rigid and semiflexible gastroscopes of the 1930s and 1940s offered a limited view of the upper gastrointestinal tract, although drawings revealed that the early endoscopists identified the "visible vessel" in patients presenting with upper gastrointestinal bleeding.[38 49] The advent of fibreoptic endoscopy in the 1970s allowed the source of bleeding to be accurately identified, and prognostic significance attached to lesions with identifiable stigmata of recent haemorrhage.[50–52] Endoscopists again reported identification of the "visible vessel".[32 53 54] Although this is a misnomer—the underlying artery in an ulcer base is generally invisible, and only the protruding clot visible—histological studies have confirmed that the endoscopic "visible vessel" does represent a small (mean diameter 0·7 mm) artery (Figure 2.2).[55]

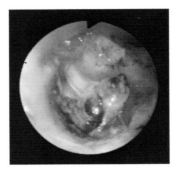

FIGURE 2.2—*Endoscopic view of a visible vessel at the base of a duodenal ulcer.*

Bleeding duodenal ulcers outnumber bleeding gastric ulcers by 1·5:1,[56] but there is an increasing incidence of gastric ulcer bleeding, with NSAID intake as an important cause. At least 30% of all ulcer bleeds may be attributed to NSAIDs, often after only short term use.[57] The underlying ulcer vessel pathology is similar in classic peptic ulcer disease and NSAID-induced ulceration, but gastric ulceration predominates in the NSAID group.[58]

Ulcer vessel pathology

Major peptic ulcer bleeding occurs when an artery in the ulcer base is eroded.[59] Usually these arteries are small (less than 1 mm in diameter) and lie in the submucosa (60% of cases) or subserosa (40%). In ulcers involving the posterior duodenal bulb or high lesser gastric curve, however, the main trunk or branches of the gastroduodenal or left gastric artery may be involved (Figure 2.3). In a prospective study of 27 patients with major gastric ulcer haemorrhage, who all underwent partial gastrectomy for continuing bleeding,[55] there was endoscopic evidence of a "visible vessel" in every patient. The vessel was a small artery (mean diameter 0·66 mm); range 0·1–1·8 mm) in 26 of the 27 cases (96%), confirming the adverse prognostic significance of the endoscopic "visible vessel".

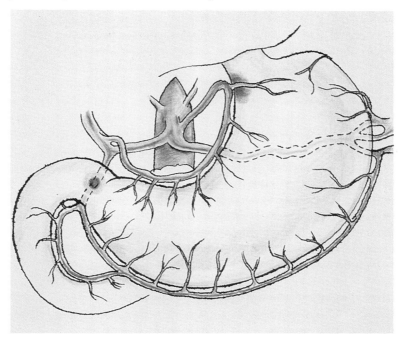

FIGURE 2.3—*Major haemorrhage occurs more often in ulcers situated in the posterior duodenal bulb or high lesser gastric curve (areas shaded green) because of the proximity of major vessels (gastroduodenal or left gastric artery).*

In the same study, histological examination confirmed aneurysmal dilation of the vessel wall in 14 (52%) of the vessels. In addition, arteritis with polymorphonuclear cell infiltrate and fibrinoid necrosis was seen in 24 (83%) of the vessels. This inflammation was usually localised to the vessel wall closest to the ulcer floor, suggesting that direct chemical attack by acid or pepsin may have been the initiating factor (Figure 2.4). Although these eroded arteries were diseased in more than 80% of the patients studied, rebleeding occurred in only 58% of endoscopically confirmed visible vessels. Recanalised thrombus was seen in about 25% of cases, suggesting that bleeding was intermittent.

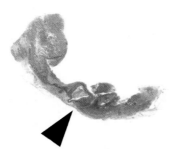

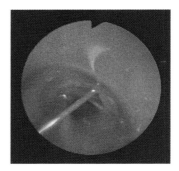

FIGURE 2.4——*A large (3 mm) eroded subserosal artery in a gastric ulcer base from a patient with major upper gastrointestinal bleeding. This artery shows intimal thickening and arteritis in the wall next to the ulcer base.*

FIGURE 2.5—*Arterial spurting from a Dieulafoy lesion high on the lesser gastric curve. The bleeding was controlled by endoscopic therapy.*

As these vessels so often showed extensive arteritis and necrosis, they would not be expected to undergo the normal haemostatic mechanisms of vessel contraction and retraction. Nevertheless, the rebleeding rate from "visible vessels" averages only 50% in other published series,[32 60] suggesting that a significant percentage of even these diseased, aneurysmally dilated vessels may undergo haemostasis.

Pathological evidence therefore indicates that ulcer haemorrhage, even from necrotic aneurysmal arteries, may be intermittent.

Pathophysiology of uncommon causes of haemorrhage

Dieulafoy's lesion

Dieulafoy's lesion usually presents with massive haemorrhage from a large artery lying close beneath the gastric mucosa (Figure 2.5). It was first described by Gallard[61] and later by Dieulafoy.[62] The lesion may well be under diagnosed because the bleeding source may be a tiny mucosal breach of 2–5 mm, and therefore hard to identify.

In 80% of cases the abnormal submucosal vessel lies within 6 cm of the oesophagogastric junction.[63] The tortuous enlarged artery may be up to 3 mm in diameter.[64 65] Unlike bleeding ulcer vessels, Dieulafoy vessels show no evidence of vasculitis, atheroma or aneurysm formation, suggesting a different pathogenesis. Associated abnormal veins and internal vessels indicate that the lesion may be a developmental anomaly similar to an arteriovenous malformation.[66] Bleeding occurs from the segment of the dilated submucosal vessel that passes into the mucosa for a few millimetres and becomes eroded.[67 68] Minor mucosal trauma, whether physical or chemical, may lead to torrential haemorrhage uncontrolled by the normal defence mechanisms.

Arteriovenous malformations

Arteriovenous malformations may be non-hereditary or hereditary.

Non-hereditary arteriovenous malformations are either primary or secondary; the latter are associated with systemic disease, such as systemic sclerosis and the CREST syndrome (calcinosis, Raynaud's phenomenon, sclerodactyly and telangiectasia).[69 70]
Primary vascular malformations of the stomach are rare. Histologically, they may be capillary, cavernous or mixed. Capillary lesions may be solitary and nodular, 1–3 mm in diameter, with submucosal clusters of tortuous capillaries and venules. Superficial mucosal ulceration may lead to haemorrhage.[71] Cavernous haemangiomas are more commonly solitary or diffuse lesions that may be considerably larger than capillary lesions, often protruding into the lumen;[71] they appear as distended submucosal vessels in histological specimens.[72]

Hereditary haemorrhagic telangiectasia (Osler–Weber–Rendu syndrome) presents as an autosomal dominant disease with telangiectasia throughout the gastrointestinal tract[73] (Figure 2.6). Multiple mucosal and submucosal telangiectasia present on angiography as a mesh of small vessels with arteriovenous shunts and early venous drainage.

Gastric antral vascular ectasia

Gastric antral vascular ectasia (GAVE) is diagnosed endoscopically from segmented meshes of reddened antral mucosa leading to the pylorus (Figure 2.7)—"watermelon" or "tiger-stripe" stomach. The pathogenesis of the syndrome is unclear, but it is often associated with achlorhydria and hypergastrinaemia and may have an autoimmune basis.[74] Histologically, the vascular "stripes" are meshes of dilated vessels; thrombosis of capillaries in the lamina propria is associated with fibromuscular hyperplasia.

Pathophysiology of Variceal Haemorrhage

Obstruction of the portal venous blood flow causes portal hypertension. Portal venous pressure may rise from the normal 7 mm Hg to 20–30 mm Hg, triggering the development of collateral vessels that attempt to decompress the portal system. Venous collateral vessels (varices) form between the portal systems among the coronary and short gastric veins, the intercostal, oesophageal and azygos veins, the haemorrhoidal veins, the paraumbilical plexus and in the retroperitoneum.

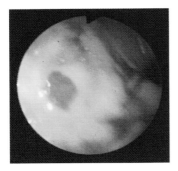

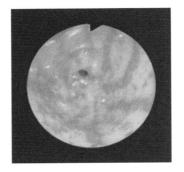

FIGURE 2.6—*Endoscopic appearances of gastric telangiectasia in a patient with hereditary haemorrhagic telangiectasia. Multiple such lesions were present throughout the stomach.*

FIGURE 2.7—*Gastric antral vascular ectasia: the characteristic endoscopic view of the antrum, with prominent meshes of reddened mucosa.*

Oesophageal varices

Oesophageal varices are clinically the most important, because of their tendency to produce major haemorrhage. The normal and abnormal venous anatomy of the lower oesophagus have been well described by high resolution vascular casts.[75] Intraepithelial channels in the distal oesophagus drain into a superficial plexus of veins that is also connected to larger deep intrinsic veins. These deep veins communicate with adventitial veins through perforating veins that traverse the muscular layers of the oesophageal wall.

With increasing portal presure all these intercommunicating veins dilate, but the most extreme dilation occurs in the deep intrinsic veins; these are recognised endoscopically as oesophageal varices. The varices lie in the lamina propria, which allows them to dilate freely and bulge into the oesophageal lumen. The true situation may be more complex, with both dilation of both the normal superficial venous network and the intercommunicating veins.[76]

Factors related to variceal bleeding

Gastro-oesophageal reflux may damage the lower oesophageal mucosa and promote variceal bleeding,[77] but studies have indicated a similar prevalence of acid reflux or disturbed oesophageal motility in patients with oesophageal varices and controls.[78 79] Histological assessment of lower oesophageal mucosa from recently transected oesophageal varices revealed no significant inflammation.[80]

Portal venous pressure Although there is no clear correlation between portal pressure and risk of variceal haemorrhage, portal pressure measured by wedged hepatic venous pressure is of predictive value in the early phase of variceal haemorrhage.[81][82] Patients who die within 2 weeks of presentation have significantly higher portal pressures than do those who survive, suggesting an aetiological role for elevated pressure in variceal bleeding.[81][83]

Variceal size. Larger varices are more likely to bleed than are smaller ones,[83][84] but size does not show a clear correlation with portal pressure.[85] It is likely therefore that other local factors play a part in variceal formation and bleeding tendency.

Variceal wall tension. Oesophageal varices bulge into the lumen of the oesophagus, and the surface tension in their walls is greater than that in supported vessels. The surface tension may be estimated by applying Laplace's law, $T = PD/W$, where T is the tension, P is the transmural pressure, D is the variceal diameter and W the wall thickness. A sudden increase in variceal pressure may cause the surface tension to increase rapidly, leading to rupture of the varix.[86] The combination of large varices with high pressure and increased variceal wall tension is more frequent in varices that have recently bled, suggesting that it has a role in the pathophysiology of variceal bleeding.[86][87]

In conclusion, varices may bleed when there is a combination of high portal pressure, large varix size, reduced support for the varix and increased surface tension in the varix wall.

Key points

- Haemostasis in the upper gastrointestinal tract is inhibited by gastric acid, pepsin and fibrinolysis in the lumen of the stomach and duodenum, and by the vascularity and motility of their walls

- Upper gastrointestinal haemorrhage appears to induce local protective responses, such as:
  —inhibition of acid secretion and gastric motility
  —local changes in mucosal haemostasis
  —a hypercoagulable state

- NSAIDs damage the gastric mucosa by local irritant action and inhibition of prostaglandin synthesis

- Major peptic ulcer bleeding occurs when there is erosion of an artery in the ulcer base. The bleeding vessel is often inflamed and necrotic, suggesting chemical attack by acid or pepsin, and aneurysmally dilated. Bleeding may be intermittent

- Oesophageal varices develop in response to portal hypertension. They bulge unsupported into the lumen of the oesophagus, and larger varices bleed more easily than smaller ones

References

1 Bodi T, Wirts CW, Tocantins LM. Local environmental factors affecting haemostasis in bleeding from the upper gastrointestinal tract. In: Bodi T, ed. *Progress in haematology.* New York: Grune and Stratton, 1956:221–48.

2 Whittle BJR, Kauffman GL, Moncada S. Haemostatic mechanisms, independent of platelet aggregation, arrest gastric mucosal bleeding. *Proc Natnl Acad Sci* 1986;**83**:5683–7.

3 McLean KR, Veloso H. Change of shape without aggregation caused by ADP in rabbit platelets at low pH. *Life Sci* 1967;**6**:1983–4.

4 Rogers AB. The effect of pH on human platelet aggregation induced by epinephrine and ADP. *Proc Soc Exp Biol Med* 1972;**139**:1100–9.

5 Green WF, Kaplan MM, Curtis LE, Levine PH. Effect of acid and pepsin on blood coagulation and platelet aggregation: a possible contribution to prolonged gastroduodenal haemorrhage. *Gastroenterology* 1978;**74**:38–43.

6 Chaimoff C, Creter D, Djaldetti M. The effect of pH on platelet and coagulation factor activities. *Am J Surg* 1973;**136**:257–9.

7 Rune SJ. Problems associated with in situ measurements of duodenal pH. In: Domschke W, Wormsley KG, eds. *Magen Und Magenkrankheiten.* Stuttgart: Georg Thieme Verlag, 1981:150–61.

8 Hannibal S, Rune SJ. Duodenal bulb pH in normal subjects. *Eur J Clin Invest* 1983;**13**: 455–60.

9 Bendsten F, Rosenkilde-Gram B, Tage-Jensen U, Ovensen L, Rune SJ. Duodenal bulb acidity in patients with duodenal ulcer. *Gastroenterology* 1987;**93**:1263–9.

10 Berstad A. Management of acute upper gastrointestinal bleeding. *Scand J Gastroenterol* 1982;**17 (suppl 75)**:103–8.

11 Etherington DJ, Taylor WH. Nomenclature of pepsins. *Nature* 1967;**216**:279–80.

12 Taylor WH. Pepsins of patients with peptic ulcer. *Nature* 1970;**227**:76–7.

13 Etherington DJ, Taylor WH. The pepsins from human gastric mucosal extracts. *Biochem J* 1970;**118**:587–94.

14 Etherington DJ, Roberts NB, Taylor WH. The collagen degrading activity of purified human pepsins 1 and 3. *Clin Sci* 1980;**58**:30.

15 Allen A, Garner A. Gastric mucus and bicarbonate secretion and their possible role in mucosal protection. *Gut* 1980;**21**:249–62.

16 Piper DW, Fenton DB. pH stability and activity curves of pepsin with special reference to their clinical importance. *Gut* 1965;**6**:506–8.

17 Pearson JP, Ward R, Allen A, Roberts NB, Taylor WH. Mucus degradation by pepsin: comparison of mucolytic activity of human pepsin 1 and pepsin 3: implications in peptic ulceration. *Gut* 1986;**27**:243–8.

18 Cox HT, Poller L, Thomson JM. Gastric fibrinolysis. A possible aetiological link with peptic ulcer. *Lancet* 1967;**1**:1300–2.

19 Cox HT, Poller L, Thomson JM. Evidence for the release of gastric fibrinolytic activity into peripheral blood. *Gut* 1969;**10**:404–7.

20 Nilsson IM, Bergentz SE, Hedner U, Kullenberg K. Gastric fibrinolysis. *Thromb Diath Haemorrhag* (Stuttgart) 1975;**34**:409–18.

21 Low J, Dodds AJ, Biggs LC. Fibrinolytic activity of gastroduodenal secretions—a possible role in upper gastrointestinal haemorrhage. *Thromb Res* 1980;**17**:819–30.

22 Cormack F, Jouhar AJ, Chakrabarti RR, Fearnely GR. Tranexamic acid in upper gastrointestinal haemorrhage. *Lancet* 1973;**1**:1207–8.

23 Biggs JC, Hugh TB, Dodds AJ. Tranexamic acid and upper gastrointestinal haemorrhage—a double blind trial. *Gut* 1976;**17**:729–34.

24 Stael von Holstein CCS, Eriksson SBS, Kallen R. Tranexamic acid as an aid to reducing blood transfusion requirements in gastric and duodenal bleeding. *BMJ* 1987;**297**:7–10.

25 Buhr HJ, Encke A, Seufert RM. Untersuchungen zur lokalen fibrinoyse des magens. *Chirurg* (Berlin) 1978;**49**:431–5.

26 Wheatley KE, Poxon BA, Dykes PW, Keighley MRB. Intragastric fibrinolysis in bleeding peptic ulcer disease [abstract]. *Gut* 1987;**28**:A1402.

27 Guth PH. The gastric microcirculation and gastric mucosal blood flow under normal and pathological conditions. In: Glass G, Glass J, eds. *Progress in gastroenterology.* New York: Grune and Stratton, 1977:323–47.

28 Konturek SJ. Gastric secretion: physiological aspects. In: Duthie HL, Wormsley KG, eds. *Scientific basis of gastroenterology.* Edinburgh: Churchill Livingstone, 1979:133–62.

29 Jacobson ED, Swan KG, Grossman MI. Blood flow and secretion in the stomach. *Gastroenterology* 1967;**52**:414–20.
30 Guth PH. Stomach blood flow and acid secretion. *Ann Rev Physiol* 1982;**44**:3–12.
31 Kiel JW, Riedel GL, Shepherd AP. Autoregulation of canine gastric mucosal blood flow. *Gastroenterology* 1987;**93**:12–20.
32 Wara P. Endoscopic prediction of major rebleeding: a prospective study of stigmata of haemorrhage in bleeding ulcer. *Gastroenterology* 1985;**88**:1209–14.
33 Pique JM, Leung FW, Tan HW, Livingston E, Scremin OU, Guth PH. Gastric mucosal and blood flow response to stimulation and inhibition of gastric acid secretion. *Gastroenterology* 1988;**95**:642–50.
34 Houghton LA, Read NW, Heddle R, *et al.* Motor activity of the gastric antrum, pylorus and duodenum under fasted conditions and after a liquid meal. *Gastroenterology* 1988;**94**: 1276–84.
35 Bodi T, Kazal LA. Some aspects of the pathophysiology and the multiple contributory factors in haemorrhage from the upper gastrointestinal tract. *Am J Gastroenterol* 1965;**44**: 202–23.
36 Mallory GK, Weiss J. Haemorrhage from lacerations of the cardiac orifice of stomach due to vomiting. *Am J Med Sci* 1929;**178**:506–15.
37 Meulengracht E. Treatment of haematemesis and melaena with food. *Lancet* 1935;**ii**: 1220–2.
38 Avery Jones F. Haematemesis and melaena—with special reference to bleeding peptic ulcer. *BMJ* 1947;**2**:441–6.
39 Fullarton GM, Boyd EJS, Crean GP, Buchanan K, McColl KEL. Inhibition of gastric secretion and motility by simulated upper gastrointestinal haemorrhage—a response to facilitate haemostasis? *Gut* 1989;**30**:156–60.
40 Fullarton GM, Boyd EJS, Crean GP, McColl KEL. Effect of simulated intragastric motility and serum gastrin. *Gut* 1990;**31**:518–21.
41 Allison MC, Fullarton GM, Brown IL, Crean GP, McColl KEL. Enhanced gastric mucosal haemostasis following upper gastrointestinal haemorrhage. *Gut* 1991;**32**:735–9.
42 Blair SD, Janvrin SB, McCollum CN, Greenhalgh RM. Effect of early blood transfusion on gastrointestinal haemorrhage. *Br J Surg* 1986;**73**:783–5.
43 Lanza FL. NSAID induced gastroduodenal injury. *Gastroenterology* 1991;**101**:555–7.
44 Bardhan KD, Bjarnason I, Scott DI, *et al.* The prevention and healing of NSAID damage by misoprostol. *Br J Rheumatol* 1993;**32**:990–5.
45 Cruveilhier J. *Anatomie pathologique du corps humaine*, vol. 41. Paris: Ballière, 1839.
46 Rokitansky CF. *Handbuch der allgemeinen pathologischen Anatomie*, vol. 3. Vienna: Braunmuller & Siedel, 1842:193–4.
47 Trousseau A. *Lectures on Clinical Medicine*, vol. IV. Translated by John Rose Cormack. London: New Sydenham Society, 1889:68–9.
48 Osborn GR. The pathology of gastric arteries, with special reference to fatal haemorrhage from peptic ulcer. *Br J Surg* 1954;**41**:585–94.
49 Schindler R. *Gastroscopy.* Chicago: University of Chicago Press, 1937:156–72.
50 Cotton PB, Rosenberg MT, Waldram PPL, Axon ATR. Early endoscopy of oesophagus, stomach and duodenal bulb in patients with haematemesis and melaena. *BMJ* 1973;**2**: 505–9.
51 Forrest JAH, Finlayson NDC, Shearman DJC. Endoscopy in gastrointestinal bleeding. *Lancet* 1974;**ii**:394–7.
52 Foster DN, Miloszewski KJA, Losowsky MS. Stigmata of recent haemorrhage in diagnosis and prognosis of upper gastrointestinal bleeding. *BMJ* 1978;**1**:1173–7.
53 Griffiths WJ, Newmann DA, Welsh JD. The visible vessel as an indicator of uncontrolled or recurrent gastrointestinal haemorrhage. *N Engl J Med* 1970;**300**:1411–3.
54 Johnston JH. The sentinel clot and invisible vessel: pathologic anatomy of bleeding peptic ulcer. *Gastrointest Endosc* 1984;**30**:313–5.
55 Swain CP, Storey DW, Bown SG, *et al.* Nature of the bleeding vessel in recurrently bleeding gastric ulcers. *Gastroenterology* 1986;**90**:595–608.
56 Fullarton GM, Birnie GG, MacDonald A, Murray WR. The effect of introducing endoscopic therapy on surgery and mortality rates for peptic ulcer haemorrhage—a single centre analysis of 1125 cases. *Endoscopy* 1990;**22**:110–3.
57 Langman MJS, Weil J, Wainright P, *et al.* Risks of bleeding peptic ulcer associated with individual non-steroidal anti-inflammatory drugs. *Lancet* 1994;**343**:1075–8.

58 Allison MC, Howatson AG, Torrance CJ, Lee FD, Russell RI. Gastrointestinal damage associated with the use of non-steroidal anti-inflammatory drugs. *N Engl J Med* 1992; **327**:749–54.

59 Mackay CR. The significance of local vascular changes in bleeding peptic ulcer. *Surgery* 1954;**35**:724–33.

60 Vallon AG, Cotton PB, Laurence BH, Miro JRA, Oses JCS. Randomised trial of endoscopic argon laser photocoagulation in bleeding peptic ulcer. *Gut* 1981;**22**:228–33.

61 Gallard T. Aneurysmes miliaires de l'estomac, donnant lieu a des hematemeses mortelles. *Bull Soc Med Hôp Paris* 1884;**1**:84–91.

62 Dieulafoy G. Exulceratio simplex: l'intervention chirurgicale dans les hematemeses foudroyantes consecutives a l'exulceration simplex de l'estomac. *Bull Acad Med* 1898;**39**: 49–84.

63 Veldhuyzen van Zanten SJO, Bartelsman JFWM, Schipper MEI, Tytgat GNJ. Recurrent massive haematemesis from Dieulafoy vascular malformations—a review of 101 cases. *Gut* 1986;**27**:213–22.

64 Mortensen NJMC, Mountford RA, Davies JD, Jeans WD. Dieulafoy's disease: a distinctive arteriovenous malformation causing massive gastric haemorrhage. *Br J Surg* 1983;**70**: 76–8.

65 Sarles HE Jr, Schenkein JP, Hecht RM, Sanowski RA, Miller P. Dieulafoy's ulcer: a rare cause of massive gastric haemorrhage in an 11 year old girl: case report and literature review. *Am J Gastroenterol* 1984;**79**:930–2.

66 Eidus LB, Rasuli P, Manion D, Heringer R. Caliber persistent artery of the stomach (Dieulafoy's vascular malformation). *Gastroenterology* 1990;**99**:1507–10.

67 Goldman RL. Submucosal arterial malformation ("aneurysm") of the stomach with fatal haemorrhage. *Gastroenterology* 1964;**79**:589–94.

68 Juler GL, Labitzke HG, Lamb R, Allen R. The pathogenesis of Dieulafoy's gastric erosion. *Am J Gastroenterol* 1984;**79**:195–200.

69 Rosekrans PCM, de Rooy DJ, Bosman FT, Eulderink F, Cats A. Gastrointestinal telangiectasia as a cause of severe blood loss in systemic sclerosis. *Endoscopy* 1980;**12**: 200–4.

70 Kolodny M, Baker WG Jr. CRST syndrome with persistent gastrointestinal bleeding. *Gastrointest Endosc* 1986;**15**:16–7.

71 Gentry RW, Dockerty MB, Claggett OT. Collective review: vascular malformation and vascular tumours of the gastrointestinal tract. *Int Abstr Surg* 1949;**88**:281–323.

72 Bongiovi JJ Jr, Duffy JL. Gastric haemangioma associated with upper gastrointestinal bleeding. *Arch Surg* 1967;**95**:93–8.

73 Osler W. On a family form of receiving epistaxis associated with multiple telangiectasia of the skin and mucous membranes. *Bull Johns Hopkins Hosp* 1901;**12**:333.

74 Quintero E, Pique JM, Bombi JA, *et al.* Gastric mucosal vascular ectasias causing bleeding in cirrhosis: a distinct entity associated with hypergastrinemia and low levels of pepsinogen 1. *Gastroenterology* 1987;**93**:1054–61.

75 Kitano S, Terblanche J, Kahn D, *et al.* Venous anatomy of the lower oesophagus in portal hypertension: practical implications. *Br J Surg* 1986;**73**:525–53.

76 Hashizume M, Kitano S, Sugimuchi K, Sucishi K. Three dimensional view of the vascular structure of the lower oesophagus in clinical hypertension. *Hepatology* 1988;**8**:1482–7.

77 Liebowitz HR. Pathogenesis of oesophageal varix rupture. *JAMA* 1961;**175**:874–9.

78 Eckardt VF, Grace ND. Gastroesophageal reflux and bleeding oesophageal varices. *Gastroenterology* 1979;**76**:39–42.

79 Heil T, Mattes P, Loeprecht H. Gastroesophageal reflux: an aetiological factor for bleeding in oesophageal varices? *Br J Surg* 1980;**67**:467–8.

80 Spence RAJ, Sloan JM, Johnston GW. Histologic factors of the oesophageal transection ring as clues to the pathogenesis of bleeding varices. *Surg Gynecol Obstet* 1984;**159**:253–9.

81 Ready JB, Rector WG. Stratification of risk of continued bleeding and early rebleeding from oesophageal varices by measurement of portal pressure within 24 hours of index haemorrhage [abstract]. *Gastroenterology* 1989;**96**:A649.

82 Paquet KJ. Endoscopic haemostasis in upper gastrointestinal bleeding. *J Gastroenterol Hepatol* 1989;**4**:385–6.

83 Vinel JP, Cassigneul J, Leuade M, *et al.* Assessment of short-term prognosis after variceal bleeding in patients with alcoholic cirrhosis by early measurement of portohepatic gradient. *Hepatology* 1986;**6**:116–7.

84 North Italian Endoscopic Club for the Study and Treatment of Oesophageal Varices. Prediction of the first variceal hemorrhage in patients with cirrhosis of the liver and esophageal varices. *N Engl J Med* 1989;**319**:983–99.

85 Garcia-Tsao G, Groszmann RJ, Fisher RL, *et al.* Portal pressure, presence of gastroesophageal varices and variceal bleeding. *Hepatology* 1985;**5**:419–24.

86 Rigau J, Bosch J, Bordas JM, *et al.* Endoscopic measurement of variceal pressure in cirrhosis: correlation with portal pressure and variceal haemorrhage. *Gastroenterology* 1989; **96**:873–80.

87 Polio J, Groszmann RJ. Haemodynamic factors involved in the development and rupture of oesophageal varices: a physiological approach to treatment. *Semin Liver Dis* 1986;**6**: 318–31.

3: Clinical diagnosis: patterns, symptoms and signs of gastrointestinal bleeding

A I MORRIS

Gastrointestinal bleeding can be overt or occult, acute or chronic, and the symptoms and signs associated with the bleed will depend not only upon the severity of the bleed but also upon the site of origin. The convention is to define gastrointestinal bleeding by the nature of its presentation, and the anatomical site from which it originates.

Symptoms of Gastrointestinal Bleeding

Acute overt upper gastrointestinal bleeding

Overt bleeding from the upper gastrointestinal tract usually presents as a frank haematemesis or melaena. Occasionally it can be of sufficient severity to present as bright red rectal bleeding. An elderly or arteriosclerotic patient experiencing a sudden brisk bleed may present with a syncopal episode before the bleeding becomes apparent. Overt bleeding may not be recognised if the patient is blind or, as many do, fails to recognise melaena as being altered blood. A patient who vomits "coffee grounds" also may not interpret this as the result of bleeding.

If a patient presents with acute abdominal pain associated with bleeding, the doctor should be alert to the possibility of either a bleeding, perforated ulcer or, particularly if there is jaundice or abnormal liver function tests, haemobilia.

It is rare for patients to suffer repeated acute gastrointestinal bleeds without seeking medical advice, or for an acute bleed to remain occult.

Chronic occult upper gastrointestinal bleeding

Occult bleeding usually presents as anaemia with symptoms of tiredness breathlessness or oedema, or is found on routine blood testing—perhaps prior to blood donation or as part of a routine health check.

Acute overt lower gastrointestinal bleeding

Rectal bleeding is the normal presentation of acute overt bleeding from the lower gastrointestinal tract. The site of bleeding will to some extent determine the colour of the blood—bright red blood usually comes from the left side of the colon, and darker blood from more proximal sites. The rate of blood loss may be slow enough on the right side to give rise to melaena stools, or brisk enough to present as frank bright red blood. Haemorrhoidal bleeding tends to be separate from the motion or may drip into the lavatory pan, but this history cannot be relied upon. Any rectal bleeding must be investigated. It is rare for colonic bleeding to be of sufficient severity to cause syncope, but severe bleeding in patients with angiodysplasia, diverticular disease or colitis may give rise to hypotension and shock.

Chronic overt and occult lower gastrointestinal bleeding

Chronic bleeding from the lower gastrointestinal tract may be overt, with continued passage of obvious blood per rectum or, if of small volume, may be occult. It is not uncommon for patients to ignore rectal bleeding, especially if it is of small volume. It should never be assumed, as it often is by both patient and doctor, that the cause is haemorrhoidal, because haemorrhoids are common and may coexist with other more serious disorders.

Causes of Upper Gastrointestinal Bleeding

Acute bleeding

The causes of acute upper gastrointestinal bleeding will vary according to the age and the ethnic and geographic origin of the patient. Common and rare causes are listed in Box 3.1. Where alcoholic liver disease or hepatitis B are prevalent, varices will be more common. Tumours of the upper gastrointestinal tract are rare in children. In an individual patient there may be more than one potential site for haemorrhage. An example of this is acute bleeding in an alcoholic patient with cirrhosis, who may bleed from varices, peptic ulceration, portal hypertensive gastropathy or gastritis, all of which are associated with the alcoholic liver disease, or from a coincidental oesophageal or gastric malignancy.

37

Box 3.1   Causes of acute upper gastrointestinal bleeding

Common causes
- Duodenal ulceration
- Gastric ulceration
- Oesophagitis, gastritis and duodenitis
- Varices
- Mallory–Weiss tear

Less common causes
- Gastro-oesophageal cancer
- Leiomyoma
- Portal hypertensive gastropathy
- Dieulafoy lesion

Rare causes
- Aortoduodenal fistula (after aortic graft insertion)
- Bleeding diathesis
- From posterior nasopharynx
- Angiodysplasia
- Telangiectasia
- Ehlers–Danlos syndrome
- Pseudoxanthoma elasticum
- Hepatobiliary disease
- Pancreatic disease
- Foreign body
- Factitious bleed

Chronic bleeding

Common and uncommon causes of chronic bleeding from the upper gastrointestinal tract are listed in Box 3.2.

Box 3.2   Causes of chronic upper gastrointestinal bleeding

Common causes
- Chronic peptic ulceration
- Severe oesophagitis, gastritis, duodenitis
- Gastro-oesophageal cancer
- Portal hypertensive gastropathy
- Telangiectasia
- Angiodysplasia and vascular ectasia

Uncommon causes
- Leiomyoma
- Hiatus hernia

Causes of Lower Gastrointestinal Bleeding

See the Boxes 3.3–3.5 for common, less common and rare causes of acute lower gastrointestinal bleeding, and overt and occult causes of chronic bleeding. Note that bleeding may also originate from the small intestine.

Box 3.3   Causes of acute lower gastrointestinal bleeding

Common causes

- Haemorrhoids and fissure in ano
- Diverticular disease
- Colonic cancer
- Colonic polyps

Uncommon causes

- Inflammatory bowel disease (ulcerative colitis, Crohn's disease)
- Infective colitides
- Angiodysplasia
- Ischaemic colitis

Rare causes

- Solitary rectal ulcer
- Lymphoma
- Intussuception
- Tuberculosis

Box 3.4   Causes of chronic lower gastrointestinal bleeding

Overt bleeding

- Haemorrhoids and fissure in ano
- Colonic cancer
- Colonic polyps
- Inflammatory bowel disease
- Angiodysplasia

Occult bleeding

- Colonic cancer
- Colonic polyps
- Inflammatory bowel disease (Crohn's disease)
- Angiodysplasia

Box 3.5   Causes of small intestinal bleeding

Acute causes

- Crohn's disease
- Small bowel tumours
- Angiodysplasia
- Meckel's diverticulum
- Intussuception
- Dysentery

Chronic causes

- Crohn's disease
- Small bowel tumours
- Angiodysplasia
- Meckel's diverticulum
- Infestation (worms)

Physical Signs of a Clinically Significant Bleed

Signs of acute blood loss

The main physical signs of an acute bleed are those associated with the normal homeostatic responses to loss of intravascular fluid volume. These physiological signs form the basis for the assessment of the severity of the bleed.

Tachycardia and a fall in mean arterial blood pressure are the classic signs that, in conjunction with a history of blood loss, should alert the doctor to a bleed of some severity. Tachycardia, as an initial protective reflex to maintain the cardiac output, may be present for some time before the blood pressure drops. Another factor that may elevate the pulse rate in such a patient is the fright associated with the loss of blood and the fear of the unknown (the cause of the bleed, type of treatment and prognosis).

Pallor, sweating and cold peripheries may indicate a significant bleed but like tachycardia may occur for other reasons, such as fluid depletion (after profound vomiting or diarrhoea or both, or an Addisonian hypoadrenal crisis) or cardiac disease (myocardial infarction, cardiogenic shock, tachyarrhythmias).

Assessment of the extent of unobserved and unmeasured blood loss may be difficult, if not impossible, by such indirect means, particularly in patients with other diseases or conditions, such as cardiac failure. If there is doubt about the severity of blood loss, or if over-transfusion may be hazardous—as in patients with an acute myocardial infarct or heart failure—measurement of the central venous pressure provides the best assessment of the circulating blood volume.

Sudden loss of a large volume of blood may induce syncope, and many patients with a profound bleed become drowsy and confused because of a combination of impaired cerebral perfusion and hypoxia.

Signs of chronic blood loss

The signs of chronic blood loss are those associated with chronic iron deficiency. (Remember, however, that iron deficiency has causes other than gastrointestinal bleeding, such as a poor diet, malabsorption and other factors such as multiple pregnancies). Pallor of the mucous membranes is a poor guide to the presence of anaemia, but the presence of glossitis (Figure 3.1) angular stomatitis (Figure 3.2) and koilonychia (Figure 3.3) should suggest chronic iron deficiency. Chronic anaemia may cause congestive cardiac failure and present with dyspnoea and oedema.

Signs associated with specific causes of blood loss

When a patient is admitted with a gastrointestinal haemorrhage it is sensible to search for physical signs associated with conditions that might have predisposed him or her to such a bleed.

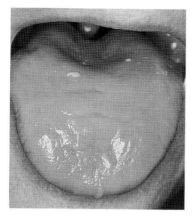

FIGURE 3.1—*Glossitis caused by iron deficiency anaemia.*

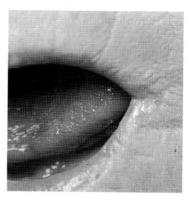

FIGURE 3.2—*Angular stomatitis caused by iron deficiency anaemia.*

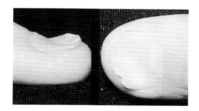

FIGURE 3.3—*Koilonychia: a sign of chronic iron deficiency anaemia.*

Hepatological signs

The presence of any of the peripheral signs of chronic liver disease should suggest the presence of oesophageal varices. More specific signs of portal hypertension, such as splenomegaly, ascites or a caput medusae, make the likelihood of variceal bleeding even greater. Even if the patient appears to have had only a small bleed, without cardiovascular effects, such signs should encourage early endoscopy. The risk of rebleeding and death is much higher if the initial bleeding was variceal.

Dermatological signs

Apart from signs of bleeding diatheses, the skin should be examined for telangiectasia (Figure 3.4) or the lesions of the Ehlers–Danlos syndrome or pseudoxanthoma elasticum. Bullous lesions in the mouth, such as those of pemphigoid and pemphigus as well as ulcerative lesions affecting the lips and mouth in the Stevens–Johnson syndrome or toxic epidermal necrolysis, may be associated with ulceration in the oesophagus and gastrointestinal bleeding.

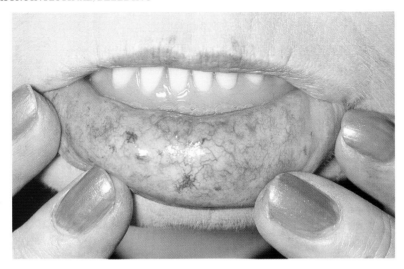

FIGURE 3.4—*Hereditary haemorrhagic telangiectasia: telangiectasia on the lip.*

Rheumatological/locomotor signs

In any patient with an overt arthritic complaint (Figure 3.5), be it acute or chronic, the ingestion of non-steroidal anti-inflammatory drugs should be suspected as the cause of a gastrointestinal bleed.

Rarely arteritis involving the gastrointestinal tract can bleed, in such conditions as systemic lupus erythematosus, polyarteritis nodosa and Behçet's syndrome.

Haematological signs

Petechial haemorrhages (Figure 3.6), bruising or bleeding from the gums or other signs of a generalised bleeding diathesis must never be assumed to be the sole cause of a gastrointestinal bleed. The bleed might have a separate, local gastrointestinal cause, such as an ulcer, rather than being the result of a generalised bleeding tendency related to thrombocytopenia or other abnormalities of the clotting system.

Vascular signs

A history of abdominal aortic surgery and the insertion of an aortic graft should always alert one to the possibility of an aortoduodenal fistula. An abdominal scar in association with an acute bleed is an indication for an early computed tomography scan or arteriography or both; these investigations should not be delayed by an endoscopy, which often detects no lesion or just a red spot at the site of the fistula.

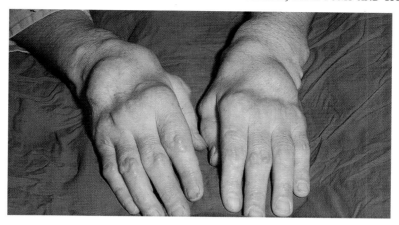

FIGURE 3.5—*Patients with rheumatoid arthritis may suffer chronic blood loss from lesions caused by non-steroidal anti-inflammatory drugs.*

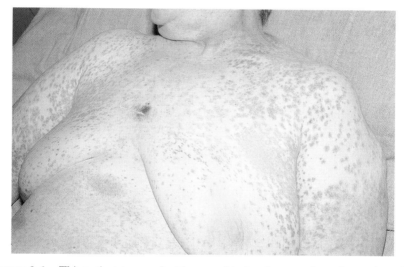

FIGURE 3.6—*This patient presented with a petechical rash, anaemia and gastrointestinal blood loss. She had drug induced aplastic anaemia and was bleeding from mucosal petechiae.*

Investigation of Gastrointestinal Bleeding

Investigation of gastrointestinal haemorrhage is discussed elsewhere in this volume, but some general comments will be made here on the investigation of bleeding from less common sites.

Although most gastrointestinal bleeds originate from above the second part of the duodenum, or from below the ileocaecal valve, within easy

43

reach of conventional endoscopy, a small cohort of patients either bleed overtly from a site within the gastrointestinal tract between these points, or present with anaemia, a positive occult blood test and negative routine endoscopy.

Before deciding on what method of investigation is appropriate for such patients, a careful history and examination is required to avoid missing such conditions as hereditary telangiectasia (Figure 3.4) and pseudoxanthoma elasticum. Bleeding from the hepatobiliary tract and pancreas, although rare, must be considered in patients with diseases of these organs. In any case of gastrointestinal bleeding of obscure cause, it is possible that:

- The lesion has been missed
- The bleeding is intermittent or
- The lesion has not been reached or considered.

Enteroscopy

Development of a variety of enteroscopes for viewing the small bowel has allowed the gastroenterologist to look beyond the range of conventional endoscopy and, depending upon the type of enteroscope, may also permit haemostatic therapy to be delivered. The handling characteristics of the push enteroscope permit detailed examination of the jejunum and, in some cases, the upper ileum. A push enteroscope has a full sized biopsy channel that allows a variety of haemostatic procedures to be carried out under direct vision deep in the small bowel. The sonde type of enteroscope enables intubation of the entire small bowel, but is time consuming to use, offers limited views and lacks a therapeutic channel for the delivery of haemostatic treatment.

Enteroscopy or angiography?

In patients with severe, overt bleeding, angiography probably has a more important role than enteroscopy, whereas in the patient who presents with obscure bleeding and anaemia, enteroscopy should be the first choice.

Contrast barium radiology of the small bowel has a more limited role, but should be considered for those patients in whom endoscopy does not permit full visualisation of the ileum.

Angiography is particularly helpful in elucidating the cause of hepatobiliary and pancreatic bleeding.

Panendoscopy on the operating table, with transillumination of the bowel, remains the last option in seeking the cause of obscure gastrointestinal bleeding; in selected cases and experienced hands, the procedure has a good diagnostic return.

Key points

- Gastrointestinal bleeding (GIB) is defined by the nature of its presentation and its site of origin:
  —acute overt upper GIB (frank haemetemesis or melaena)
  —chronic occult upper GIB (anaemia with tiredness, breathlessness or oedema)
  —acute overt lower GIB (rectal bleeding)
  —chronic overt and chronic occult lower GIB (continued passage of blood per rectum)

- An individual patient may bleed from more than one site

- Classic signs of a severe bleed are tachycardia and a fall in mean arterial pressure

- Gastrointestinal haemorrhage should prompt a search for physical signs of a predisposing condition such as liver disease, telangiectasia, NSAID use, abdominal aortic surgery

- Enteroscopes allow visualisation of the small bowel and delivery of haemostatic therapy under direct vision

Further Reading

1 Davies GR, Benson MJ, Geitner DJ, Van Someren RMN, Rampton DS, Swain CP. Diagnostic and therapeutic push type enteroscopy in clinical use. *Gut* 1995;**37**:346–52.
2 Lewis MPN, Khoo DE, Spencer J. Value of laparotomy in the diagnosis of obscure gastrointestinal haemorrhage. *Gut* 1995;**37**:187–90.
3 Morris AJ. Endoscopy of the small bowel. (1966) In Cotton PB, Tytgat GNJ, Williams CB, ed. *Annal of Gastrointestinal Endoscopy.* 9th edition. London, Rapid Science Publishers.
4 Pennazio M, Arrigoni A, Risio M, Spandre M, Rossini FP. Clinical evaluation of push type enteroscopy. *Endoscopy* 1995;**27**:164–70.

4: Endoscopic technique in the bleeding patient

PAUL SWAIN

Endoscopy in patients with gastrointestinal bleeding is sometimes more difficult than routine diagnostic endoscopy. The patients tend to be more frightened. They are more likely to be shocked. Some patients with bleeding will have severe associated cardiopulmonary diseases that increase the risk of endoscopy. Patients bleeding because of liver disease may be encephalopathic; alcoholic patients may be difficult to sedate.

Endoscopy may take longer, because it can be harder to define the bleeding site and treatment of the lesion takes extra time. It may have to be done out of hours, with the assistance of a less experienced nurse. The endoscope is more likely to become blocked.

If the patient is shocked or has clearly had a substantial bleed it can be helpful to examine the stomach for a succussion splash, which will give some indication that a large volume of blood is likely to be encountered. If the patient has had aortic graft surgery it is important to reach the third part of the duodenum, as this is the common site at which grafts erode into the duodenum.

Explanation and consent

If there is a chance that therapeutic endoscopy will be used the patient should be informed of the possible risks and benefits of this and a statement to this effect should be included in the consent form. In patients with shock and a substantial bleed it makes sense to obtain their consent for operative treatment as well as endoscopy, so that they can go quickly to theatre if necessary.

Sedation and monitoring

Discriminating use of sedation is required in some groups of patients with gastrointestinal bleeding. Very elderly patients, those with cardiopulmonary disease, and patients with liver failure require smaller doses or no sedation. Pulse oximetry, with supplementary oxygen saturation, expert oropharyngeal suction and careful observation of the patient's clinical condition are especially helpful during the endoscopy. Alcoholic patients tend to be poorly responsive to benzdiazepines and can become disinhibited during endoscopy. Patients who have delirium tremens, or who are fighting drunk, are usually best left to be endoscoped the next morning unless they are bleeding substantially.

Choice of endoscope

The choice of endoscope usually depends on what is available.

Video endoscopes are useful for teaching, photography, making video recordings and demonstrating therapeutic practice with bleeding patients,

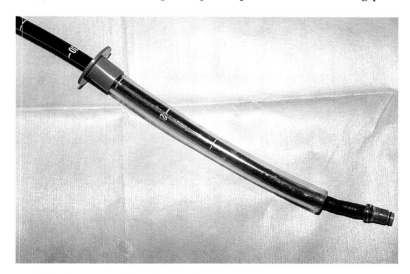

FIGURE 4.1—*An oro-oesophageal overtube.*

but sometimes give poor images, especially in patients with major bleeding. This is mainly because of the CCD (charge-coupled device) chip quenching response to the red colour of blood and the greater absorption of light by blood. If the view is inferior it is best to change to a conventional non-video fibreoptic endoscope.

Large diameter endoscopes have bigger light bundles and larger channels, and therefore some advantages. They offer a clearer, better lit view and allow more rapid suction of blood and the passage of larger therapeutic accessories. Large diameter biopsy channel endoscopes are probably necessary if bipolar or heater probes are to be used to best effect, because the small diameter probes are less effective than their larger diameter counterparts at haemostasis.

Double channel endoscopes allow suction to be maintained while therapy is delivered. They can be helpful with patients who have major bleeding, but it can be difficult to pass them, especially in small elderly women. Large diameter endoscopes (>11 mm) cannot be used for banding of varices with the devices as configured at present, because once the banding device has been attached to the tip of the endoscope it cannot be passed through the overtube.

A side-viewing duodenoscope gives better views of the medial wall of the duodenum, especially in the second part, and is useful if haemobilia is suspected or if bleeding is seen to be coming from the distal bulb or second part of the duodenum.

Use of an overtube, airway or nasogastric tube

The passage of an oro-oesophageal overtube (see Figure 4.1) provided it passes the cricopharyngeus easily, can be an asset to the endoscopy of patients with substantial bleeding and a stomach full of blood. It protects the airway if the patient vomits up large quantities of blood, allows aspiration of stomach and oral secretions separately and facilitates the frequent removal and reinsertion of the endoscope for cleaning and attachment of therepeutic accessories, such as banding for varices. If an overtube is being used it is helpful to soak it in hot water; this makes it more pliable and lubricates the plastic, making it easier to insert. The passage of a guide wire, with the subsequent use of a dilator that fits the overtube, is also helpful, especially if there is resistance to passage at the cricopharyngeus.

Endotracheal intubation

Occasionally it may be necessary to pass an endotracheal tube, especially for endoscopy in patients in a hepatic coma. All endoscopists must be trained to pass an endotracheal tube in patients with incipient aspiration or who have been over sedated without waiting for an anaesthetist to arrive. More commonly patients receiving intensive care have to be endoscoped with an airway in situ. Occasionally the endotracheal tube with a well distended balloon, combined with the fact that the patient is lying on his or her back, can make oesophageal intubation difficult.

Avoidance of nasogastric tubes

Nasogastric tubes are used routinely in some countries and accident and emergency units to see if there really is blood in the stomach and to select patients requiring early endoscopy. It is usually more unpleasant to have a nasogastric tube passed than to have an endoscopy, and nasogastric tubes can cause misleading erosions and oesophagitis, and rarely precipitate bleeding from ulcers or varices. Some patients have a particularly bad time when inexperienced staff try to pass them. If patients need to have a tube down, it might as well be an endoscope. I think that the use of nasogastric tubes in gastrointestinal bleeding is an example of thoughtless cruelty to patients and can give misleading appearances. Although it is usually possible to do an endoscopy with a nasogastric tube in situ, it is important to cap off the end of the tube so that intragastric air does not escape. Nasogastric tubes usually come out when the endoscope is withdrawn, even if the endoscope is well lubricated. It is usually best to take the nasogastric tube out before the endoscopy or to use it as a marker for the oesophageal orifice and remove it as soon as the oesophagus is intubated.

Avoiding blockage of the endoscope

Endoscope blockage is more likely to occur during endoscopy of bleeding patients than during routine endoscopy. Check that the endoscope is blowing well before starting by placing the tip under water and covering the blowing valve. Use inflation and washing rather than suction to improve visualisation of an area. Avoid using the suction channel if clots are seen. If the views are poor remove the endoscope and check that it is still blowing. Check that the blowing function is working well after the endoscopy, then flush the system and use the clearance valves, especially if the endoscope is to be cleaned by less experienced staff out of hours. The commonest cause of a poor view during endoscopy for bleeding is blockage of the blowing channel.

Use of an ancillary washing facility

A means to wash blood away is the single most useful endoscopic accessory for the diagnosis of bleeding site at endoscopy. It is useful for clearing loose blood clot away to allow a view of the mucosal surface. It is essential for the diagnosis of oozing, which can only be made securely by seeing a point that looks as if it might be oozing, washing the blood away and watching to see that blood really is coming from the bleeding point. Some thermal devices, such as bipolar probe and heater probe, have pumps that can wash the bleeding point through a small channel in the probe, using the biopsy channel (see Figure 4.2). These work well and are worth having for this facility alone. A hand powered washing catheter can be readily improvised from a cannula used for endoscopic retrograde choloangiopancreatography, or the ulcer can be washed by attaching a large syringe to the biopsy channel. We made a cheap endoscopic washing pump from a car windscreen wiper pump and a cannula. It can help to put some silicone oil in the washing liquid to reduce bubbling.

What to do if there is a lot of blood

Don't panic. Tell the nurse at the patient's head to be ready with suction, and keep the patient well over in the left lateral position. Encourage the patient not to retch. Most retching settles once the endoscope is in the stomach and if the movements of the endoscope are gentle. Inflation of the stomach will lift the lesser curve of the stomach away from the dependent pool of blood, substantial bleeding from gastric ulcers is likely to derive from ulcers high on the posterior aspect of the lesser curve (see Figure 4.3). The endoscope can be slipped along the lesser curve into the antrum,

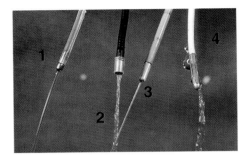

FIGURE 4.2—*Washing facilities in action: (1) "dry" monopolar, (2) "liquid" monopolar, (3) bipolar electrocoagulation probes, (4) heater probe.*

which is usually relatively free of blood because with the patient in the left lateral position it is sloping upwards. It is usually easy to identify the pylorus and enter the duodenum. Active bleeding in the bulb is usually cleared quickly by peristaltic duodenal activity. Endoscopic difficulty in this area usually results from large floppy clots. These can prolapse through the pylorus, cover the ulcer and be difficult to clear.

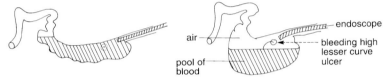

FIGURE 4.3—*Inflation of the stomach lifts a high lesser curve ulcer out of the pool of blood in the stomach.*

Never try to roll the patient over with the endoscope in place as this can cause aspiration and rarely improves the view. If you are suspicious that bleeding is coming from high on the greater curve, take the endoscope out, turn the patient carefully over and position him or her to lie facing the endoscopist, so that the greater curve is uppermost by reversing the head–feet orientation of the patient. Major bleeding is uncommon from sites high on the greater curve of the stomach, and is usually associated with angiodysplasia, leiomyoma or cancer. See Box 4.1 for the key points when there is a lot of blood.

Box 4.1   When there is a lot of blood

- Ensure that assistant is ready with suction
- Keep patient well over in the left lateral position
- Encourage the patient not to retch
- Inflate
- Slip the endoscope along the lesser curve into the antrum and so to the pylorus
- To see the greater curve, always remove the endoscope before turning the patient

---

Getting covered with blood

Endoscoping patients with gastrointestinal bleeding can be a messy business. Wearing aprons and protective clothing is sensible. Eye protection is important, especially when endoscoping HIV positive patients who are bleeding. The risk of eye splash is higher with optical endoscopes than it is with video types, because the eye is closer to the biopsy channel.

Hepatitis B protection

Hepatitis B vaccination should be an essential precaution for doctors and nursing or endoscopy associate staff who are endoscoping bleeding patients.

A plan of endoscopy for a bleeding patient

A systematic approach is essential.

- Have a check list of diagnoses that are being excluded as the endoscopy proceeds.
- Look at the pharynx: a lot of blood here but little in the oesophagus may indicate a nasal, throat or bronchial source. The mid-oesophagus is sometimes poorly examined in bleeding patients by endoscopists in a hurry to reach the stomach and duodenum: check for varices (see Figure 4.4).

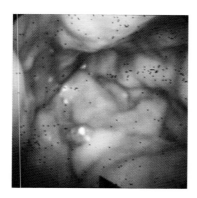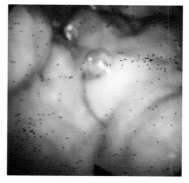

FIGURE 4.4—*Oesophageal varices.*

- Try to see the cardio-oesophageal junction before crossing it; look especially at the 1 o'clock position, which is the common site for Mallory-Weiss tear (see Figure 4.5).
- If an ulcer is present, try to assess whether there are stigmata of recent bleeding and then whether there is a vessel to be seen. If unsure, try to wash the ulcer.
- Check that the difficult areas have been seen, especially the posterior duodenal bulb, the second part of the duodenum and under the angulus;

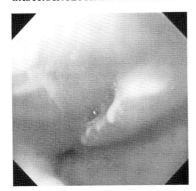

FIGURE 4.5—*A Mallory-Weiss tear.*

examine the high posterior lesser curve and the cardia fully with a J manoeuvre.

- If one ulcer or lesion is seen do not allow this finding to prevent a full examination of the upper gastrointestinal tract for another lesion.
- Ask yourself if the findings fit with the clinical story. If there has been a big bleed and the endoscopic findings are trivial, have another look around.
- Check that the endoscope is inflating well throughout the examination and change it if the view is inferior.

What to do if you are sure there has been upper gastrointestinal bleeding but no source is obvious

Change from a video to an optical endoscope. Schedule a repeat endoscopy once the patient has been transfused if the patient is severely anaemic. Always cross the pylorus at least twice, because the endoscope commonly fails to visualise ulcers just inside the bulb, positioned posteriorly; it is usually pointing at the anterior wall as the pylorus is crossed.

Catches for the unwary endoscopist

- About 50% of Mallory-Weiss tears are missed on the first pass into the stomach. This is because the stomach may need to be inflated to open up the folds at the cardio-eosophageal junction before this lesion can be well seen.
- Multiple ulcers can cause diagnostic problems. A prepyloric ulcer can be associated with a large duodenal ulcer. Usually the duodenal ulcer will be the significant source of bleeding. Occasionally there are two or more ulcers high on the lesser curve. The bleeding is most likely to be coming from the largest, and usually the most proximal, ulcer.
- The diagnosis of early varices is more difficult than non-endoscopists or inexperienced operators realise. If you are uncertain, withdraw the

endoscope about 3 cm from the cardio-oesophageal junction and look for the cordlike appearance. Overinflating the oesophagus can flatten varices. They do not always have a blue colour and sometimes appear whiter or browner than the oesophageal mucosa.

- Rarities cause difficulty because of inexperience. Dieulafoy ulceratio simplex usually is found within 3 cm of the cardia (at the classic site for high lesser curve gastric ulcers). The appearance is of a visible vessel high on the lesser curve with minimal surrounding ulceration. Solitary gastric angiomas can occur at the junction of gastric body and fundus on the greater curve and may be hidden under a pool of blood. "Watermelon" stomach is often mistaken for gastritis. Oesophageal apoplexy, with a huge blue haematoma dissecting the oesophageal mucosa, is puzzling when first encountered. Gastric angiomas can be mistaken for suction artefacts.

- Diagnosis of bleeding from angiomas or aneurysms in the duodenum requires a clear endoscopic view, and recognitions of abnormal pulsation. The diagnosis of heamatobilia, i.e. bleeding from the biliary tract or wirsungorrhagia, i.e. bleeding from the pancreatic duct, requires patience, a washing facility and sometimes a side-viewing endoscope.

- Severe anaemia makes endoscopy difficult because the pale, anaemic mucosa is difficult to distinguish from superficial ulcers and erosions. Transfusing the patient and scheduling a repeat endoscopy can help to make the diagnosis. Repeat endoscopy later if the first attempt is limited by the volume of blood in the stomach.

Conclusion

Diagnostic endoscopy in gastrointestinal bleeding is an exciting and rewarding part of gasteroenterology. The occasional technical difficulties that can test the endoscopist's skill can usually be overcome with care.

Key points

- Endoscopy in the presence of gastrointestinal bleeding is likely to be more difficult than routine diagnostic endoscopy

- Consent should be obtained for both endoscopy and operative treatment, to allow rapid transfer of the patient to theatre if necessary

- Video endoscopes often give a poor image in patients with major bleeding

- The commonest cause of a poor view during endoscopy for bleeding is blockage of the blowing channel

- A means to wash away blood is the most useful accessory to facilitate diagnosis

- Hepatitis B vaccination is essential for all staff who endoscope bleeding patients

---

Part III
Management of upper gastrointestinal haemorrhage

5: Endoscopic stigmata of recent bleeding

PAUL SWAIN

The appearance of a vessel in the floor of an ulcer in patients dying from bleeding peptic ulcer was described by Cruveilhier in 1830[1] and Rokitansky in 1848[2] in textbooks of pathology. Pioneer endoscopists Gutzeit and Tietge, using rigid endoscopes in Germany in the 1930s, first used the term "stigmata" to indicate spots of blood adherent to the gastric mucosa.[3] Schindler, who pioneered tip deflectable rigid gastrointestinal endoscopy in Germany and America in the 1930s–50s, considered the prognostic significance of a vessel visible in an ulcer that had recently bled.[4]

During the early era of flexible endoscopy in the 1970s there was excitement and interest in the high incidence of recurrent bleeding when active bleeding, especially spurting, was seen in an ulcer at endoscopy.[5] Observation of blood in the stomach or adherent to an ulcer was taken to indicate that the endoscopically observed ulcer was the source of bleeding.

The phrase "stigmata of recent haemorrhage" was reintroduced and popularised in 1978 by Foster, who suggested not only that the presence of blood adherent to an ulcer indicated that it had recently bled but that this finding carried a risk of further bleeding of 42%.[6] In 1979 a study by Griffiths published with a colour illustration in the *New England Journal of Medicine* attracted attention because of the suggestion that the finding of a "visible vessel" was associated with 100% (28/28) incidence of recurrent bleeding.[7] In 1981 another *New England Journal* article, by Storey,[8] analysed the rebleeding rates in patients with a visible vessel prospectively and found a rebleeding rate of around 50% in the course of randomised trials of endoscopic therapy (Table 5.1).

Recognition of the visible vessel was important for those conducting trials of endoscopic therapy. Some endoscopists had been trying to stop bleeding by burning the whole of an ulcer floor or around the rim of the ulcer; identification of the visible vessel allowed the treatment to become more focussed and, perhaps in consequence, the results of trials improved after this observation became generally known to endoscopists. Many subsequent series, mainly drawn from the control group in randomised trials of endoscopic treatment, have documented an incidence of rebleeding with a non-bleeding visible vessel of about 45%. The frequency with which

TABLE 5.1—*Clinical course in patients with peptic ulcer, according to features of ulcer at endoscopy.**

Ulcer feature	Total	Further bleeding	Urgent surgery	Death
			No. of patients (%)	
Visible vessel	93	54 (58)	48 (52)	16 (17)
Stigmata of bleeding other than a visible vessel	36	2 (6)	1 (3)	1 (3)
No stigmata of bleeding	107	0	0	0

* Ulcers inadequately visualised at endoscopy or treated with argon or Nd: YAG laser are not considered in this table (data from studies[8,14,18,25]).

TABLE 5.2—*Incidence of rebleeding from peptic ulcers with a non-bleeding visible vessel reported in various studies; modified from Johnston[17]*

Author	n	Rebleeding (%)	Author	n	Rebleeding
Griffiths	28	100	Swain	31	48
MacLeod	12	100	Laine	37	41
Papp	16	81	O'Brien	43	37
Panes	21	71	Buset	46	37
Jensen	22	55	Moreto	15	33
Swain	24	54	Wara	39	31
Freitas	17	53	Krejs	15	13
Vallon	16	50	Chang-Chien	19	0
Bornman	10	50			

n, no. of patients.

visible vessels are seen varies widely from series to series[9–25] (4–39%) and there are series[10 11] in which the rebleeding incidence is much higher (100%)[24 25] or much lower (13%, 0%) than the median (Table 5.2). There are a variety of ways of classifying stigmata of recent haemorrhage seen at endoscopy (see Box 5.1).

Box 5.1   Classification of stigmata of recent bleeding[14 18]

- Visible vessel with spurting arterial bleeding
- Non-bleeding visible vessel
- Minor stigmata of recent haemorrhage with active bleeding (oozing)
- Minor stigmata of recent haemorrhage without bleeding
- Overlying clot with active bleeding
- Overlying clot without bleeding
- Clean ulcer floor

Forrest classification of stigmata of recent bleeding (as developed in the German literature)

Ia   Spurting bleeding

continued

Ib	Non-spurting active bleeding
IIa	Visible vessel (no active bleeding)
IIb	Non-bleeding ulcer with overlying clot (no visible vessel)
IIc	Ulcer with hematin-covered base
III	Clean ulcer ground (no clot, no vessel)

Forrest IIa may be subdivided into (i) red or dark blue hemispheric protruding lesion and (ii) pulsatile pseudoaneurysm
NB: this classification is not mentioned as such in Forrest's 1974 article[3]

Definition of terms

Spurting (see Figure 5.1):

Usually endoscopically obvious bleeding, with blood pulsing in a jet or arc usually from right to left in the stomach. A string of clot can mimic spurting bleeding, and transmitted cardiac pulsation can move pools of blood in a way that looks like arterial bleeding.

Oozing:

Non-pulsatile bleeding that is often overdiagnosed, because endoscope contact with granulation tissue on an ulcer edge can cause oozing. Careful endoscopic washing is usually needed to confirm the diagnosis. It is difficult to be sure that oozing is spontaneous if the ulcer is spotted on a pull-back rather than the first pass.

Visible vessel (see Figure 5.2):

A protruding red, blue, black or even white mound, situated in the floor of an ulcer in a patient with a recent gastrointestinal bleed, that is resistant to endoscopic washing. Aneurysmal pulsation is occasionally seen. No other area in the ulcer floor looks as if it has bled. Endoscopic or tissue movement is required to confirm the raised appearance, because endoscopic vision is uniocular.

Minor stigmata (see Figure 5.3):

Pigmented red, blue or black non-protruding macules, smaller than 0·5 mm, in the floor of the ulcer, which are resistant to endoscopic washing.

Clot (see Figure 5.4):

Red or black material in the ulcer floor, may be loose and easy to wash away. Clot can be like a large floppy bag adherent to the vessel or the ulcer floor, obscuring the features of the ulcer crater; it may become enmeshed in the ulcer floor.

Other "stigmata":

The presence, colour and volume of blood in the lumen has rarely been considered for its prognostic significance. No blood in the lumen probably

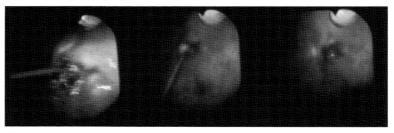

Figure 5.1

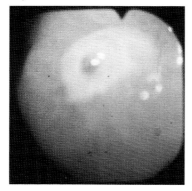

Figure 5.2

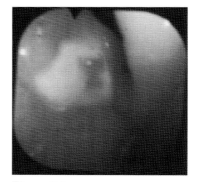

Figure 5.3

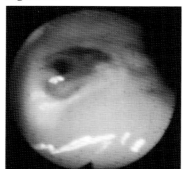

Figure 5.4

FIGURE 5.1—*Spurting stopped by laser.*
FIGURE 5.2—*A visible vessel.*
FIGURE 5.3—*A minor stigma (flat red spot).*
FIGURE 5.4—*An adherent clot.*

indicates a lower risk of bleeding than a large volume. Bright red blood may indicate a higher risk of further bleeding. Patients with large clot forming a tense cast of the stomach tend to do badly.

Colour of visible vessels

The colour that makes the vessel visible is derived from haemoglobin. Arteries without blood in them are transparent.[26] The initial red colour of the visible vessel seen at endoscopy is usually that of fresh clotted blood adherent to the vessel that may protrude into the floor of the ulcer from a rent in the vessel side. The clot darkens as it oxidises speeded by the presence of acid. Later many of the red cells enmeshed in the clot are lysed, leaving a slowly whitening plug of fibrin and platelets. The remaining brown, discoloured clot is subsequently cleared by fibrinolytic mechanisms including pepsinogen. Small amounts of blood may become enmeshed by granulation tissue, probably accounting for minor stigmata of haemorrhage or spots.

The floor of a chronic ulcer is usually white if there is scar tissue and pale pink if it is an acute ulcer without scar tissue.

Colour and prediction of rebleeding

Can observation of the colour of the visible vessel at endoscopy improve predictions of further bleeding?

In Wara's study,[23] when a vessel was associated with oozing or fresh clot, the incidence of further bleeding was higher (42%) than when a "bare" visible vessel was seen or one associated with black slough (18%) (Table 5.3). Chang-Chien[25] described a low incidence of further bleeding with black vessels (0%). Lin[27] reported visible vessel rebleeding rates of 10/33 (30%) for red or dark red vessels, 4/12 (33%) for black and 5/8 (63%) for white vessels. Endoscopists may disagree when asked to choose the colour of stigmata.[28]

TABLE 5.3—*Incidence and predictive value of stigmata of recent bleeding; from Wara*[23]

Stigma of haemorrhage	Incidence (%)	Major rebleeding (%)	Rebleeding potential
Arterial bleeding	23/303 (8)	23/23 (100)	High
Visible vessel	31/303 (10)	13/31 (42)	Moderate
Oozing (no visible vessel)	62/303 (20)	12/62 (31)	Moderate
Clot (no visible vessel)	79/303 (24)	19/79 (24)	Equivocal
"Bare" visible vessel or with old stigmata	22/303 (7)	4/44 (18)	Low
Minor stigmata with no visible vessel	56/303 (18)	5/56 (9)	Low
No stigmata	30/303 (10)	0/30 (0)	None

Freeman[29] has developed a colour based macroscopic classification of visible vessels seen at endoscopy:

1. Clear, pale or translucent vessels (perhaps correlating pathologically with a vessel without clot extending above the ulcer surface).
2. A vessel with an attached clot protruding above the ulcer surface (red/purple).
3. A "sentinel" clot (black) (compare Johnston[9 30]) with protruding clot and the vessel well below the surface of the ulcer.

Ten out of eleven (91%) patients with vessels rebled while 0/7 patients with "sentinel clot" appearance rebled. These patients had daily endoscopy and no endoscopic treatment.

This suggestion that a "white" vessel has a high incidence (91%) of further bleeding is a controversial idea, because pigmentation was initially part of the definition of a visible vessel, and Johnston[9] has suggested that the white "sentinel" clot or visible vessel is a late stage indicating healing and disappearance of the vessel. Perhaps Freeman's "white" vessel could represent a stage at which the red cells in the clot have been removed and fibrinolysis is about to remove the fibrin clot, leaving the eroded vessel underneath dangerously exposed.

Other features increasing the chance of further bleeding

Some series have suggested that there is an additive effect when clinical and endoscopic features are combined to predict further bleeding. For example, endoscopic stigmata with hypotension had a rebleeding rate of 67%, while those without hypotension but similar stigmata had a rebleeding incidence of 27% in a series reported by Brearley[31] and these observations have been supported by data from the series of Bornman[17] and Braniki.[32] By using selection criteria for major haemorrhage, including shock and a substantial transfusion requirement, MacLeod found that all ulcer patients with a demonstrable artery (visible vessel) rebled.[10 33] Rebleeding is more likely at certain locations, especially the posterior duodenal bulb (gastroduodenal artery) or high lesser curve (left gastric artery),[34] while pre-pyloric ulcers appear to have a better prognosis.[23] Positive Doppler signal over a vessel suggests an increased chance of further bleeding (Beckely, Fullarton).[35 36] Large ulcer size in two series of Matthewson and Braniki[32 37] and a large visible vessel appearance in Papp's series[11] have been associated with, a high rebleeding rate. Garrigues has suggested that computer analysis of clinical factors is as reliable as the presence of stigmata in prediction of rebleeding and that combining the two does not improve prediction,[38] while Pimpl suggested that scoring systems based on a combination of endoscopic and clinical measurements enhance prediction.[39]

Common questions asked about stigmata

Why are there differences in the reported incidence of bleeding?

Differences in definition may be relevant. Our group included spurting and active bleeding from a protrusion in an ulcer in our definition of a visible vessel, which will tend to increase the rebleeding rate.[14 18] If selection criteria require shock or high transfusion requirement before inclusion then rates are likely to be high, as in MacLeod's series.[10 33]

The use of an endoscopic washing technique is likely to increase the yield of vessels observed under loose clot. Two studies[24 25] with an unusually low incidence of further bleeding did not use washing.

The need to choose a randomisation envelope saying "non-bleeding visible vessel 'yes' or 'no' ", and the need to focus endoscopic therapy somewhere in the ulcer base forces decision making, which is not always easy.

The learning curve of endoscopic therapy means that those who burn or inject ulcers learn rather quickly what is a vessel. If you burn a small clot away and see a clean ulcer floor, there was no vessel, but if you poke a mound and it spurts, you learn to recognise and respect the appearance of a visible vessel.

There is a subjective element in the reporting. Data from two groups suggest that, if definitions are agreed, some degree of concordance can be achieved on what is meant by a non-bleeding vessel when videotapes are reviewed blindly.[29][40]

Stigmata of haemorrhage are found more frequently at early endoscopy, performed soon after hospital admission, than at 1 or 2 days later. The incidence and risk of rebleeding is likely to vary depending how soon patients are endoscoped.

There are likely to be true differences between series reflecting geographic and other patterns of referral with gastrointestinal bleeding. For example, our patients in London[14][18] were on average 20 years older than patients with bleeding peptic ulcer in Hong Kong,[40] which is likely to influence outcome but may influence differences in observations of stigmata of recent haemorrhage.

Is treatment of the non-bleeding visible vessel valuable?

Several randomised controlled trials have prospectively treated non-bleeding visible vessels. Laine's study of bipolar electrocoagulation, for example (38 bipolar treated v 37 control patients) showed an 18% v 41% rebleeding rate (p<0·05) with a significantly lower requirement for urgent surgery, shorter hospital stay and reduced cost.[19] Our group showed a reduction in rebleeding rate both with argon and Nd:YAG laser with non-bleeding visible vessels.[14][18] Buset, using a Nd:YAG laser, reported significantly less rebleeding in the groups with gastric ulcer with a non-bleeding vessel, but not in duodenal ulcers.[21] Some groups do not recommend injection for non-bleeding visible vessel.[41] There are trials that show significant benefit for treatment of this group using injection of adrenalin and polidocanol.[12][42] Meta-analysis of the data on treatment of non-bleeding visible vessel suggests significant reduction in rebleeding rate and urgent surgery rates after laser, thermal probe, and injection treatments.[43]

On the debit side, treatment of non-bleeding visible vessel sometimes precipitates further bleeding (with an average reported incidence of 20%; most will stop with further treatment). Although endoscopic treatment improves the hospital course of most patients with a non-bleeding visible vessel, it can worsen the course of an individual patient. Some would argue that such patients are particularly closely observed in hospital and will have early surgery, but it is possible that some patients who might have settled if managed conservatively have died because treatment precipitated bleeding.

Can stigmata of recent haemorrhage indicate that an ulcer seen at endoscopy is definitely the source of major haemorrhage?

It seems probable that, if a patient is admitted with gastrointestinal bleeding and an ulcer with stigmata of recent haemorrhage is seen, then that ulcer is the likeliest source of bleeding provided that another source, for example varices, is not found.

Most ulcers probably bleed a small amount[44] and do not present with haematemesis and melaena; some will present with anaemia. We have shown that about 25% of ulcers seen at routine endoscopy in patients without manifest bleeding have minor stigmata of recent haemorrhage, with red or black spots adherent to the ulcer floor. In this series visible vessels were not seen in patients with peptic ulcers who had not been admitted because of manifest bleeding.[45]

How do stigmata and visible vessels correlate with pathological studies of bleeding ulcer?

Vessels have been reported as protruding from bleeding ulcers in post-mortem series since 1830.[1 2 46 47] Surgical series also report the appearance of vessels visible in the floor of ulcers.[48-52] One series tried to correlate the endoscopic appearance of a visible vessel with the pathological findings in patients who rebled and had a bleeding gastric ulcer resected at surgery.[27] About one-third of ulcers with visible vessels have a structure protruding above the surface of the ulcer that is recognisable as an artery, which may or may not have adherent clot. In another third, the protrusion is a clot with the vessel structure identifiable below the ulcer. Sometimes the clot forms a pseudoaneurysmal roof over a breach in the side of the vessel. In the remainder, no protrusion was seen and the clot or protruding vessel seen at endoscopy has presumably fallen off with further bleeding before surgery.

Fibrinoid necrosis, aneurysm (true or false), loose intimal thickening and recanalisation of thrombus were commonly found in the artery, indicating the range of pathological changes seen in the vessel.

The size of vessels eroded ranges from 0·1 mm to 3·45 mm. It is likely that bleeding from large vessels is more likely to continue and may be harder to stop using endoscopic methods. Although major bleeding in peptic ulcer patients stems from erosion of a single, medium sized artery, about a quarter of the patients also have erosion of an accompanying vein and the same percentage have erosion of other smaller arterial vessels.[26]

Which patients with which stigmata should have treatment?

There is little doubt that spurting arterial haemorrhage requires treatment, as the risk of continued or recurrent bleeding is about 85% in several series.[14 18] Some recommend treatment of oozing lesions. If there is a visible vessel appearance with oozing this should be treated. Treating oozing in the absence of such an appearance is less certainly of value.[14 18] There is good evidence from trials that treatment of the non-bleeding visible vessel can improve outcome.[43]

There is good evidence that patients with no stigmata of haemorrhage are at low risk of further bleeding.[14 18 23 26] Such patients do not need treatment and can probably be sent home early if they have no other problems. The frequency and incidence of further bleeding with stigmata of recent haemorrhage in two large series is indicated in Tables 5.3 and 5.4.

TABLE 5.4—*Stigmata of haemorrhage and rebleeding in 370 patients; from Swain et al.*[14 18]

Stigma	Incidence (%)	Rebleeding (%)
Spurting arterial bleeding	30 (8)	85
Visible vessel	95 (26)	51
Adherent clot obscuring ulcer floor	68 (18)	41
Other stigmata	45 (12)	5
No stigmata	132 (36)	0

Conclusions

Stigmata of recent haemorrhage, especially the identification of a bleeding or non-bleeding visible vessel, seem a useful aid to selecting patients for close observation and endoscopic treatment. If rebleeding prediction rates of 85% for spurting arterial bleeding and 45% for a non-bleeding visible vessel hold true for most endoscopists, then these odds seem good enough to be the basis for endoscopic treatment policies. Endoscopic treatments have proved reasonably but not perfectly safe. Patients found to have ulcers without stigmata can be discharged early with consequent cost savings. Closer observation of stigmata or their combination with other clinical or endoscopic features may further refine their predictive capacity. It may not be possible to predict rebleeding much more precisely. Any gambler who is offered a certainty needs to be on his guard and no tests can predict outcome with 100% accuracy. It would be valuable if more photographs, videos and teaching material were available, so that more endoscopists could learn to recognise these appearances before embarking on treatment.

Key points
- Do not let the finding of one bleeding lesion prevent a full examination of the upper gastrointestinal tract
- Stigmata of recent haemorrhage are found more often when endoscopy is carried out soon after admission, rather than 1 or 2 days later
- Stigmata can predict the risk of rebleeding, and identify patients who need close observation and endoscopic treatment.

1 Cruveilhier J. *Anatomie pathologique du corps humaine*. Paris: Balliere, 1829: 42.
2 von Rokitansky CF. *Handbuch der allgemeinen pathologischen Anatomie*, 3 vols. Vienna: Braunmuller and Siedel, 1842–1846; vol 3, 193–4. For an English translation, see von Rokitansky CF. *A manual of pathological anatomy*, 4 vols. London: Sydenham Society, 1839–54; vol 2, 33–4. Translated from the German by Edward Sieveking.
3 Gutzeit K, Tietge H. *Die Gastrokopie*. Berlin: Urban & Schwarzenberg; 1933.
4 Schindler R. *Gastroscopy*. The University of Chicago Press, Chicago; Illinois 1937.
5 Forrest JAH, Finlayson N. Endoscopy in gastrointestinal bleeding. *Lancet* 1974;2:394–7.
6 Foster DN, Miloszewski K, Losowsky MS. Stigmata of recent haemorrhage in diagnosis and prognosis of upper gastrointestinal haemorrhage. *BMJ* 1978;1:1173–7.
7 Griffiths WJ, Neumann DA, Welsh JD. The visible vessel as an indicator of uncontrolled or recurrent hemorrhage. *N Engl J Med* 1979;**300**:1411–3.
8 Storey DW, Bown SG, Swain CP, Salmon PR, Kirkham JS, Northfield TC. Endoscopic prediction of recurrent bleeding in peptic ulcers. *N Engl J Med* 1981;**305**:915–6.
9 Johnston JH. Endoscopic risk factors for bleeding peptic ulcer. *Gastrointest Endosc* 1990; **36**:S16–20.
10 Macleod IA, Mills PR, MacKenzie JF, Joffe SN, Russell RI, Carter DC. Neodymium yttrium aluminium garnet laser photocoagulation for major haemorrhage from peptic ulcers and single vessels; a single blind controlled study. *BMJ* 1983;**286**:345–8.
11 Papp JP. Endoscopic electrocoagulation in the management of upper gastrointestinal tract bleeding. *Surg Clin North Am* 1982;**62**:797–805.
12 Panes J, Vivier J, Forne M. Controlled trial of endoscopic sclerosis in bleeding peptic ulcers. *Lancet* 1987;2:1292–4.
13 Jensen DM, Machicado G, Kovaks T *et al*. Controlled randomized study of heater probe and BICAP for hemostasis of severe ulcer bleeding [abstract]. *Gastroenterology* 1988;**94**: A208.
14 Swain CP, Bown SG, Storey DW *et al*. Controlled trial of argon laser photocoagulation in bleeding peptic ulcers. *Lancet* 1981;2:1313–6.
15 Freitas D, Donato A, Monteiro JG. Controlled trial of liquid monopolar electrocoagulation in bleeding peptic ulcers. *Am J Gastroenterol* 1985;**80**:853–7.
16 Vallon AG, Cotton PB, Laurence BH *et al*. Randomized trial of endsocopic argon laser photocoagulation in bleeding peptic ulcers. *Gut* 1981;**22**:228–233.
17 Bornman PC, Theodorou NA, Shuttleworth RD *et al*. Importance of hypovolaemic shock and endoscopic signs in predicting recurrent haemorrhage from peptic ulceration: a prospective evaluation. *BMJ* 1985;**291**:245–7.
18 Swain CP, Kirkham JS, Salmon PR *et al*. Controlled trial of Nd-YAG laser photocoagulation in bleeding peptic ulcer. *Lancet* 1986;1:1113–6.
19 Laine L. Multipolar electrocoagulation in the treatment of peptic ulcers with non-bleeding visible vessels. *Ann Intern Med* 1989;**110**:510–4.
20 O'Brien JD, Day SD, Burnham WR. Controlled trial of small bipolar probe in bleeding peptic ulcers. *Lancet* 1986;1:464–7.
21 Buset M, Des Marez B, Vandermeeren A *et al*. Laser therapy for non-bleeding visible vessels in peptic ulcer hemorrhage: a prospective randomized study. *Gastrointest Endosc* 1988;**34**:173.
22 Moreto M, Zaballa M, Ibanez S *et al*. Efficacy of monopolar electrocoagulation in the treatment of bleeding gastric ulcer: a controlled trial. *Endoscopy* 1987;**19**:54–6.
23 Wara P. Endoscopic prediction of major rebleeding – a prospective study of stigmata of hemorrhage in bleeding peptic ulcer. *Gastroenterology* 1985;**88**:1209–4.
24 Krejs GJ, Little KH, Westergaard LT *et al*. Laser photocoagulation for the treatment of acute peptic ulcer bleeding: a randomized controlled clinical trial. *N Engl J Med* 1987; **316**:1614–8.
25 Chang-Chien C, Wu C, Chen P *et al*. Different implications of stigmata of recent haemorrhage in gastric and duodenal ulcers. *Dig Dis Sci* 1988;**33**:400–4.
26 Swain CP, Storey DW, Bown SG *et al*. Nature of the bleeding vessel in recurrently bleeding gastric ulcer. *Gastroenterology* 1986;**90**:595–608.
27 Lin HJ, Perng CL, Lee SD. The predictive factors of rebleeding in peptic ulcer with non-bleeding visible vessel: a prospective observation, with emphasis on the size and colour of the vessel [abstract]. *Gastroenterology* 1992;**102**:A113.
28 Laine L, Freeman M, Cohen H. Interobserver agreement for stigmata of recent haemorrhage: a prospective evaluation in 202 endoscopists. *Gastrointest Endosc* 1993;**39**: 281.

29 Freeman ML, Cass OW, Peine CJ, Onstad GR. The non-bleeding visible vessel versus the sentinel clot: natural history and risk of rebleeding. *Gastrointest Endosc* 1993;**39**:359–66.

30 Johnston JH. The sentinel clot and invisible vessel: pathologic anatomy of bleeding peptic ulcer. *Gastrointest Endosc* 1984;**30**:313–5.

31 Brearley S, Hawkes PC, Dykes PW *et al*. Per-endoscopic bipolar diathermy coagulation of visible vessels using a 3.2 mm probe – a randomized clinical trial. *Endoscopy* 1987;**19**: 160–3.

32 Braniki FJ, Coleman SY, Lam TCF *et al*. Hypotension and endoscopic stigmata of recent haemorrhage in bleeding peptic ulcer: risk models for rebleeding and mortality. *J Gastro Hepatol* 1992;**7**:184–90.

33 MacLeod IA, Mills PR. Factors identifying the probability of further haemorrhage after acute upper gastrointestinal haemorrhage. *Br J Surg* 1982;**69**:256–8.

34 Swain CP, Salmon PR, Northfield TC. Does ulcer position influence presentation or prognosis of acute gastrointestinal bleeding? [abstract] *Gut* 1986;**27**:A632.

35 Beckley DE, Casebow MP. Prediction of rebleeding from peptic ulcer: experience with an endoscopic Doppler device. *Gut* 1986;**27**:96–9.

36 Fullarton GM, Murray WR. Prediction of rebleeding in peptic ulcers by visual stigmata and endoscopic ultrasound criteria. *Endoscopy* 1990;**22**:68–71.

37 Matthewson K, Pugh S, Northfield T. Which peptic ulcer patients bleed? *Gut* 1988;**29**: 70–4.

38 Garrigues V, Ponce J, Martinez F, Sala T, Pertejo V, Berenguer J. Does endoscopy improve prediction of the prognosis in upper gastrointestinal bleeding. *J Clin Gastroenterol* 1992; **15**:8–11.

39 Pimpl W, Boeckl O, Waclamiczek HW *et al*. Estimation of the mortality rate in patients with severe gastroduodenal hemorrhage with aid of a scoring system. *Endoscopy* 1987;**19**: 101–6.

40 Chung SCS, Leung JWC, Lo KK, So LYS, Li AKC. Natural history of the sentinel clot; and endoscopic study [abstract]. *Gastroenterology* 1990;**98**:A31.

41 Chung SCS, Leung JWC, Sung JY *et al*. Injection or heat probe for bleeding ulcer. *Gastroenterology* 1991;**100**:33–7.

42 Rutgeerts P, Gevers AM, Hiele M, Broeckeart L, Vantrappen G. Endoscopic injection therapy to prevent rebleeding from peptic ulcers with a protruding vessel: a controlled comparative trial. *Gut* 1993;**34**:348–50.

43 Cook DJ, Guyatt GH, Salena BJ, Laine LA. Endoscopic therapy for acute nonvariceal upper gastrointestinal hemorrhage: a meta-analysis. *Gastroenterology* 1992;**102**:139–48.

44 Swain CP. When and why do ulcers bleed and what can be done about it? *Aliment Pharmacol Therap* 1987;**1**:455–67S.

45 Kalabakas A, Xourgias B, Karamanolis D *et al*. Incidence and significance of stigmata of recent haemorrhage in ulcer patients without clinical evidence of recent bleeding. *Gut* 1990;**31**:A1206.

46 Osborne GR. The pathology of gastric arteries with special reference to fatal haemorrhage from peptic ulcer. *Br J Surg* 1954;**41**:585–9.

47 Swain P, Kalabakas A, Grandison A *et al*. Size and pathology of vessel and ulcer in patients with fatal bleeding from duodenal ulcer [abstract]. *Gastroenterology* 1990;**96A**:133.

48 Dieulafoy G. Exulceratio simplex. *Bull Acad Med* 1889;**39**–40:49–82.

49 Bolton C. *Ulcer of the stomach*. London: Edward Arnold, 1913.

50 Tixier L, Clavel C. Les grands hemorrhage gastroduodenales. Paris: Masson et Cie, Libraire de l'Academie de Medicin,1933:27.

51 Meulengracht E. Fifteen years' experience with free feeding of patients with bleeding peptic ulcer: fatal cases. *Arch Intern Med* 1947;**80**:697–708.

52 Chalmers TC, Zamcheck N, Curtens GW *et al*. Fatal gastrointestinal haemorrhage. Clinicopathological correlations in 101 patients. *Am J Clin Pathol* 1952;**22**:634–45.

6: Acute resuscitation

G R LIPSCOMB AND W D W REES

All patients admitted with gastrointestinal bleeding are at risk of hypovolaemia, inadequate treatment of which remains an important cause of preventable death. Certain factors associated with higher mortality must be monitored and treated in such patients.

Box 6.1 Cardiovascular response to gastrointestinal bleeding

Loss not exceeding 20% of blood volume

- About 10% of total blood volume can be lost without significant effect on arterial blood pressure or cardiac output. Further loss results in a gradual decrease in both; after loss of 35–40%, cardiac output falls to near zero.

- In the absence of tissue injury, low levels of acute blood loss result in a progressive rise in heart rate and systemic vascular resistance. This response maintains arterial blood pressure near to prehaemorrhage levels, while selective changes in systemic vascular resistance ensure perfusion of essential organs by reducing flow through splanchnic, muscular and dermal circulations. Venous reservoirs also constrict, helping to maintain adequate venous return.

- These cardiovascular responses to hypovolaemia are triggered by decreased vagal tone and increased sympathetic activity, and are mediated by the baroreflex, the sensitivity of which is increased by haemorrhage.

Loss exceeding 20% of blood volume

- As blood loss increases, so does vagal tone, which may cause significant slowing of the heart rate. This is associated with a fall in blood pressure, because of decreased systemic vascular resistance, and hence syncope.

- These hypotensive and bradycardic responses are started by the activation of cardiac C-fibre afferents, the receptors of which are thought to occur mainly in the left ventricle where they are stimulated by distortion of the left ventricular wall during vigorous contraction.

- As blood loss increases to above 30% of blood volume, heart rate may again increase. Simple measurement of vital signs is therefore a poor indicator of blood volume loss.

continued

- Decreased blood flow through the aortic and carotid bodies activates chemoreceptors that produce a vagally mediated bradycardia, sympathetically mediated vasoconstriction and increased respiration. The tachypnoea reduces the reflex bradycardia mediated by cardiac C-fibre afferents and therefore, during the hypotensive phase following severe haemorrhage, stimulation of arterial chemoreceptors may prevent further falls in the blood pressure and pulse.

- During severe hypovolaemia, flow through the cerebral and coronary circulations is preserved. This is mainly because increased sympathetic activity fails to cause significant vasospasm in these circulations and local autoregulation maintains normal flow even when other vascular beds are under perfused.

- If blood loss continues, coronary blood flow will decrease to a rate to below that required for adequate myocardial function. This leads to diminished cardiac output, further cardiovascular deterioration, and death.

Evaluation of Blood Loss

Evaluation of the volume of blood lost is an important and often difficult aspect of the initial assessment of acute gastrointestinal bleeding. The history and direct measurement of blood loss may contribute little information and measurement of the vital signs (pulse, blood pressure, and postural changes in pulse and blood pressure) is the most important first step.

Bleeding history

"Coffee ground" haematemesis or melaena alone is less predictive of significant haemorrhage than red haematemesis and melaena occurring together.[1] Melaena represents degradation of haemoglobin by colonic bacteria and may develop in either upper or lower gastrointestinal bleeding. As little as 50–100 ml of blood introduced into the upper gastrointestinal tract can produce melaena, which is not an accurate indicator of either the site or degree of blood loss.[2] Haematochaesia (passage of blood per rectum) may be caused by upper or lower gastrointestinal bleeding but when caused by upper gastrointestinal bleeding is usually associated with hypovolaemia.

Stomach contents

Some authors advocate early nasogastric intubation to assess the nature of gastric contents.[3] This has some prognostic value, as mortality increases from 6% when a clear aspirate is obtained to 18% when bright red blood is present.[4] Nasogastric intubation can also indicate the site of bleeding. Bleeding from the upper gastrointestinal tract is indicated by a positive aspirate, but not excluded by a negative result. However, nasogastric tubes are uncomfortable, they can cause oesophageal and gastric trauma, and may clog when large clots are present. On balance, nasogastric intubation is best avoided.

Vital signs

Measurement of vital signs in isolation, may not provide an accurate reflection of blood loss. The physiological response to hypovolaemia (see Box 6.1) includes bradycardia or tachycardia and hypotension is a late feature, especially in the young who are able to preserve cardiovascular stability despite large losses. Vital signs may also be influenced by other medical disorders or drug therapy, such as preceding hypertension treated by betablockers. Nevertheless a pulse rate in excess of 100 beats per min, systolic blood pressure below 100 mm Hg and a drop in diastolic blood pressure of more than 10 mm Hg on standing or sitting all indicate significant blood loss, see Box 6.2. These signs are often associated with pallor and sweating. The shock index (pulse rate/systolic pressure) reflects actual volume deficit better than do its individual components.[5] Most patients with a volume loss of less than 25% have a shock index below 1·0, which increases to 1·0 with 25–33% loss and to above 1·0 with greater loss.

Central venous pressure and volumetric analysis

Acute blood loss decreases venous return, causing a fall in central venous pressure (CVP). There is a significant correlation between CVP and the extent of blood loss[5] and its measurement is often useful in monitoring patients with hypovolaemia. More invasive monitoring using pulmonary wedge pressures and oxygen transport gives accurate information about volume depletion but during the early stages of assessment and resuscitation such measures are not feasible. Volumetric analysis using tracer dilutional techniques such as erythrocytes labelled with $^{99}Tc^m$ or indocyanine green, or ^{125}I-labelled albumin can also provide accurate estimations of blood volume in haemodynamically stable patients, but is also inappropriate during acute resuscitation.

Haematocrit

Haematocrit, often measured as part of the routine full blood count at initial presentation, bears little relation to the degree of blood loss. Because haemorrhage involves loss of whole blood the haematocrit remains constant despite reduced intravascular volume; it declines only over the next 72 h as intravascular volume is restored.

Box 6.2   How much blood has been lost?

- Initial assessment of blood loss depends on a combination of the history and regular recording of pulse, blood pressure and postural changes in blood pressure and pulse.
- Volume deficit is well reflected by the shock index (pulse rate/systolic blood pressure).

continued

Signs of significant blood loss

- Pulse >100 beats/min
- Systolic blood pressure <100 mmHg
- Diastolic blood pressure drop on sitting or standing >10 mmHg
- Pallor and sweating
- Shock index ⩾ 1

Assessment of Individual Risk

Early identification of patients at high risk of dying from their bleed is essential. The mortality rate rises with age, the presence of serious concomitant disease and signs of hypovolaemia at presentation.[67] Risk can be assessed from the history and examination, with particular emphasis on cardiovascular status.

Healthy patients under 60 years of age with no underlying disease have a mortality rate of 2–3% whereas that in older patients is two to four times higher. Older patients are also more likely to have underlying renal, pulmonary and cardiac disease that increases mortality to 22–28%.[8] First presentation with bleeding oesophageal varices is associated with a mortality of 30–40% and jaundice with a mortality of over 40%. Most patients do not fall into these high risk groups and overall mortality is around 5%.

Depending on the cardiovascular status of the patient, assessment and resuscitation may need to be performed at the same time. In most cases a brief but thorough history, examination and routine blood tests should establish the presence of concomitant disease and other risk factors (see Box 6.3). Physicians are often poor at predicting the cause of bleeding on purely clinical grounds, although peptic ulceration is likely in patients taking NSAIDs who have dyspepsia, and a Mallory–Weiss tear in those with repeated vomiting or retching preceding haematemesis. History of preceding liver disease suggests varices, although in 50% of those with alcoholic liver disease the bleed is non-variceal. A previous history of peptic ulceration or variceal bleeding obviously suggests recurrent disease. Unfortunately, many patients have no symptoms or physical signs to suggest the underlying cause of gastrointestinal bleeding.

Box 6.3   Factors associated with a high risk of mortality from gastrointestinal bleeding

Age

- >60 years

Presence of hypovolaemia

- Systolic blood pressure less than 100 mmHg   *continued*

- Diastolic blood pressure falls on sitting/standing
- Pulse >100 bpm
- Shock index $\geqslant 1$

Haemoglobin on presentation

- <10 g/dl

Presence of severe concomitant disease

- Cardiovascular
- Respiratory
- Renal
- Hepatic

Symptoms of gastrointestinal bleed

- Bright red haematemesis and melaena

Physical examination

The main aim of initial physical examination is to evaluate the patient's respiratory and haemodynamic status. Ideally a complete examination should be performed, including a rectal examination, and it is important to check for postural hypotension. For the patient "in extremis", however, resuscitation takes precedence over a thorough examination.

Often there will be few clues to the cause of the bleeding. Varices caused by chronic liver disease are suggested by the presence of jaundice, spider naevi, a liver flap and hepatosplenomegaly. A rectal polyp or carcinoma may be felt on rectal examination and carcinoma of the stomach may present with an epigastric mass. Occasionally, rare causes of gastrointestinal bleeding are diagnosed from classical external appearances; for example, hereditary haemorrhagic telangectasia or the CREST syndrome (calcinosiscutis, Raynaud's phenomenon, oesophageal involvement, sclerodactyly, telangectasia).

Precise diagnosis is usually not essential to initial management. Patients judged to be at high risk should, after appropriate resuscitation, be admitted to a high dependency ward.

Initial Management

For most patients with gastrointestinal bleeding, simple supportive measures are adequate. However, the management of a 70 year old obtunded patient with jaundice and bleeding oesophageal varices will clearly be different from that of a fit, young patient with a history suggestive of a Mallory–Weiss tear. In the accident and emergency department, an experienced triage nurse can assess whether the patient needs immediate resuscitation.

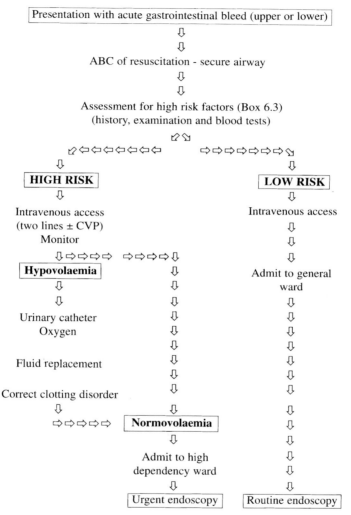

FIGURE 6.1—*Immediate steps in the management of acute gastrointestinal bleeding. CVP: central venous pressure.*

Immediate management steps[10] are summarised in Figure 6.1 and comprise: initial assessment; assessment of cardiorespiratory status; airway protection if appropriate; assessment of volume loss; fluid replacement therapy; documentation of risk factors; diagnosis of the site of bleeding.

Initial resuscitation requires speedy decisions and efficient actions. The "ABC" of resuscitation (airway, breathing, and circulation) may play a crucial part in the first few minutes; Airway protection will take priority in

73

a few patients who present with vomiting and decreased conscious level, and who are at risk of aspiration and subsequent pneumonia. Such patients require oropharyngeal suction to clear the airway of blood and vomit and insertion of an airway. Patients unable to protect their own airway require a cuffed endotracheal tube and may also need mechanical ventilation. Arterial blood gases should be taken from all patients with respiratory difficulty, and oxygen given at appropriate concentration using a mask, nasal cannulae or endotracheal tube.

Once respiratory problems have been assessed and dealt with, blood loss and patient risk factors can be quickly evaluated. Most patients are haemodynamically stable, with little risk of further bleeding or death. Venous access should be established during or shortly after the initial assessment, and at the same time blood taken for urgent full blood count, blood grouping and cross-match, prothrombin time, urea and electrolytes and liver function tests (although the latter may not be required urgently). Those patients who are at high risk should have a 12-lead electrocardiogram and be admitted to a high dependency ward.

Patients with signs of hypovolaemia

The priority in patients with signs of hypovolaemia is to restore intravascular volume. Adequate intravenous access should be established using two large bore intravenous cannulas. If it is difficult to establish peripheral intravenous access, or if the patient has significant cardiovascular disease, a central venous line should be inserted to allow more accurate assessment of fluid replacement. The patient should be catheterised, to allow monitoring of renal function, and given supplementary oxygen. He or she should be monitored using pulse oximetry and ECG, and the urinary catheter removed and oxygen discontinued when the patient is haemodynamically stable.

Initial fluid replacement is with isotonic saline or a synthetic colloid until cross matched whole blood is available. Human albumin should be administered only after 2–3 l of crystalloids, to avoid undue reduction of colloid pressure, or in a hypoproteinaemic patient with oedema. Saline should be avoided in patients with decompensated liver disease, as it leads to accumulation of ascites.

An individual's requirement for blood or blood products depends on several factors, these include: initial blood loss, coagulation defects and concomitant disease. The minimum aim is to restore normal systolic blood pressure, maintain a urine output of at least 30 ml/h and a haematocrit of 0·32.

The initial full blood count and clotting studies may detect abnormalities that need correction. Prolongation of the prothrombin time and partial thromboplastin time may reflect underlying liver disease, anticoagulant administration or absence of specific clotting factors. If the prothrombin time or partial thromboplastin time exceed the normal range by more than

1·5 times they should be corrected as soon as possible using fresh frozen plasma. If the patient has a specific clotting disorder, such as von Willebrand's disease or haemophilia, the appropriate factors should be replaced.

Thrombocytopenia of less than $50 \times 10^9/l$ should be corrected by platelet transfusion, although if underlying disease results in abnormalities of platelet function, transfusion may be indicated at levels higher than $50 \times 10^9/l$.

Massive transfusion, defined as transfusion equivalent to the patient's total blood volume, may result in coagulation defects, because factors V and VIII decay during storage. Coagulation should be monitored by repeated full blood count and clotting studies during and after transfusion, and any defects that develop treated with fresh frozen plasma. There is no place for routine administration of fresh frozen plasma, platelets or calcium without clinical indication.[9]

Many empirical therapies for acute gastrointestinal bleeding have been tried, including intragastric instillation of cold saline, gastric acid suppression, antifibrinolytic agents and various vasoactive drugs. None of these is of certain benefit to the heterogenous group of patients that presents with haematemesis and melaena. However, early intervention with vasoactive drugs is effective in certain groups. In particular, early treatment of patients who have bleeding oesophageal varices (with octreotide and somatostatin) has been shown to arrest bleeding in 70–80% of cases, decrease rebleeding and reduce mortality (see Chapter 7). If such haemostasis is achieved, subsequent diagnostic and therapeutic endoscopic evaluation is made easier. Both octreotide and somatostatin have few side effects, and patients at high risk of bleeding from the consequences of portal hypertension should be started on such treatment pending endoscopic confirmation. We would recommend a 50 µg bolus of intravenous octreotide followed by an intravenous infusion (50 µg/h in 5% dextrose) until endoscopy.

Stable patients should be transferred to a high dependency area for close monitoring by experienced nursing and medical staff, and referred for endoscopy to determine the precise site and cause of bleeding. Ideally patients should be admitted to a combined medical/surgical unit for continued care, as such an approach has been shown to improve mortality.[11] Repeated measurements of blood pressure, pulse and, if appropriate central venous pressure are used to calculate subsequent transfusion requirements.

Patients without signs of hypovolaemia

Patients may present with signs and symptoms of gastrointestinal bleeding but not of hypovolaemia. If they have no high risk factors, were previously fit, and have a haemoglobin greater than 10 g/dl, venous access should be established with a single intravenous cannula before transfer to a general ward for monitoring to detect continued bleeding or rebleeding. An early diagnostic endoscopy may then be arranged.

References

1 Wara P, Stodkild EH. Bleeding pattern before admission as guideline for emergency endoscopy. *Scand J Gastroenterol* 1985;**20**:72–8.

2 Daniel WA, Egan S. The quantity of blood required to produce a tarry stool. *JAMA* 1939;**113**:2232.

3 Lieberman D. Gastrointestinal bleeding: initial management. *Gastroenterol Clin North Am* 1993;**22**:723–36.

4 McLoughlin WD, Kolts BE, Achem SR. Nasogastric lavage compared to the outcome in 101 patients seen in an emergency room for upper gastrointestinal haemorrhage [abstract]. *Gastroenterology* 1987;**92**:1529.

5 Burri C, Henkemeyer H, Passler H. Evaluation of acute blood loss by simple haemodynamic parameters. *Progr Surg* 1973;**11**:109–27.

6 Morgan AG, McAdam WAF, Walmersley GL, *et al.* Clinical findings of early endoscopy and multivariate analysis in patients bleeding from the upper gastrointestinal tract. *BMJ* 1977;**2**:237–40.

7 Clason AE, McCoud DAD, Elton RA. Clinical factors in the prediction of further haemorrhage or mortality in acute upper gastrointestinal haemorrhage. *Br J Surg* 1986;**73**:1985–7.

8 Silverstein FE, Gilbert DA, Tedesci FJ, *et al.* The national ASGE survey on upper gastrointestinal bleeding II. Clinical prognostic factors. *Gastrointest Endosc* 1981;**27**:80–93.

9 Blood Transfusion Task Force. Transfusion for massive blood loss. *Clin Lab Haematol* 1988;**10**:265–73.

10 Lennard-Jones JE, Hopkins A, Arthur MJP, *et al.* Upper gastrointestinal haemorrhage: guidelines for good practice and audit of management. *J Roy Coll Physicians Lond* 1992;**26**(3):281.

11 Holman RAE Davis M, Gough KR, Gartell P, Britton DC, Smith RB. Value of a centralised approach in the management of haematemesis and melaena: experience in a district general hospital. *Gut* 1990;**31**:504–8.

7: Pharmacotherapy of acute upper gastrointestinal haemorrhage

G R LIPSCOMB AND W D W REES

Over the past 20 years many pharmacological approaches to the treatment of gastrointestinal bleeding have been explored. The principal drugs used are listed in Box 7.1. Many trials have been too small to assess effects of drug therapy on mortality, and have had broad entry criteria such as "haematemesis and melaena" with little regard for the pathological cause of bleeding. The effect of individual drugs on specific end points, such as mortality, caused by a variety of disease processes, has been difficult to interpret. Morbidity end points, such as surgery rates, incidence of rebleeding and transfusion requirements, are therefore used to evaluate drug success or failure. However, accurate endoscopic diagnosis has made it possible to evaluate the efficacy of drugs in specific causes of gastrointestinal bleeding, giving rise to some optimism for the treatment of certain groups of patients.

Box 7.1 Principal drugs used in the treatment of acute gastrointestinal bleeding. See text for comments on their effectiveness

Peptic ulcer bleeding

- Acid inhibiting drugs (H_2 antagonists and proton pump inhibitors)
- Antifibrinolytic agents (tranexamic acid, aminocaprioic acid)
- Agents to reduce splanchnic blood flow and gastric activity (somatostatin and octreotide)

Bleeding oesophageal varices

- Vasoactive drugs (vasopressin and terlipressin)
- Somatostatin and octreotide

continued

Prophylaxis of variceal bleeding
- Beta-blockers
- Sclerotherapy
- Isosorbide-5-mononitrate

Treatment for Bleeding Peptic Ulcers

Pharmacotherapy may be expected to influence the outcome of peptic ulcer bleeding in three ways:

- Decreasing gastric acid production, thus producing a more favourable environment for peptic ulcer healing and clot formation
- Reducing fibrinolysis at the ulcer site
- Decreasing splanchnic blood flow.

Several studies have evaluated candidate drugs but have often recruited relatively small numbers of patients and produced conflicting results. Meta-analysis of such published work has proved a useful if sometimes controversial tool with which to evaluate the overall effect of drugs on the outcome of gastrointestinal bleeding.

Acid inhibiting drugs

Reduction of gastric acid levels, using H_2 receptor antagonists or proton pump inhibitors, enhances peptic ulcer healing. Platelet function and haemostasis are impaired in an acidic environment, so decreasing acid output should also expedite clotting, thus decreasing blood loss and subsequent rebleeding. These combined actions should decrease the need for surgical intervention and reduce overall mortality. A meta-analysis of studies involving H_2 antagonists has been performed by Collins and Langman.[1] They examined data from 27 randomised studies involving more than 2500 patients who were treated with either cimetidine or ranitidine; they concluded that treatment reduced bleeding rates from gastric ulcers, with a marginal effect on surgery rates and mortality. Individual studies were too small to allow firm conclusions to be drawn. In the largest single study, more than 1000 patients with bleeding peptic ulcers were treated with intravenous famotidine, which had no effect on rebleeding rates, mortality or surgery.[2]

Proton pump inhibitors produce more profound acid suppression and faster ulcer healing than do H_2 antagonists,[3] and intravenous omeprazole rapidly increases intragastric pH.[4] The value of high dose intravenous and oral omeprazole has been examined in a double blind placebo controlled trial of 1147 subjects with upper gastrointestinal bleeding of varied aetiology.[5] Forty five per cent of the patients had peptic ulcers, overall mortality was low and omeprazole failed to reduce mortality, rebleeding or transfusion requirements.

These limited observations provide little support for the routine use of acid inhibiting drugs in the immediate management of haematemesis and melaena, even that caused by peptic ulceration. However, it seems sensible to start ulcer patients on appropriate ulcer healing agents as soon as the diagnosis has been made, to enhance re-epithelialisation.

Antifibrinolytic agents

In contrast to acid inhibitors, antifibrinolytic agents have no effect on ulcer healing and have not been widely used by gastroenterologists in the treatment of gastrointestinal bleeding. Several studies have examined the effects of antifibrinolytics, especially tranexamic acid, on upper gastrointestinal bleeding. Tranexamic acid inhibits plasminogen and plasminogen activators found in gastric and duodenal mucosa and reduces the fibrinolytic action of pepsin. Aminocaproic acid has a similar action and blocks conversion of plasminogen to plasmin, a powerful fibrinolytic enzyme. Unfortunately, these studies have been too small to show a definite effect, the largest being on 516 patients.[6] A meta-analysis of six randomised placebo controlled studies involving 1267 patients, of which 43–88% were bleeding from peptic ulcers,[7] showed a 40% decrease in mortality, a 20–30% decrease in rebleeding and a 30–40% decrease in the need for surgery. However, in the largest study included in the meta-analysis, the active and placebo groups were not well matched with regard to age, a potentially confounding factor, and although there was a decrease in mortality there was no decrease in rebleeding or transfusion requirements. Consequently the results of the meta-analysis are not conclusive, and the value of tranexamic acid and other fibrinolytic agents remains in doubt.

Somatostatin and octreotide

Somatostatin is a naturally occurring hormone that decreases splanchnic blood flow and inhibits output of gastric acid, pepsin and gastrin.[8–10] A synthetic analogue, octreotide, has been developed that has a similar activity profile but a longer half life (100 min versus 3 min).

Several small studies have reported a beneficial effect of somatostatin on upper gastrointestinal bleeding.[11–13] These studies, all of fewer than 100 patients, concluded that somatostatin reduced the frequency of recurrent bleeding and need for operation in patients admitted with haematemesis and melaena. A larger placebo controlled study involving 630 patients with haematemesis and melaena (45% related to peptic ulcer) showed no difference in rebleeding and surgery rates.[14] A multi-centre double-blind controlled study of octreotide in the treatment of 241 patients with bleeding gastric or duodenal ulcer also showed no difference in cessation of bleeding, prevention of rebleeding, surgery rates or transfusion requirements.[15] All the patients in this study had endoscopically confirmed actively bleeding peptic ulcers, and would be expected therefore to have a high risk of continued bleeding and rebleeding and a low placebo response rate.

Theoretically this should have amplified any differences between active and placebo groups, but the 70% placebo response rate observed was similar to that of other studies, and subgroup analysis showed no benefit. Somatostatin and octreotide therefore cannot be recommended for the routine treatment of acute peptic ulcer bleeding.

Oesophageal Varices

Oesophageal varices are the site of bleeding in about 10% of patients presenting with upper gastrointestinal haemorrhage.[16] As portal pressure increases, an important pressure gradient develops between the inferior vena cava and portal vein. When this gradient exceeds 12 mm Hg clinically relevant portal hypertension develops, leading to variceal haemorrhage.

In patients with chronic liver disease it is essential to stop bleeding as soon as possible, to minimise the risk of precipitating encephalopathy or hepatorenal syndrome. Diagnostic and therapeutic endoscopy are also easier and more effective when haemostasis has been achieved. Several drugs have been used to treat acutely bleeding oesophageal varices, including vasopressin, terlipressin, somatostatin, octreotide, and metoclopramide. Several trials have also studied primary and secondary prevention of bleeding from oesophageal varices using beta-blockers and nitrates. The experimental design of such trials is fraught with problems. In patients with chronic liver disease the most important predictor of final outcome is the severity of underlying disease,[17] which is usually classified using the Child's score. Comparison between studies is therefore difficult because the inclusion and exclusion criteria vary according to the aetiology and severity of the liver disease. Furthermore, most studies recruit a small number of patients and compare endpoints such as rebleeding and transfusion requirements rather than mortality.

Treatment of Bleeding Oesophageal Varices

Therapy aimed at reducing or stopping active variceal bleeding works by decreasing portal pressure.

Vasopressin and terlipressin

Vasoactive drugs have been used in the treatment of bleeding oesophageal varices for 40 years and vasopressin, a synthetic nine-amino peptide, is the most widely used, even though it has a short half life. Vasopressin causes an increase in mesenteric vascular resistance and hence a fall in portal venous blood flow and pressure. Increased peripheral vascular resistance and a decreased cardiac output are the main adverse haemodynamic consequences. Transient myocardial ischaemia, myocardial infarction, and cardiac dysrythmias have all been reported and vasopressin treatment is contraindicated in patients with significant ischaemic heart disease.

Increased gut motility with diarrhoea is common, and there are reports of bowel, limb, and cerebral ischaemia.

These multiple side effects of vasopressin have led to the concomitant use of nitrates and prompted the development of chemical analogues. Concomitant administration of intravenous, sublingual or transdermal glyceryl trinitrate decreases portal pressure and ameliorates the peripheral vasoconstriction caused by vasopressin,[18 19] allowing increased doses of vasopressin to be used. Terlipressin is the triglycyl synthetic analogue of vasopressin, over which it has several distinct advantages. Given as an intravenous bolus, it has a considerably longer half life of 4 h and fewer cardiovascular side effects.

Many studies comparing vasopressin with placebo have demonstrated at best a modest effect on haemostasis, and no effect on mortality. Side effects were prominent, although the addition of intravenous or sublingual glyceryltrinitrate decreased cardiovascular side effects and enabled higher doses of vasopressin to be used. Combined treatment thus produces fewer systemic complications and more effective control of bleeding. Terlipressin, with its longer half life and decreased systemic side effects, is superior to placebo[20] and when combined with glyceryltrinitrate is as effective as balloon tamponade at controlling acute bleeding.[21]

Metoclopramide

Pharmacological constriction of the lower oesophageal sphincter decreases blood flow in submucosal varices, and may be expected to decrease bleeding from this area. A small double blind, placebo controlled study involving 22 patients has shown that bleeding from oesophageal varices stopped after 15 min in 10 out of 11 patients given intravenous metoclopramide compared with 4 out of 11 patients given placebo.[22] Short term haemostasis may not prolong survival but aids endoscopy and subsequent therapeutic manoeuvres. However, these observations need to be further evaluated in larger studies before recommendations can be made.

Somatostatin and octreotide

Somatostatin acts on the smooth muscle of splanchnic vessels to decrease blood flow and thus portal pressure. It has no adverse effects on the systemic circulation and a good side effect profile. Several studies have shown that somatostatin stops variceal haemorrhage in about 80% of cases. Its half life is only 1–2 min and administration has to be monitored carefully, because interruption of the infusion results in sudden loss of efficacy. Octreotide is a synthetic analogue of somatostatin, with which it shares four amino acids. Its main advantages are a longer half life (1–2 h) and subcutaneous route of administration.

An initial placebo controlled study of somatostatin[23] showed no benefit, but was complicated by a much higher placebo response rate (83%) than that found in most similar studies (30–40%). Octreotide and somatostatin have been compared with vasopressin,[24-27] injection sclerotherapy[28 29] and terlipressin combined with nitroglycerine.[30] Although the trials differ in protocol, aetiology of participants' liver disease and drug dosages, somatostatin appears to be more effective than vasopressin and lacks the latter's adverse side effect profile. Compared to injection sclerotherapy, somatostatin and octreotide achieved similar high rates of haemostasis (77–84%) and octreotide is as effective as terlipressin and transdermal nitroglycerine in the emergency control of acute variceal bleeding. An advantage of early administration of somatostatin or octreotide is that the haemostasis produced in most patients allows easier endoscopy and sclerotherapy. Large controlled studies comparing octreotide with newer methods of treating actively bleeding varices, such as band ligation and injection of thrombin, are awaited.

In summary, octreotide is an attractive option for drug treatment of acutely bleeding varices. Various treatment regimens have been advocated but the authors recommend that octreotide should be started as soon as variceal bleeding is suspected (for dosage, see p. 75). If subsequent endoscopy shows another cause of bleeding, the octreotide can be stopped.

Primary and Secondary Prevention of Bleeding Oesophageal Varices

Seventy per cent of patients with varices never bleed, but those who do have significant morbidity and a high mortality. Rebleeding occurs in 50–80% of patients. Prophylaxis with sclerotherapy or drugs is not without risk and ideally would be reserved for those individuals at high risk of bleeding.

Who is likely to bleed?

The predictive value of several factors, including variceal size, severity of liver disease and wedged hepatic pressures, has been assessed. In isolation, none of these appears to predict the risk of variceal bleeding. The best prognostic index, produced by the North Italian Endoscopy Club (NIEC), is based on three independent risk factors: modified Child classification, size of varices and the presence and grade of red wale markings (longitudinal dilated venules resembling whip marks) seen at endoscopy.[17] The index has been tested prospectively, and identified a group of patients with a 65% chance of bleeding within 1 year. All these patients were in Child class C and all had large varices with severe red wale markings. Patients in Child class A, with small varices and no red wale markings, had a 2% risk of bleeding within 1 year. The NIEC index can be used to identify the 20% of patients who are at greatest risk of bleeding and therefore most likely to benefit from prophylaxis.

Beta-blocker prophylaxis

Beta-blockers, the drugs most commonly used in prophylaxis, decrease portal pressure when given in a dose that reduces the resting pulse by 25% or to 55 beats per min (whichever is lower). They are generally safe to use in the presence of liver disease but may cause fatigue, bronchospasm and impotence. However, the reduction of pulse rate by 25% or to 55 beats per min does not necessarily indicate an adequate fall in portal pressure. Some authorities have recommended invasive monitoring of patients undergoing initial beta-blockade, to determine when portal pressure has fallen to below 12 mm Hg before instituting long term beta-blocker therapy.[31] The non-selective beta-blocker propranolol has been most widely used, although nadolol and metoprolol have also been investigated. Nadolol may be preferable to propranolol because it has a longer half life, is less lipophilic and is not metabolised by the liver.

A meta-analysis was carried out of six studies of primary prevention and 19 of secondary prevention that involved 1877 patients, of whom 967 were randomised to receive a beta-blocker.[32] The authors showed that propranolol reduced the risk of bleeding or rebleeding by 40% and decreased mortality by 25% in both primary and secondary prevention. Further analysis, using stricter criteria, showed a reduction in rebleeding but not mortality.[33] These results compare favourably with those for sclerotherapy, which decreases the risk of rebleeding by as much as 50% and mortality by 25%.[34] Prophylactic injection sclerotherapy and beta-blocker have been compared in several studies.[35-37] The most recent involved 116 patients, and this compared propanolol at a dose that decreased resting pulse by 25% or to 55 beats per min with weekly sclerotherapy until variceal obliteration. Rebleeding occurred in 63% of those taking propanolol and in 45% of the sclerotherapy group. No differences were found in hospital admission requirements, survival, or causes of death. Complications were more severe in the sclerotherapy group. A meta-analysis of eight earlier studies compared beta-blockers with sclerotherapy in the prevention of rebleeding in 648 patients, with follow up periods of 11–36 months.[38] This showed no difference in rebleeding rates or mortality. Seven further studies involving 347 patients have compared sclerotherapy with sclerotherapy plus beta-blockers in the prevention of rebleeding.[39-45] The follow up periods varied from 6 to 24 months, and the results showed that addition of a beta-blocker to injection sclerotherapy conferred no advantage for either rebleeding or mortality rates.

Nitrate prophylaxis

Nitrates have been used primarily in combination with vasopressin and terlipressin in the treatment of acute bleeding oesophageal varices. However there has been considerable interest in the use of nitrates per se in the prevention of bleeding oesophageal varices. Nitrates produce a dose dependent venous and arterial vasodilation, the systemic effects of which are valuable in the treatment of angina and hypertension. These actions also decrease portal pressure, and in a prospective controlled study comparing isosorbide-5-mononitrate (20 mg three times daily) and propranolol (median dose 40 mg twice daily) nitrates were shown to be a safe and effective alternative to beta-blockers.[46] Isosorbide-5-mononitrate and propranolol prevented primary bleeding at 2 years in 82% and 85% of cases respectively. Because isosorbide-5-mononitrate is not metabolised by the liver it is not contraindicated in patients with severe hepatic dysfunction, and provides a valuable alternative to beta-blockade in this group.

Portal Hypertensive Gastropathy

Portal hypertensive gastropathy is responsible for up to 20% of upper gastrointestinal bleeding in patients who have portal hypertension. There is little correlation between the degree of portal hypertension and severity of gastropathy, which occurs mainly in patients who have cirrhosis and are treated with variceal sclerotherapy. Bleeding is usually chronic and occult but can present with haematemesis and melaena. The mucosal abnormalities are diffuse and rarely amenable to endoscopic therapy, so treatment is aimed at decreasing portal pressure.

The value of propranolol has been examined in a placebo controlled study of 54 patients with cirrhosis and acute or chronic bleeding from severe portal hypertensive gastropathy.[47] Propranolol was given at a dose of 20–160 mg twice daily that reduced resting pulse rate by 25% or to 55 beats per min; at 30 months the actuarial percentage of patients free of rebleeding was significantly higher in the propranolol group than in the placebo group (52% versus 7%). Survival was slightly, but not significantly, higher in the propranolol group.

Gastritis

Haemorrhagic and erosive gastritis is implicated as a cause of upper gastrointestinal bleeding in approximately 20% of cases. It is not usually associated with major life threatening haematemesis because gastritis is a mucosal disorder, whereas the arteries and veins that cause major haemorrhage are submucosal. The major factors pre-disposing to gastritis are non-steroidal anti-inflammatory drugs, alcohol and stress.

Most information about drug therapy for gastritis comes from studies that have included gastritis as a cause of haematemesis and melaena. Treatment with H_2 blockers, proton pump inhibitors, antifibrinolytic agents and vasoactive drugs have not been shown to decrease mortality.

Gastropathy caused by non-steroidal anti-inflammatory drugs

Acute exposure to non-steroidal anti-inflammatory drugs (NSAIDs) causes gastric damage in up to 100% of patients.[48] However mucosal adaptation occurs in response to repeated dosing and only 30% of patients on long term treatment with an NSAID have erosions or peptic ulcers. Prophylactic therapy with proton pump inhibitors, H_2 antagonists and misoprostil decreases the incidence of gastric damage,[49-51] but only misoprostil decreases the incidence of both gastric and duodenal ulcers.[52]

A double blind placebo controlled study of 8843 patients with rheumatoid arthritis compared NSAIDs treatment with and without concomitant administration of misoprostol.[53] Ten different NSAIDs were used and misoprostol was given at an initial dose of 100 µg four times daily for 10 days before being increased to 200 µg for 6 months. A total of 67 patients (25 in the NSAID/misoprostol group and 42 in the NSAID/placebo group) developed significant gastrointestinal adverse effects, including perforation, gastrointestinal haemorrhage and gastric outlet obstruction. This is an important observation, because the study is the first to show a significant reduction in the complications of NSAID induced gastropathy. It also suggests that the reduction in endoscopically proven gastroduodenal ulceration noted in many previous smaller studies may translate into a reduction in significant gastrointestinal side effects.

Stress gastropathy

Bleeding caused by stress gastropathy is an important complication in patients with critical illness, and occurs in up to 50% of patients admitted to intensive therapy units. The bleeding is normally detected by nasogastric aspiration and is usually of small volume.

Several drugs have been used in the management of stress gastro-pathy,[54 55] but none has been shown to reduce mortality once bleeding has developed. However, prophylactic treatment with antacids, H_2 blockers or sucralfate decreases the incidence of bleeding.[56] Critically ill patients are often unable to maintain a low gastric pH, so cytoprotective agents have a theoretical advantage over drugs that neutralise or inhibit the production of gastric acid. Furthermore, gastric acid is a natural barrier against bacterial overgrowth and its reduction leads to a higher incidence of nosocomial pneumonia in this group of patients.[56]

Sucralfate, a chemical complex of sucrose octasulphate and aluminium hydroxide, is a weak antacid; it increases mucosal blood flow and promotes mucosal regeneration. A study comparing sucralfate (1 g four times daily) and H_2 antagonists with and without antacids in 130 patients being ventilated[56] demonstrated no significant difference in bleeding rates (27·2% versus 36·7%). However the sucralfate group had significantly lower concentrations of Gram negative bacilli in their gastric aspirate and half the rate of pneumonia when compared with those in the H_2 blocker/antacid group. Sucralfate suspension is therefore the prophylactic agent of choice in this group of patients.

Vascular Abnormalities

Angiodysplasia may occur in isolation or as part of a syndrome such as hereditary haemorrhage telangiectasia (Osler–Weber–Rendu) syndrome or the CREST syndrome. The distinctive bright red lesions are usually detected at endoscopy and present most often with occult blood loss. Occasionally they cause acute gastrointestinal bleeding and the usual treatment is endoscopic coagulation or surgical resection. However, a small double blind, placebo controlled, crossover study has shown that oral oestrogen/progesterone therapy decreases transfusion requirements in patients with recurrent bleeding from gastrointestinal vascular malformations.[57] Ten patients with a history of recurrent bleeding over more than 1 year and multiple vascular malformations detected at endoscopy received 0·05 mg ethinyloestradiol and 1 mg norethisterone or placebo, with crossover of medication after 6 months. All patients on placebo and only two patients in the active treatment group needed transfusion. Transfusion requirements also fell significantly from 10·9 to 1·1 units of packed cells per patient per 6 months when patients were on active treatment. These observations indicate that oral oestrogen/progesterone therapy may be useful in patients with severely bleeding gastrointestinal vascular malformations.

Conclusion

No single agent "blanket therapy" in all patients with upper gastrointestinal bleeding can be recommended. Effective pharmacotherapy depends on accurate diagnosis of the cause of bleeding. No treatment has been shown to be effective in the acute treatment of bleeding peptic ulcers. Vasoactive drugs, particularly somatostatin and octreotide, are useful in the treatment of gastro-oesophageal varices. Prophylaxis is effective against bleeding oesophageal varices (beta-blockers and nitrates), NSAID gastropathy (misoprostil and acid inhibition) and stress gastropathy (sucralfate). More effective targeting of patients at risk of gastrointestinal bleeding or rebleeding will improve the value of prophylaxis.

Key points

Peptic ulcer bleeding
- There is little evidence to support the use of acid inhibiting drugs
- The value of tranexamic acid and other fibrinolytic agents remains in doubt
- Routine use of somatostatin and its synthetic analogue octreotide, agents that reduce splanchnic blood flow and inhibit gastric activity, cannot be recommended for acute peptic ulcer bleeding

Bleeding oesophageal varices
- Terlipressin, a synthetic analogue of vasopressin, when combined with
  continued

---

glyceryl trinitrate, is as effective as balloon tamponade at controlling acute bleeding

- Octreotide is the most attractive option for the drug treatment of acutely bleeding oesophageal varices.

Prevention of variceal bleeding

- Prophylaxis with beta-blockers should be considered for most patients at risk of bleeding varices
- Injection sclerotherapy and beta-blockade reduce rebleeding and mortality rates to a similar extent. Combining the two confers no additional benefit
- Isosorbide-5-mononitrate is a safe and effective alternative to beta-blockers, valuable for patients with severe hepatic dysfunction

Portal hypertensive gastropathy

- Propranolol significantly reduces rebleeding and slightly improves survival

NSAID gastropathy

- Concomitant administration of the cytoprotectant misoprostil reduces the incidence of gastric and duodenal ulcers and their complications

Stress gastropathy

- Sucralfate suspension is the prophylactic agent of choice in this group

Vascular abnormalities

- Oral oestrogen/progesterone therapy may be useful in patients with severely bleeding vascular malformations

References

1 Collins R, Langman M. Treatment with histamine H_2 antagonists in acute upper gastrointestinal bleeding. *N Engl J Med* 1985;**313**:660–6.
2 Walt RP, Cottrell J, Mann SG, Freemantle M, Langman MJS. A randomised double blind controlled trial of intravenous famotidine infusion in 1005 patients with peptic ulcer bleeding [abstract]. *Gut* 1991;**32**:A571–2.
3 Cooperative Study Group. Double blind comparative study of omeprazole and ranitidine in patients with duodenal or gastric ulcers: a multicentre study. *Gut* 1990;**31**:653–6.
4 Walt RP, Reynolds JR, Langman MJS, *et al*. Intravenous omeprazole rapidly raises intragastric pH. *Gut* 1985;**26**:902–6.
5 Daneshmend TK, Hawkey CJ, Langman MJS, Logan RFA, Long RG, Walt R. Omeprazole versus placebo for acute upper gastrointestinal bleeding. Results of a randomised double blind controlled study. *BMJ* 1992;**304**:143–8.
6 Barer D, Ogalvie A, Henry D, *et al*. Cimetidine and tranexamic acid in the treatment of acute upper gastrointestinal bleeding. *N Engl J Med* 1983;**308**:1571–5.
7 Henry DA, O'Connell DL. Effects of fibrinolytic inhibitors on mortality from upper gastrointestinal haemorrhage. *BMJ* 1989;**298**:1142–6.
8 Bloom SR, Russell RCG, Barros D'Sa AAJ, *et al*. Inhibition of gastrin and gastric acid by growth hormone inhibiting hormone. *Gut* 1975;**16**:396.
9 Schrumpf E, Vatn MH, Hanssen KF, Myren J. A small dose of somatostatin inhibits the pentagastrin stimulated gastric secretion of acid, pepsin and intrinsic factor in man. *Clin Endocrinol* 1978;**9**:8391–5.
10 Sonnenberg GE, Keller U, Perruchoud A, Burckhardt D, Gyr K. Effect of somatostatin

on splanchnic haemodynamics in patients with cirrhosis of the liver and in normal subjects. *Gastroenterology* 1981;**80**:526–32.

11 Coraggio F, Scarpato T, Spina M, Lombardi S. Somatostatin and ranitidine in the control of iatrogenic haemorrhage of the upper gastrointestinal tract. *BMJ* 1984;**289**:224.

12 Magnusson I, Ihre T, Johannson C, Seligson U, Torngren S, Uvnasmobergk. A randomised double blind trial of somatostatin in the treatment of massive upper gastrointestinal haemorrhage. *Gut* 1985;**26**:221–6.

13 Kayasseh L, Gyr K, Keller U, Stalder GA, Wall M. Somatostatin and cimetidine in peptic ulcer haemorrhage. *Lancet* 1980;**i**:844–6.

14 Sommerville KW, Henry DA, Davies JG, Hine KR, Hawkey CJ, Langman MJS. Somatostatin in the treatment of haematemesis and melaena. *Lancet* 1985;**i**:130–2.

15 Christiansen J, Ottenjann R, Von Arx F, *et al*. Placebo-controlled trial with the somatostatin analogue SMS 201-995 in peptic ulcer bleeding. *Gastroenterology* 1989;**97**:568–74.

16 Silverstine FE, Gilbert DA, Tedesco FJ, *et al*. The National ASGE Survey on upper gastrointestinal bleeding 1. Study design and baseline data. *Gastrointest Endosc* 1981;**27**: 73–9.

17 The Northern Italy Endoscopy Endoscopic Club for the Study and Treatment of Oesophageal Varices. Prediction of the outcome in variceal haemorrhage in patients with cirrhosis of the liver and oesophageal varices: a prospective multi-centre study. *N Engl J Med* 1988;**319**:983–9.

18 Tsai YT, Lay CS, Lai KH, *et al*. Controlled trial of vasopressin plus nitroglycerine versus vasopressin alone in the treatment of bleeding oesophageal varices. *Hepatology* 1986;**6**: 406–9.

19 Soderlund C, Magnusson I, Torngren S, Lundell L. Terlipressin (triglycyl-lysine vasopressin) controls acute bleeding oesophageal varices: a double blind randomized placebo controlled trial. *Scand J Gastroenterol* 1990;**25**:622–30.

20 Fort E, Satereau D Silvain C, Ingrand P, Pellegand B, Beaumant M. A randomised trial of terlipressin plus nitroglycerine vs balloon tamponade in the control of acute variceal haemorrhage. *Hepatology* 1990;**11**:6678–81.

21 Gimson AES, Westerby D, Hegarty J, Watson A, Williams RA. A randomised trial of vasopressin and vasopressin plus nitroglycerine in the control of acute haemorrhage. *Hepatology* 1986;**6**:410–3.

22 Hoskins SW, Doss W, El-Zeiny H, Robinson P, Barsounm S, Johnson AG. Pharmacological constriction of the lower oesophageal sphincter: A simple method of arresting variceal haemorrhage. *Gut* 1988;**29**:1098–102.

23 Valenzuela JE, Schubert T, Fogel MR, *et al*. A multicentre randomised double-blind trial of somatostatin in the management of acute haemorrhage from oesophageal varices. *Hepatology* 1989;**10**:958–61.

24 Kravetz D, Bosch J, Terres J, *et al*. Comparison of intravenous somatostatin and vasopressin infusions in the treatment of acute variceal haemorrhage. *Hepatology* 1984;**4**:442–6.

25 Jenkins SA, Baxter JN, Corbett W, *et al*. A prospective randomised controlled clinical trial comparing somatostatin and vasopressin in controlling acute variceal haemorrhage. *BMJ* 1985;**219**:275–8.

26 Bagarani M, Albertini V, Anza M, *et al*. The effect of somatostatin in controlling bleeding from oesophageal varices. *Ital J Surg Sci* 1987;**17**:21–6.

27 Saari A, Klvilaakso E, Inburg M, *et al*. Comparison of somatostatin and vasopressin in bleeding oesophageal varices. *Am J Gastroenterol* 1990;**85**:804–7.

28 Shields R, Jenkins SA, Baxter JN, *et al*. A prospective randomised controlled trial comparing the efficacy of somatostatin with injection sclerotherapy in the control of oesophageal varices. *J Hepatol* 1992;**16**:128–37.

29 Sung JJY, Chung SCS, Lai CW, *et al*. Octreotide infusion or emergency sclerotherapy for variceal haemorrhage. *Lancet* 1993;**342**:637–41.

30 Silvain C, Carpentier S, Sautereau D, *et al*. Terlipressin plus transdermal nitroglycerine vs. octreotide in the control of acute bleeding from esophageal varices: a multicentre randomised trial. *Hepatology* 1993;**18**:61–5.

31 Conn HO. Sclerotherapy versus beta blockade. Unanticipated anomalies of experimental design. *Gastroenterology* 1993;**105**:1575–77.

32 Hayes PC, Davis JM, Lewis JA, Bouchieri AD. Meta-analysis of value of propranolol in prevention of variceal haemorrhage. *Lancet* 1990;**336**:153–6.

33 Pagliaro L, Burroughs AK, Sorensen TIA, *et al*. Beta-blockers for preventing variceal bleeding. *Lancet* 1990;**336**:1001–2.

34 Infante-Rivard C, Esnaola S, Villeneuve JP. Role of endoscopic sclerotherapy in the long term management of variceal bleeding: a meta-analysis. *Gastroenterology* 1989;**96**:1087–92.

35 Teres J, Bosch J, Bordas JM, *et al.* Propranolol versus sclerotherapy in preventing variceal rebleeding: a randomised controlled trial. *Gastroenterology* 1993;**105**:1508–14.

36 Westaby D, Polson RJ, Gimson AES, Hayes PC, Hallyar K, Williams R. A controlled trial of oral propanolol compared with injection sclerotherapy for long-term management of variceal bleeding. *Hepatology* 1990;**11**:353–9.

37 Fleig WE, Stange EF, Hunecke R, *et al.* Prevention of recurrent bleeding in cirrhotics with recent haemorrhage: prospective randomised comparison of propanolol and sclerotherapy. *Hepatology* 1987;**7**:355–61.

38 Pagliaro L, Burroughs AK, Sorensen TIA, *et al.* Therapeutic controversies and randomised controlled trials (RCTs): prevention of bleeding and rebleeding in cirrhosis. *Gastroenterol Int* 1989;**2**:71–84.

39 Westaby D, Melia E, Hegarty J, *et al.* Use of propanolol to reduce the rebleeding rate during injection sclerotherapy prior to variceal obliteration. *Hepatology* 1986;**6**:673–5.

40 Vickers C, Rodes J, Hillenbrand P, *et al.* Prospective controlled trial of propranolol and sclerotherapy for the prevention of rebleeding from oesophageal varices. *Gut* 1987;**28**:A1359.

41 Venel JP, Lamouliliette H, Cales P, *et al.* Propanolol reduced the rebleeding rate during injection sclerotherapy: results of a randomised study [abstract]. *Gastroenterology* 1990;**98**:644.

42 Jensen LS, Karup N. Propanolol may prevent recurrence of oesophageal varices after obliteration by endoscopic sclerotherapy. *Scand J Gastroenterol* 1990;**25**:352–6.

43 Vickers C, Rodes J, Hillenbrand P, *et al.* Prospective controlled trial of propanolol and sclerotherapy for prevention of rebleeding from oesophageal varices. *Gut* 1987;**28**:A1359.

44 Gerunda GE, Neri D, Cangrandi F, *et al.* Nadolol does not reduce early rebleeding in cirrhotics undergoing endoscopic variceal scleropathy: a multicenter randomised controlled trial. *Hepatology* 1990;**12**:988.

45 Lundell L, Leth R, Lind T, *et al.* Evaluation of propanolol for prevention of recurrent bleeding from oesophageal varices between sclerotherapy sessions. *Acta Chir Scand* 1990;**156**:711–5.

46 Angilico M, Carli L, Piat C, *et al.* Isosorbide 5 mononitrate versus propranolol in the prevention of first bleeding in cirrhosis. *Gastroenterology* 1993;**104**:1460–5.

47 Peres-Ayuso RM, Pique JM, Bosch J, *et al.* Propranolol in the prevention of recurrent bleeding from severe portal hypertensive gastropathy in cirrhosis. *Lancet* 1991;**337**:1431–4.

48 Shorrock CJ, Rees WDW. Mucosal adaptation to indomethacin induced gastric damage in man. Studies on morphology, blood flow and prostaglandin E2 metabolism. *Gut* 1992;**33**:164–9.

49 Graham DY, Agrawal NM, Roth SH. Prevention of NSAID induced gastric ulcer with misoprostol: a multicentre double blind placebo controlled trial. *Lancet* 1988;**ii**:1277–80.

50 Kitchingham GK, Prichard PJ, Daneshmend TK, Walt RP, Hawkey CJ. Human gastric mucosal bleeding induced by aspirin and its prevention by ranitidine [abstract]. *Gut* 1988;**29**:A711.

51 Daneshmend TK, Stein AG, Bhaskar NK, Hawkey CJ. Abolition by omeprazole of aspirin induced gastric injury in man. *Gut* 1990;**31**:514–7.

52 Melo Gomes JA, Roth SH, Zeeh J, Bruyn GAW, Woods EM, Geis GS. Double-blind comparison of efficacy and gastroduodenal safety of diclofenac/misoprostil, piroxicam and naproxen in the treatment of osteoarthritis. *Ann Rheum Dis* 1993;**52**:881–5.

53 Silverstein FE, Graham DY, Senior JR, *et al.* Misoprostol reduces serious gastrointestinal complications in patients with rheumatoid arthritis receiving NSAIDs. *Annals of Internal Medicine* 1995;**123**:241–9.

54 Tryba M, Burkard M. Acute treatment of severe haemorrhagic gastritis with high dose sucralfate. *Lancet* 1988;**ii**:1304.

55 Collier D, Crampton J, Everett WG. Acute haemorrhagic gastritis controlled by omeprazole. *Lancet* 1989;**ii**:776.

56 Driks MR, Craven DE, Celli BR, *et al.* Nosocomial pneumonia in intubated patients given sucralfate as compared with antacids or histamine type 2 blockers. *New Engl J Med* 1987;**317**:1376–82.

57 Van Cutsem E, Rutgeerts P, Vantrappen G. Treatment of bleeding gastrointestinal vascular malformations with oestrogen-progesterone. *Lancet* 1990;**335**:953–5.

8: Endoscopic techniques for haemostasis

A K KUBBA AND K R PALMER

In specialised centres the mortality of peptic ulcer haemorrhage lies between 2% and 6%.[1-4] No single factor is responsible for this low mortality and further reductions are unlikely because some deaths from ulcer bleeding are an agonal event in terminally ill patients or occur in frail, elderly patients who have severe coexisting diseases. Endoscopy of patients admitted to hospital because of ulcer bleeding allows the physician to make an early, accurate diagnosis, obtain prognostic information and deliver haemostatic therapy. Nevertheless it is difficult to prove that diagnostic or therapeutic endoscopy improves survival; it is likely that the best outcome is achieved by concentration of resources and expert personnel upon the critically ill patient, thus ensuring proper resuscitation and appropriate use of pharmacological, surgical and endoscopic treatments. Endoscopic therapy is only part of the management jigsaw and best therapy requires multidisciplinary care from endoscopists, surgeons, radiologists, and experts in intensive care.

Endoscopy is done after the patient has been resuscitated. Elective diagnostic endoscopy is associated with significant morbidity and mortality,[5] and risks are greatly increased when inadequately resuscitated bleeding patients are endoscoped. Many patients who present with major peptic ulcer haemorrhage are elderly, frail and have multiple diseases. Despite this, out of hours emergency endoscopy in the most severely ill patients is often undertaken by relatively inexperienced endoscopists in suboptimal surroundings, without expert nursing assistance. Centres with a special interest in gastrointestinal bleeding have properly equipped and staffed facilities that are available 24 hours a day. Although most patients can be safely endoscoped during the next working day,[6] some actively bleeding patients do require out of hours endoscopy and resources must be available to manage them.

Pathophysiology and Endoscopic Therapy

Major bleeding occurs when a peptic ulcer erodes a large artery. Branches of the gastroduodenal artery may be ruptured by posterior duodenal ulcers, and tributaries of the left gastric artery by lesser curve ulcers. Bleeding from ulcers in these sites tends to be particularly brisk.[7] The involved arteries are usually 0·1–1·8 mm in diameter, and breaches greater than 4 mm in diameter are unlikely to respond to any form of endoscopic therapy.[8]

Patient Selection

About 80% of patients stop bleeding spontaneously,[9 10] and endoscopic or surgical therapy is unnecessary and meddlesome in this group. Patients at risk of uncontrolled bleeding tend to be elderly, and to present with hypotension, tachycardia and anaemia. Mortality is high in bleeding patients who are in hospital for other reasons. The presence of other significant disease increases the risk of death, particularly if a surgical operation is necessary.[11–14] The most important prognostic factor, however, is the endoscopic findings.[9–21]

Patients who at endoscopy are found to be actively bleeding and are shocked have an 80% risk of continuing to bleed or of rebleeding during that hospital admission. The presence of a non-bleeding "visible vessel" (Figure 8.1) is associated with a 50% chance of rebleeding. The "visible vessel" represents either a pseudoaneurysm of the damaged artery or a sentinel blood clot.[22] Although adequate cleaning of the ulcer base is necessary to define the endoscopic appearances, the endoscopist must be aware that disturbing the "visible vessel" can cause brisk, active bleeding.

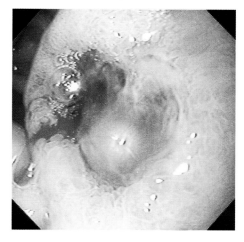

FIGURE 8.1—*Endoscopic view of a duodenal ulcer containing a "visible vessel"*.

Adherent blood clot and "oozing" have been associated with a significant risk of rebleeding by some authors;[20 21] others suggest that rebleeding is uncommon, and it is our own practice not to treat patients who have ulcers that display oozing or adherent clots. A clean ulcer base is not associated with further bleeding.

Some enthusiasts have advocated the use of endoscopic Doppler devices to identify patent arteries within and around the ulcer, and have reported that only ulcers with a positive Doppler signal should be treated.[23–25] Endoscopic stigmata of ulcer haemorrhage are ephemeral;[18] while all patients who present with ulcer haemorrhage have active bleeding at some stage, and the frequency with which stigmata are found varies with the timing of endoscopy. The timing of endoscopy is therefore an important factor when interpreting clinical trials of ulcer bleeding therapy. Nevertheless, it is generally agreed that patients who are bleeding from an ulcer and those who present with a non-bleeding visible vessel should be treated endoscopically, and those without stigmata should be managed conservatively. Surgery is carried out only when endoscopic therapy fails, when access is impossible because of profuse bleeding, or when the patient continues to bleed despite apparently adequate endoscopic therapy.

The endoscopist must know his limitations. Massive bleeding from a major artery demands early emergency surgery; the patient's operation should not be delayed by endoscopic therapy that has little chance of success. Minor bleeding will settle with supportive therapy. It is patients with moderately severe bleeding who benefit from endoscopic therapy. Because endoscopic therapy has limited value in the more profusely bleeding patients, it has little impact on hospital mortality.

End Points in Trials of Efficacy

The most important and best defined end point is death. Most published series report "hospital mortality", although surgical studies generally refer to "30 day mortality".

Only a few patients die because of peptic ulcer bleeding, so few studies include enough patients to show the impact of a therapy upon mortality. Furthermore, in some clinical trials patients randomised to conservative therapy have received active treatment for continuing bleeding or rebleeding[26]—in clinical practice it is ethically difficult to deny ill patients access to active therapy. These trials therefore show no effect upon mortality, although analysis of other end points has demonstrated efficacy of therapy.

"Rebleeding" is strongly associated with death, and the mortality of patients who rebleed in hospital is increased tenfold.[9] Rebleeding rates are therefore used in most series to define efficacy of therapy, and in many studies rebleeding and uncontrolled bleeding (bleeding that continues despite therapy) are reported together. Unfortunately it is often difficult in clinical practice to know when rebleeding has occurred. It is usual to define rebleeding as the sudden development of haematemesis or melaena or both associated with clinical shock or a rapid fall in haemoglobin concentration of at least 2 g/dl over 24 h. Rebleeding should in all cases be endoscopically confirmed.

Principles of Endoscopic Therapy

The basis of haemostatic therapy is the need to thrombose the bleeding artery, and the different approaches are listed in Box 8.1.

Box 8.1 Endoscopic treatment for bleeding ulcer

Thermal modalities

- Argon laser
- Neodymium YAG laser
- Heater probe
- Electrocoagulation

Injection therapy

- Adrenaline (vasoconstrictor)
- Sclerosants
- Alcohol
- Thrombin (clotting factor)

Other methods

- Topical sprays
- Microwave coagulation
- Mechanical devices

Thermal devices

Laser photocoagulation

The argon laser emits visible blue-green light energy. Tissue penetration is superficial and high power settings are needed to cause a tissue effect.

Experiments in a canine model of ulcer bleeding showed that haemostasis can be achieved using the argon laser with low risk of gastric perforation.[27] Three controlled clinical trials involving patients who, at endoscopy, had major stigmata of peptic ulcer bleeding were published in the 1980s[28-30] (Table 8.1). Swain *et al.*[28] selected 76 of 330 patients who presented with gastrointestinal bleeding; 52 of these were randomised to laser photocoagulation or managed conservatively. Rebleeding episodes (8 in the treated group, 17 in the controls) and hospital mortality (0 and 7, respectively) were significantly reduced in treated patients. This study, like many of ulcer bleeding, can be criticised for small patient numbers and therefore potential for a type II error and selection bias. Nevertheless, efficacy of argon laser photocoagulation was also shown by Vallon *et al.*[29] and Jensen *et al.*[30]

Further animal studies suggested that neodymium:yttrium–aluminium–garnet (Nd:YAG) laser energy might be a more appropriate haemostatic tool. The depth of penetration of the Nd:YAG beam is several millimeters, resulting in an immediate, obvious tissue effect associated with coagulation within vessels, and acute inflammation within the mucosa and

TABLE 8.1—*Controlled trials of argon laser therapy in peptic ulcer bleeding.*

Author (year)	Number randomised	Further/uncontrolled bleeding		p	Comments
		Laser	Controls		
Swain et al.[28] (1981)	76 (52 with major stigmata)	8/20	17/28	<0.05	Benefit only in patients with major stigmata
		8/19	8/16	NS	Reduced mortality in treated group (0 v 7 deaths)
Vallon et al.[29] (1981)	136 { 35 NBVV, 28 active bleeding, 73 spots	8/19	8/19	NS	Benefit only in actively bleeding patients
		5/15	9/13	<0.05	
		2/34	4/39	NS	
Jensen et al.[30] (1984)	16	2/7	7/9	NS	Overall morbidity score lower in treated patients

NBVV, non-bleeding visible vessel.

submucosa leading eventually to the formation of scar tissue.[31] Studies in mesenteric arteries demonstrated that small and medium sized breaches could be sealed, but that holes greater than 0·4 mm in diameter continued to bleed.[32] Perforation of an experimental ulcer required relatively large amounts of energy, an order of magnitude greater than those needed for arterial coagulation.[33]

These characteristics led to the view that Nd:YAG laser treatment was more suitable than argon photocoagulation but the clinical efficacy of the two modalities is very similar.

Nd:YAG photocoagulation: technical aspects Nd:YAG lasers produce infrared light energy at a wavelength of 1064 nm. Light is transmitted via flexible glass fibres using medium power settings of 50–60 W. Tissue effects around the bleeding point can be achieved without allowing the probe to touch the mucosa, although the use of contact sapphire probes and a co-optive technique allows the use of lower power settings (15–25 W). Accurate therapy depends upon assiduous cleaning of the ulcer base, and active bleeding makes it more difficult to administer optimal treatment. Standard safety precautions, for example, the use of filters and of safety locks on the doors of the endoscopy suite, must be observed to protect the endoscopist and assistants.

Clinical trials The results of several uncontrolled series suggest that Nd:YAG laser photocoagulation of bleeding ulcers is safe and effective, Kiefhaber *et al.* reporting more than 90% efficacy in 1058 treated patients.[34]

Nine controlled clinical trials of Nd:YAG laser versus conservative therapy have been published[35–44] (Table 8.2). Patient numbers in each study are small, but criteria for inclusion, particularly endoscopic findings or major stigmata of bleeding, are uniform. Meta-analysis is therefore justified and has shown that laser therapy reduces the rate of rebleeding and decreases hospital mortality.[45 46]

The best individual study is that reported by Swain *et al.*[35] Over 2 years, these authors randomised 131 patients to laser or conservative therapy. Treatment was given by one of two experienced endoscopists and objective end points were assessed by independent clinicians. Seven of 70 patients treated by laser rebled and one of these died in hospital. This contrasted with rebleeding in 27 of the 68 conservatively managed patients, eight of whom died. These differences were statistically significant. However, even in the experienced hands of these endoscopists, 19% of patients had ulcers that were inaccessible to treatment, either because bleeding was severe and obscured the ulcer or because the bleeding ulcer was awkwardly situated.

A contrasting study is that reported by Krejs *et al.*[38] This two centre American trial failed to show benefit for Nd:YAG laser therapy. Nineteen of 85 treated patients and 18 of 89 conservatively managed patients rebled and surgical operation rates, hospital mortality and transfusion requirements were virtually identical in the treatment arms.

TABLE 8.2—*Controlled trials of Nd:Yag laser photocoagulation in peptic ulcer bleeding.*

Author (year)	Number randomised		Further/uncontrolled bleeding		p	Comments
			Laser	Controls		
Swain et al.[35] (1988)	148 {	59 NBVV	4/28	15/31	<0·001	Active treatment associated with improved mortality (1/70 v 8·65, p<0·005)
		20 active bleeding	2/10	8/10	<0·002	
		69 other stigmata	1/32	6/27	NS	
Rutgeerts et al.[36] (1982)	152 {	43 active bleeding	3/17	8/26	<0·01	Rebleeding
		86 non active bleeding	5/46	15/40	0·45	Rebleeding
		23 not randomised				
MacLeod et al.[39] (1983)	45 {	20 active bleeding	6/12	8/8	NS	Failures of laser treatment associated with "inaccessibility"; see text
		25 other stigmata	6/9	0/16	NS	
Krejs et al.[38] (1987)	174 {	32 active bleeding	5/29	5/33	NS	Many exclusions because of "instability"; see text
		142 other stigmata	14/85	13/89	NS	
Mathewson et al.[37] (1990)	143		9/44	18/24	<0·05	Also included group of patients treated by heater probe
Rohde et al.[39] (1980)	105		35/62	25/43	NS	Reported in abstract form; details of therapy and randomisation unavailable
Buset et al.[40] (1988)	88		6/44	28/44	<0·05	Other end points not reported
Ihre et al.[41] (1981)	135 {	42 active bleeding	7/23	8/19		Rebleeding
		93 other stigmata	9/43	8/50		Rebleeding
Escourrou et al.[42] (1981)	83		7/40	12/43	NS	
Homer et al.[43] (1983)	42		4/21	5/21	NS	No other end points

NBVV, non-bleeding visible vessel.

The reasons for the different conclusions of these studies illustrate many of the difficulties associated with clinical trials in this field. Although both trials exclusively randomised ulcers associated with major endoscopic stigmata, actively bleeding ("unstable") patients—who comprise the highest risk category—were few in the American study, which therefore compared outcomes in relatively less severe disease. This is confirmed by the rebleeding rate being much lower in the American control groups than in the London study. Patients in the study of Krejs *et al.* were also relatively young, with a median age of only 49 years—much less than reported in all other bleeding studies. Endoscopic therapy was given by two experienced endoscopists in the London study, while many more operators took part in the American trial. It seems likely that some of the American endoscopists were still climbing their learning curve, whereas the British doctors were established experts.

The efficacy of Nd:YAG laser therapy may vary between trials, but the studies are consistent in demonstrating that treatment is safe: only one case of laser associated perforation has been reported.[38]

Current status of laser photocoagulation   Clinical trials show that both argon and Nd:YAG photocoagulation are effective treatments for bleeding peptic ulcer. Both modalities are safe and reported complications are rare. Laser therapy is at least as versatile as other endoscopic modalities, because it is also the treatment of choice for vascular anomalies[47] and is effective therapy for the Dieulafoy abnormality.[47]

Nevertheless, laser photocoagulation is little used as haemostatic therapy for bleeding ulcer, because the machines are expensive and until recently have been cumbersome and non-portable. Of all available modalities, laser is the most demanding for the endoscopist; the non-touch technique and the need to treat circumferentially around the bleeding point present great practical difficulties in many bleeding patients. This is reflected by the high levels of inaccessible ulcers reported in the clinical trials. Other endoscopic therapies are at least as effective, tend to be easier to apply, and are cheaper.

Heater probe coagulation

The heater probe comprises a portable power source and an endoscopically positioned catheter. Preset amounts of heat energy are transmitted to the Teflon coated metal tip of the catheter, and best results are obtained using larger diameter probes at medium power settings. The catheter is fitted with a powerful water jet that cleans and irrigates the bleeding point and prevents the catheter tip sticking to the ulcer crater. Tamponade can be administered to aid haemostasis, and heat can be applied by tangential application.

Haemostasis probably results from a combination of heat and pressure. Experiments in animals showed that the heater probe was more effective than injection therapy in arresting bleeding from canine arteries.[49]

Early uncontrolled series suggested that the heater probe was effective in clinical practice.[50 51] In the 1980s small, controlled series from Fullarton et al.[52] and Jensen et al.[53] confirmed that haemostasis of bleeding ulcers can usually be achieved, and that rebleeding after therapy is infrequent (Table 8.3). Tekant et al.[54] performed a much larger controlled trial in which 153 patients, who exhibited a range of endoscopic stigmata associated with peptic ulcer bleeding, were randomised to a combination of adrenaline and heater probe thermocoagulation or to no endoscopic treatment. The two groups were well matched with regard to usual risk factors for rebleeding or death, although some patients in both groups had minor stigmata, such as red or black spots, that are not regarded as having adverse prognostic significance. Haemostasis was achieved by the heater probe in all bleeding patients and rebleeding was significantly less common in treated patients (5 v 16 rebleeds, p<0·05).

Heater probe and laser coagulation have been compared in two clinical trials[55 56] but neither included sufficient patients to show differences in outcome. Pap also failed to show differences in efficacy between the heater probe and multipolar coagulation.[57]

These trials, limited as they are, show that there is little to choose between thermal methods with regard to efficacy in controlling ulcer bleeding. However, the heater probe is cheaper, and allows the user to apply tamponade and to approach the ulcer tangentially. It is therefore a better buy than a laser unit for the treatment of ulcer haemorrhage.

The more important comparison is between the heater probe and injection therapy. The first of three clinical trials that compared these approaches was reported by Lin et al.[58] One hundred and thirty seven patients who presented with bleeding or a non-bleeding visible vessel were randomised to heater probe, injections with pure alcohol or conservative (no intervention) therapy. Initial control of bleeding was better with the heater probe than with injection (98% v 67%, p<0·0004) and permanent haemostasis was achieved significantly more often in patients treated by the heater probe than in those who received an injection or conservative management (91%, 67% and 52%, respectively). The efficacy of injection treatment reported in this study is rather less than that found in most other series. No complications followed endoscopic intervention.

The second study, reported by Chung et al.,[59] randomised 132 patients who had endoscopic evidence of active bleeding to injection with dilute adrenaline or to the heater probe. Bleeding was initially controlled in 95% of injected patients and 83% of heater probe treated patients (p<0·05). The apparent advantage of the thermal method has to be weighed against the ulcer perforation that developed in two patients who received heater probe therapy. The third study, reported by Choudari et al.,[60] randomised 120 patients who presented with a range of endoscopic stigmata to 1:100 000 adrenaline plus 5% ethanolamine or heater probe coagulation. Permanent haemostasis was achieved in 87% of injected patients and 85%

TABLE 8.3—*Controlled trials of heater probe treatment in peptic ulcer bleeding.*

Author (year)	Number randomised	Rebleeding/uncontrolled bleeding			p	Comments
		Heater probe	Sham	Other endoscopic therapy		
Fullarton et al.[51] (1989)	43 { 39 active bleeding / 4 NBVV	0/18 / 0/2	21/21 / 0/2		<0·002	Heater probe treatment associated with perforation in one patient. Some "inaccessible" ulcers excluded from heater probe therapy
Jensen et al.[52] (1988)	94 { 38 active bleeding / 56 NBVV	22%	72%	44%*		Heater probe superior to other approaches. Details scanty (abstract form only)
Tekant et al.[53] (1995)	253 { 55 active bleeding / 198 other stigmata	3/31 / 2/43	4/22 / 12/72		<0·05	Heater probe combined with adrenaline injection. More shocked patients in heater probe group
Lin et al.[56] (1990)	137 { 71 active bleeding / 66 NBVV	2/29 / 2/16	15/24 / 7/22	12/28** / 3/18	<0·002	Heater probe significantly more effective in active bleeding
Chung et al.[58] (1991)	132 active bleeding	11/64	—	3/68†	<0·05	Two perforations with heater probe
Choudari et al.[59] (1992)	120 { 57 active bleeding / 63 NBVV	5/57	—	6/58†	NS	No difference in relation to endoscopic stigmata

NBVV, non-bleeding visible vessel; *BICAP; **alcohol; †adrenaline.

of heater probe treated patients. Other end points were similar in the two groups. No complication of therapy occurred in any patient.

These three studies suggest that use of the heater probe and injection with dilute adrenaline have similar efficacy and (although data are rather limited) that the heater probe is superior to injection with sclerosant. In clinical practice, however, these differences are not always clear-cut and the techniques are complementary. For example, the capacity of the heater probe to apply tamponade and its powerful irrigation channel make it suitable for the treatment of an ulcer that has a large amount of semiadherent blood clot that makes the ulcer difficult to inject. In another patient, the heater probe may be rather awkward to manoeuvre within a deformed duodenal cap, and injection treatment more easily administered. A well equipped unit should therefore have equipment and expertise for both heater probe and injection treatment.

Electrocoagulation

Electrocoagulation devices aim to stop bleeding by passing an electric current through the bleeding area.

Monopolar units have a ball tipped probe that is applied to the bleeding area, and the electrical circuit is completed through a plate attached to the patient. The earlier probes often precipitated bleeding because they adhered to the ulcer bed. They also caused unpredictable tissue damage and the tip required frequent cleaning. Newer, liquid monopolar probes have an electrical conducting fluid between the tip and the mucosa, which largely overcomes the problem of tissue adherence. The efficacy of monopolar probes has been examined in three controlled clinical trials[61-63] (Table 8.4). The largest study was reported by Freitas et al.,[61] who randomised 78 patients presenting with a range of endoscopic findings to electrocoagulation using a liquid monopolar electrode or to sham treatment. Permanent haemostasis was achieved in 19 of 36 treated patients, but in a high proportion of the control group bleeding stopped spontaneously and did not recur.

Because of these rather unimpressive results, together with the unpredictable tissue damage caused, monopolar electrocoagulation has been superseded by other contact methods, particularly the multipolar coagulation system.

Bipolar coagulation works by completing an electrical circuit between probes applied to the mucosa. No plate needs to be attached to the patient, and tissue penetration and damage are more predictable. In experimental animals, the most effective system is the multipolar electrocoagulation probe, known as BICAP.[64] The probe has three pairs of electrodes on its side and tip, and electrocoagulation occurs if any pair of electrodes are in tissue contact, allowing tangential treatment. Bursts of power (7–8 w for 1 s) are applied around the bleeding point until blanching occurs, and the probe is then directly applied to the bleeding point.

TABLE 8.4—*Controlled trials of monopolar coagulation in peptic ulcer bleeding.*

Author (year)	Number randomised	Bleeding/uncontrolled bleeding		p	Comments
		Coagulation	Controls		
Freitas et al.[60] (1985)	78 { 21 active bleeding, 57 other stigmata	2/11 3/25	6/10 8/25	<0·05	Fewer operations in endoscopically treated patients: liquid monopolar probe
Moreto et al.[61] (1987)	37	1/16	11/21	<0·05	Fewer operations in treated patients: liquid monopolar probe
Pap[62] (1982)	32	1/16	13/16	<0·05	Reduced operations rate and duration of hospital admission in treated patients: dry monopolar probe

Controlled clinical trials with BICAP have reported varying outcome (Table 8.5). O'Brien et al.[65] randomised 204 patients who were found at endoscopy to have a bleeding ulcer or a non-bleeding visible vessel to BICAP treatment or sham treatment. Seventeen of 101 treated patients continued to bleed or rebled, whereas only 34 of 103 sham treated patients did so (p<0·01). The greatest benefit was found in the subset of patients who had active bleeding; haemostasis was achieved in 24 of 40 patients with spurting haemorrhage while spontaneous haemostasis occurred in only 8 of 13 actively bleeding controls. These authors, and others, comment that bleeding can be precipitated by application of the probe. This can usually, but not invariably, be stopped by further BICAP treatment; catastrophic bleeding has followed BICAP therapy.

Brearley et al.[66] tested the BICAP in 41 bleeding patients and found no benefit for active treatment. Similar lack of benefit was reported by Goudie et al.[67] and by Kernohan et al.[68] In contrast, Laine reported two trials in which prognosis was improved using BICAP. In the first of these the performance of the probe was examined in 44 patients who presented with severe gastrointestinal bleeding from a range of causes.[69] Twenty four of these patients were bleeding from peptic ulcers. The 10 treated ulcer patients required less blood transfusion than did the 14 control ulcer subjects. The length and cost of the hospital stay were also reduced in the treated group. This small study is insufficient to confirm efficacy, but benefit was also reported in a larger study performed by the same author.[70] In a clinical trial involving 75 patients who exclusively had non-bleeding visible vessels within ulcers, patients were randomised to BICAP or sham treatment. Rebleeding occurred in 18% of treated patients compared with 41% of controls; blood transfusion requirements and need for surgery were lower in the BICAP group. Subsequently Laine[71] and Waring et al.[72] reported similar outcome for patients treated using BICAP or injection sclerotherapy.

It therefore appears that European experience of BICAP is disappointing compared to that reported in the US. The reasons for these differences may relate to trial design; certainly the numbers of patients included in European trials are greater than those reported by Laine. It is possible that the expertise of a single therapeutic endoscopist is a factor in the American studies. Another important factor is probe size, which was larger in the series reported by Laine (3·2 v 2·3 mm); this may have allowed better tamponade and more effective coagulation. Technical details are often scantily reported in these papers, but it does appear that Laine applied more electrical treatment than was given in the European studies.

In summary, it is probable that electrocoagulation is of modest benefit in ulcer bleeding. It may be most suitable for active bleeding. The probe can precipitate active haemorrhage, and at least one patient has sustained ulcer perforation after BICAP therapy.

TABLE 8.5—*Controlled trials of multipolar coagulation in peptic ulcer bleedings.*

Author (year)	Number randomised		Rebleeding/uncontrolled bleeding		p	Comments
			BICAP	Control		
O'Brien et al.[64] (1986)	204 {	61 active bleeding 143 other stigmata	6/40	13/21	<0·05	7F probe used. More patients in treated group with active bleeding; one perforation
Goudie et al.[66] (1984)	46		7/21	5/25	NS	2·3 mm probe used. Bleeding precipitated by BICAP in one patient
Kernohan et al.[67] (1984)	45		9/21	7/24	NS	"Inadequate coagulation" reported in 10 patients randomised to BICAP
Laine[68] (1987)	44	active bleeding	2/21	10/13	<0·0001	Included patients bleeding from several sources (24 ulcers). Reduced blood transfusions, operative intervention and hospital stay in treated patients
Laine[69] (1989)	75 NBVV		7/38	15/37	<0·05	Less operative intervention and cost in BICAP group

NBVV, non-bleeding visible vessel.

Injection therapy

Injection therapy is widely used as first line treatment for peptic ulcer bleeding. Clinical trials show that it is as effective as other options and that treatment is safe and cheap.

Many questions remain unanswered, however; these include the mechanism of action, the optimum injection solution and whether injection should be combined with other approaches, including thermal coagulation.

Mechanisms of injection therapy

It is not clear how injection therapy (Figure 8.2) stops bleeding and prevents rebleeding. Operative specimens are rarely available after injection therapy, and it is difficult to differentiate the effects of treatment from the histological characteristics of a chronic ulcer. Inflammation, vasculitis and thrombosis of vessels are inherent features of peptic ulcer. Furthermore, an appropriate reproducible animal model of bleeding peptic ulcer is unavailable.

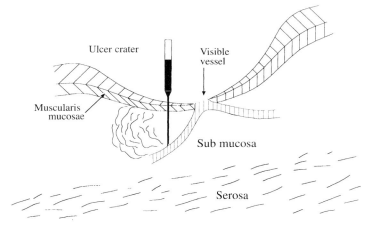

- The ulcer bleed is caused by erosion of a major submucosal artery and disruption of the muscularis mucosae
- The serosa is rarely involved
- Injection is usually directed beside the visible vessel to induce tamponade, vasoconstriction or sclerosis of the vessel

FIGURE 8.2—*Possible mechanisms for haemostasis following injection treatment of bleeding ulcer.*

Injection therapy may stop ulcer bleeding by one or all of the following mechanisms.

Tamponade Injection of fluid into a fibrotic, rigid ulcer causes compression of the bleeding vessel. This hypothesis is supported by the results of the clinical trial reported by Lin *et al.*[73] in which injections of saline or dilute dextrose into bleeding ulcers were more effective than conservative therapy and had similar efficacy to injections of absolute alcohol. Similar conclusions were reported by Fleig et al.,[74] who showed that endoscopic injection of water stopped bleeding and prevented ulcer bleeding.

In animal models of gastrointestinal bleeding it is not possible to show that haemostasis can be achieved by injection of inert fluids;[49 75] the tamponade effect is limited in these models, however, because they do not exhibit chronic ulceration and fibrosis.

In spite of observations reported in clinical trials, it seems unlikely that an intramucosal injection or an injection into the ulcer can generate enough pressure to compress arterial bleeding.

Nevertheless, this mechanism may contribute to the efficacy of injection therapy. Larger clinical trials are needed to examine the effect of injection therapy using inert substances.

Vasoconstriction Dilute adrenaline stops active bleeding in models of gastrointestinal bleeding[49 75] and in clinical practice.[76 77] It is presumed to act by causing vasoconstriction of the bleeding artery, although atheromatous change in the vessel, perivascular fibrosis and inflammation may reduce the capacity of the artery to contract. Most endoscopists inject relatively large volumes of dilute adrenaline and tamponade may also be important. Blanching around the injected area occurs at the time of adrenaline injection; the gastric mucosa of dogs looked "cyanotic" when injected with dilute adrenaline.[49] In these experiments histological examination showed that inflammation is localised to the injected area and that necrosis and vascular changes rarely occur after injection of adrenaline.

Whether adrenaline injection achieves haemostasis entirely by causing vasoconstriction is unclear. In clinical trials an injection of dilute adrenaline not only stops active bleeding, but also largely prevents rebleeding,[78 79] suggesting that it may thrombose the ruptured artery. The effect is likely to be simply a consequence of vasoconstriction, but adrenaline may also induce alteration of platelet function[80 81] and stimulate the coagulation cascade.

Sclerosants Polidocanol, ethanolamine and sodium tetradecyl sulphate are widely used sclerosants. Differing concentrations of polidocanol injected into the gastric mucosa of dogs caused extensive necrosis and deep ulcers in a dose dependent manner.[49 82] Venous thrombosis invariably follows sclerosant injection but endarteritis and arterial thrombosis occur less often;[49 75 82] in a rabbit model, ethanolamine injections were not associated with thrombosis of major arteries.[75]

Sclerosant injections are less effective than thermal methods for stopping experimental bleeding from the gastric mucosa. In the rabbit stomach, sclerosant injections temporarily increased the rate of bleeding while adrenaline injections had prompt haemostatic activity.[75]

105

A clinical trial has reported that sclerosant injections are useful in stopping active bleeding,[83] but most authorities consider that if sclerosants have a role it is likely to be in prevention of rebleeding rather than treating active bleeding.

Alcohol Injection of 98% ethanol causes profound dehydration of tissues, leading to vigorous inflammation, extensive necrosis and ulcer formation.[49 82] Surrounding areas are congested and hyperaemic and blood vessels are partially thrombosed, yet often permeable. In experimental models active bleeding is rarely stopped by alcohol injection, in contrast with the efficacy of adrenaline and laser treatment.[49]

Clotting factors Injections of bovine thrombin initiate the clotting cascade, and have been shown to arrest bleeding from peptic ulcers in several small studies.[84-87] No study has been large enough, however, to allow their efficacy to be compared with that of other modalities.

Controlled clinical trials of injection therapy

Many uncontrolled trials carried out in the 1980s suggested that injection therapy improved outcome in patients who presented with major ulcer bleeding. Inclusion criteria for these studies were often poorly defined, and they are subject to the usual criticisms of open trials, but their conclusions have largely been confirmed by randomised controlled clinical trials.

Relatively few studies have compared injection with no injection in matched groups of patients; however, clear advantage for injection has emerged, and it can be argued that trials that include a no-treatment control arm are unethical.

The optimum injection regimen is one that stops bleeding, prevents rebleeding and has no complications. Many combinations of injection solutions have been tested, but none fulfils all these requirements.

Dilute adrenaline Professor Chung's group from Hong Kong have pioneered the use of dilute adrenaline. In a controlled trial patients who presented with bleeding ulcers were randomised to endoscopic injection with 1:10 000 adrenaline or were managed without endoscopic therapy[76] (Table 8.6). Injected patients required significantly less blood transfusion, fewer emergency surgical operations and shorter hospital stay than did conservatively managed patients. "Rebleeding" is not reported in this paper, and mortality was similar in both groups.

Several groups subsequently carried out trials in which adrenaline injection was followed by injection of a sclerosant.[26 88-90] There was a preconception, supported by experiments in animal models, that adrenaline alone would not cause thrombosis of the bleeding artery. While adrenaline should stop active haemorrhage by causing vasoconstriction, the argument ran, a sclerosant is necessary to induce vascular damage and promote intra-

TABLE 8.6—*Dilute adrenaline injection versus conservative treatment in peptic ulcer bleeding.*

Author (year)	Number randomised	Operation for failed haemostasis		p	Comments
		Injected	Controls		
Chung *et al.*[75] (1988)	68 active bleeding	4/34	14/34	<0·02	Initial haemostasis in all injected patients; shorter hospital stay and reduced blood transfusion in the treated group

arterial thrombosis. To test this assertion, two clinical trials compared outcome in patients treated with dilute adrenaline with that in matched patients treated by a combination of adrenaline and a sclerosant. Chung et al.[79] randomised 200 actively bleeding patients to injection with 1:10 000 adrenaline (99 patients) or to adrenaline followed by 3% sodium tetradecyl sulphate (101 patients). The groups were well matched in all relevant respects. Initial haemostasis was achieved in almost all patients; the only failures were those in whom torrential bleeding prevented visualisation and injection of the bleeding ulcer; when injection was achieved initial haemostasis always followed. After initial control of bleeding only two patients in each group rebled in hospital. Similar conclusions were reached by Choudari and Palmer,[78] who randomised 107 patients who presented with a range of major endoscopic stigmata to injection with 1:100 000 adrenaline or to adrenaline plus an injection of 5% ethanolamine. Permanent haemostasis was achieved in 85% of patients in both groups.

These two studies clearly show that the addition of a sclerosant to an injection of adrenaline is unnecessary. This suggests that, in clinical practice, adrenaline does induce thrombosis of the bleeding vessel, and highlights the deficiencies in animal models of ulcer bleeding.

Other series have compared the outcome of patients treated by injection therapy with that of patients treated using thermal methods. Loizoa et al.[91] randomised 42 patients to 1:10 000 adrenaline or a combination of adrenaline and Nd:YAG laser photocoagulation. This small study failed to show significant differences between the treatments, but there was a tendency for combination therapy to be more effective, as suggested by rebleeding rates of 25% after injection alone and 14% after laser coagulation and injection. Carter et al.[92] compared adrenaline injection with Nd:YAG laser therapy. Permanent haemostasis was achieved in 96% of laser treated patients and 81% of injected patients, but this apparent difference was not statistically significant because of small sample size (44 patients).

The minimum effective concentration of adrenaline is not known. The Hong Kong group have used a concentration of 1:10 000, while we in Edinburgh have favoured a 1:100 000 solution. The results of endoscopic therapy are similar in trials reported by these two centres. Significant and potentially important increases in plasma adrenaline concentrations follow endoscopic injection with 1:10 000 adrenaline solutions,[93] and could have adverse effects in patients who have coexisting cardiac diseases. For this reason we favour more dilute injections, although in clinical practice no significant complications have been reported following adrenaline treatment.

Dilute adrenaline is the injection treatment of choice for active ulcer bleeding, and clinical trials show it to be at least as effective as any other approach. For patients with non-bleeding visible vessels there seems little to choose between adrenaline and alternative therapies. Combination of adrenaline injection with a thermal coagulation is attractive, because the bleeding source is treated by several approaches. Few clinical trials have adopted this approach, although Chung et al.[94] and Tekant et al.[54] have shown that combination of adrenaline and the heater probe is safe and effective. Studies powerful enough to prove that combination treatment is better than that with any single agent will require large patient numbers and almost certainly multicentre participation.

Sclerosants   A range of sclerosing agents have been injected directly into and around bleeding ulcers to try and stop active bleeding and prevent rebleeding. These include 1% polidocanol, 5% ethanolamine and 3% sodium tetradecyl sulphate.   Several uncontrolled trials[95 96] performed in the early 1980s suggested that injection of these agents was effective and safe. There are however no controlled trials in which outcome has been assessed in patients randomised to sclerosants or to conservative (no injection) treatment.

Several trials have compared the efficacy of sclerosant injection with that of other haemostatic methods. For example, Benedetti et al.[84] randomised patients presenting with bleeding from a range of sources to injection with 1% polidocanol or to thrombin injection and showed similar haemostatic effect for these treatments. Strohm et al.[97] randomised patients to one of four treatment arms (fibrin glue, 1% polidocanol, dilute adrenaline or adrenaline plus polidocanol) and showed little advantage for any one approach. These two trials have insufficient power to demonstrate that polidocanol injection is better than other approaches, but low rebleeding following 1% polidocanal injection in patients who have had endoscopic stigmata of major bleeding suggests that this agent is effective. Finally, Rutgeerts et al.[98] showed that injection of polidocanol is as effective as Nd:YAG laser photocoagulation therapy in patients with ulcer bleeding.

More studies have examined the effectiveness of combination adrenaline and sclerosant regimens (Table 8.7). The controlled trial reported by Panes et al.[88] involved 113 patients who were randomised to a combination of 1:10 000 adrenaline plus 1% polidocanol or to no injection. Recurrent bleeding occurred in 5·5% of injected patients, compared with 43% of controls (p<0·001), with corresponding reduction in the need for emergency surgery and blood transfusion and duration of hospital stay. Rajgopal and Palmer[26] subsequently showed that the combination of 1:100 000 adrenaline plus 5% ethanolamine reduced rebleeding rates (12·5 *v* 47%, p<0·001) in patients who had a range of major endoscopic stigmata. In this study some control patients were injected when they rebled; most then avoided emergency surgery, but this questionable defect of trial design resulted in loss of potential difference in other possible end points. Moreto et al.[99] showed in a small clinical trial (38 patients) that haemostasis was achieved in patients treated by a combination of ethanolamine plus thrombin injections (one of 19 treated patients developed uncontrolled bleeding, compared to further bleeding in eight of 19 controls).

The role of the sclerosant in these trials is difficult to interpret for two major reasons. Firstly, the trials suffer from the common problem of

TABLE 8.7—*Controlled trials of adrenaline plus sclerosant versus conservative treatment in peptic ulcer bleeding.*

Author (year)	Number randomised	Rebleeding/uncontrolled haemorrhage		p	Comments
		Injection	Control		
Raigopal and Palmer[26] (1991)	109 { 9 active bleeding, 100 other stigmata	7/52	25/53	<0·001	1 in 100 000 adrenaline plus 5% ethanolamine. Some control patients injected after rebleeding
Panes et al.[87] (1987)	113 { 28 active bleeding, 46 oozing/clot, 39 NBVV	3/15, 0/22, 8/18	10/13, 14/24, 15/21	<0·01, <0·05, <0·01	1 in 10 000 adrenaline plus 1% polidocanol. Reduced transfusion need in injected patients
Balanzo et al.[88] (1988)	72	7/36	15/36	<0·05	1 in 10 000 adrenaline plus 1% polidocanol. Reduced surgical intervention and transfusion needs in injected group
Oxner et al.[89] (1992)	93 { 5 active bleeding, 88 other stigmata	8/48	21/45	<0·05	1 in 10 000 adrenaline plus 1% polidocanol. Fewer deaths in injected patients (4 v 9; NS)

NBVV, non-bleeding visible vessel.

small sample size. Secondly, the sclerosant has invariably been injected in combination with another agent that has proven therapeutic value. To try and define the role of the sclerosants, three studies have compared outcome in patients randomised to adrenaline injection with that in those receiving a combination of adrenaline injection with that in those receiving a combination of adrenaline and a sclerosant.

As previously described, the trials reported by Chung et al.[79] and by Choudari and Palmer[78] showed little advantage for combination therapy over an injection of adrenaline alone. A third study reported by Villanueva et al.[100] showed similar outcome following injection with adrenaline plus polidocanol or treatment with adrenaline alone (Table 8.8). No study has compared haemostasis in patients treated by dilute adrenaline with that achieved by injection of a sclerosant alone.

Sclerosant injections have been associated with serious complications. These presumably occur when the injection causes extensive thrombosis of arteries serving the upper gastrointestinal tract. Levy et al.[101] reported a fatal case of gastric antral necrosis following injection with a combination of adrenaline and sodium tetradecyl sulphate. Similar complications complicating sclerosant injections have been reported by several authors.[102 103] Luman et al.[104] reported common bile duct stricturing causing obstructive jaundice after repeated injection of a posterior duodenal ulcer with adrenaline and 5% ethanolamine.

Because sclerosants appear to offer no advantage over injection with adrenaline alone, and because of these unusual but potentially serious side effects, we do not believe that sclerosants have a role as injection therapy for bleeding ulcers.

Alcohol The efficacy of injections of 98% ethanol has been examined in several clinical trials (Table 8.9). Sugawa et al.[105] reported effective haemostasis in bleeding ulcers and this was confirmed in a randomised trial performed by Pascu et al.[106] More recently, Lazo et al.[107] reported a study of 39 patients who were found at endoscopy to have non-bleeding visible vessels within the ulcer base. Twenty five patients were treated by injection and 14 acted as non-injected controls. Rebleeding was significantly less common in the injected group (8 v 57%, p<0·01). Lin et al.[73] reported that alcohol injection stopped active bleeding and prevented rebleeding in 86% of patients whose ulcers were injected with alcohol, although a similar proportion of ulcers treated with 3% sodium chloride (68%), 50% dextrose (78%) and normal saline (78%) also achieved permanent haemostasis.

As already stated,[49 82] injection of alcohol into the gastric mucosa of dogs causes deep ulcers and such ulcers are also common in the human oesophagus after injection sclerotherapy for varices. It is perhaps not surprising, therefore, that ulcer perforation has been reported following alcohol injection into a bleeding ulcer.[73]

One small study[107] has compared the efficacy of alcohol injection with dilute adrenaline injection therapy, but had insufficient power to detect

TABLE 8.8—*Combination of adrenaline plus sclerosant versus adrenaline alone in peptic ulcer bleeds sodium tetradecyl sulphate.*

Author (year)	Number randomised		Rebleeding/uncontrolled haemorrhage		p	Comments
			Combination	Adrenaline alone		
Chung et al.[78] (1993)	200	active bleeding	14/98	16/98	NS	Numbers refer to operations for further bleeding. Injection with 1 in 10 000 adrenaline ± STD
Choudari and Palmer[77] (1994)	107 {	57 active bleeding	6/28	7/29	NS	1 in 100 000 adrenaline + 5% ethanolamine
		50 NBVV	1/24	1/26	NS	
Villanueva et al.[99] (1993)	63		8/33	4/30	NS	1 in 100 000 adrenaline ± 1% polidocanol

TABLE 8.9—*Controlled trials involving alcohol injection of peptic ulcer bleedings.*

Author (year)	Number randomised	Number rebleeding/ uncontrolled bleeding		p	Comments
		Alcohol	Control		
Pascu et al.[105] (1989)	143	2/65	10/78	<0·05	"Rebleeding" relates to need for surgical intervention. Reduced mortality in injected patients
Lazo et al.[106] (1992)	39 NBVV	2/52	8/14	<0·001	Reduced need for surgical intervention in treated patients
Chiozzini et al.[107] (1989)	53 { 6 active bleeding, 47 other stigmata	2/16	5/19	NS	15 further patients randomised to 1 in 100 000 adrenaline (2 rebled)

NBVV, non-bleeding visible vessel.

TABLE 8.10—*Controlled trials involving thrombin injection of peptic ulcer bleeding.*

Author (year)	Number randomised	Uncontrolled haemorrhage or rebleeding		p	Comments
		Thrombin	Other		
Balanzo et al.[84] (1990)	64	6/32	5/32 (thrombin plus 1 in 100 000 adrenaline)	NS	
Benedetti et al.[83] (1991)	82 { 20 active bleeding, 62 NBVV	9/10	9/10 (polidocanol)	NS	
		2/16	1/16 (polidocanol)	NS	
Moreto et al.[98] (1992)	38	1/19	8/19 (no injection)	<0·005	Thrombin injected with 5% ethanolamine

NBVV, non-bleeding visible vessel.

113

any differences. A much larger study is needed. The evidence that alcohol stops active bleeding and prevents rebleeding is more convincing than that for the sclerosants ethanolamine, polidocanol and sodium tetradecyl sulphate. The potential for side effects induced by injection is probably higher for alcohol than for adrenaline, and this may deter such a study.

Thrombin Direct injection of thrombin into a bleeding ulcer may be the most effective method of sealing the bleeding vessel. Groitl and Scheele[86] injected bovine thrombin into ulcers of 11 patients; it halted active bleeding and prevented rebleeding. They also suggested that the agent may have value in sealing anastomotic leakage.

Balanzo et al.[85] randomised 64 patients who presented with active ulcer bleeding to 1:10 000 adrenaline or to 1:10 000 adrenaline plus thrombin. Permanent haemostasis was achieved in 81 and 84% respectively of the two groups. Benedetti et al.[84] randomised 82 consecutive patients who presented with peptic ulcer bleeding to 1% polidocanol or thrombin injections. Primary haemostasis was achieved in 90% of patients injected with polidocanol and 87% of those treated with thrombin. Permanent haemostasis (after repeated injection in rebleeding patients) was achieved in all but two cases (Table 8.10).

Thrombin injection therefore does seem at least as effective as other modalities, although the clinical trials have insufficient power to show whether it is any better (or worse) than other approaches. A trial that could define such differences would be extremely large, because standard injection treatment is relatively effective and at least some of the failures of each modality result from inaccurate localisation of the injected material rather than differences in the capacity of these materials to thrombose vessels.

A particular risk of thrombin injection is that it could precipitate extensive intravascular thrombosis. In clinical practice this has not been observed in patients injected for peptic ulcer or variceal bleeding. Bovine thrombin also carries the theoretical risk of inducing anaphylaxis, and it may be unwise repeatedly to inject the same patient with this material.

Other approaches to the bleeding ulcer

Endoscopic haemostasis has been attempted by topical application of a range of substances, including collagen haemostat,[109] clotting factors,[110] and cyanoacrylate tissue glues.[111] Experience in animals and man is limited, but has largely been disappointing.

Mechanical approaches have included metal clips,[112] rubber band ligation[113] and sewing.[114] Each has its advocates but none can be recommended in clinical practice.

A microwave coagulation method has been devised for endoscopic use. Microwave energy produces heat dielectrically, molecular motion being produced by ultra-high frequency excitation. The electrical fluid is well localised to the tip of the electrode and risk of ulcer perforation is theoretically low. In experimental models microwave coagulation performs as well as the heater probe and the BICAP, and better than injection with adrenaline and 1% polidocanol.[115] One prospective clinical trial[116] involving 127 patients, who presented with a range of endoscopic findings associated with peptic ulcer bleeding, randomised patients to endoscopic sclerosis using adrenaline or polidocanol or to microwave coagulation. No complications occurred in either group and rebleeding, surgical operation and transfusion rates were similar in both groups.

The main drawback of the microwave coagulation probe is its adherence to the bleeding point. This can be usually overcome by applying a dissociation electrical current, but serious further bleeding can be precipitated. A no-contact method with sparking across to the bleeding point has been studied in experimental animals, but not yet applied to man.[117]

Failures of Endoscopic Therapy

It can be argued that endoscopists can adversely affect outcome for patients in whom endoscopic therapy fails. Repeated endoscopy, transfusion of large volumes of blood and delayed surgical operation all increase the risk of death for patients in whom attempted endoscopic haemostasis fails. Unfortunately, we cannot predict those patients in whom endoscopic treatment will fail. Clearly patients with the most active, profuse haemorrhage are the least likely to respond to non-operative approaches, both because massive bleeding can make administration of endoscopic therapy impossible and because large holes in major arteries are unlikely to respond to any endoscopic therapy. It is patients who are shocked with active bleeding from a posterior duodenal ulcer who tend to comprise the failures in clinical trials.[118-120] Nevertheless, even in such patients, our own group reported a 75% success rate with treatment by injection or heater probe coagulation.[118]

One approach in the highest risk patients is early repeat endoscopy, with further treatment even in the absence of rebleeding. Villanueva et al.[121] suggest that such a policy might improve outcome.

The best policy to adopt when patients rebleed after endoscopic treatment is not clear. Many endoscopists tend to retreat such patients, while others believe that rebleeding is an indication for surgical intervention. Clinical trials do not tell us when to operate, and although an aggressive, early surgical approach has been reported to be best for elderly patients who present with major ulcer bleeding,[122] we have no data supporting this for patients receiving endoscopic therapy.

No study has compared surgical with endoscopic therapy. Most trials of endoscopic therapy define the need for a surgical operation as a treatment failure. An alternative view is that endoscopic control of bleeding facilitates safe, early elective surgery. A successful outcome in an individual patient often depends upon a combination of endoscopic and surgical approaches, and good management requires a team approach.

Key points

- Bleeding arteries are usually 0·1–1·8 mm in diameter. Breaches of more than 4 mm in diameter are unlikely to respond to endoscopic therapy
- Endoscopic treatments are useful only in the management of moderately severe bleeding
- Rebleeding increases ten-fold the risk of death, and therefore most trials of endoscopic therapies use rebleeding rates to define efficacy
- The principle of haemostatic endoscopic therapy is to thrombose the bleeding artery
- Laser photocoagulation (both argon and Nd:YAG) is safe and effective, and the treatment of choice for vascular anomalies
- Heater probe coagulation is as effective as laser, cheaper, and allows the user to apply tamponade and approach the ulcer tangentially
- Electrocoagulation is of only modest benefit, and can cause active haemorrhage
- Injection therapy is widely used as first-line treatment for active ulcer bleeding, and dilute adrenaline is the agent of choice
- Injection of sclerosants has no role in active bleeding; injection of alcohol or thrombin can be effective
- Successful outcome often depends on a combination of endoscopic and surgical approaches

---

References

1 Jeans PL, Padbury RTA, Touli J. A prospective evaluation of the management of bleeding peptic ulcer. *Aust NZ J Surg* 1991;**61**:187–91.
2 Hunt PS, Korman MG, Hansky J, Schmidt GT, Hillman HS. Acute gastric ulceration: a prospective study of incidence and results of management. *Aust NZ J Med* 1980;**10**:305–8.
3 Zimmerman J, Siguencia E, Tsvang E, Beeri R, Arnon R. Predictors of mortality in patients admitted to hospital for acute gastrointestinal haemorrhage. *Scand J Gastroenterol* 1995;**30**:327–31.
4 Bramley PN, Masson J, Walsh D. The impact of a specialised bleeding unit serving Grampian region: the way forward? *Gut* 1993;**34**:560–3.
5 Quine MA, Bell GD, McLoy RF, Charlton JE, Devlin HB, Hopkins A. Prospective audit of upper gastrointestinal endoscopy in two regions of England: safety, staffing and sedation methods. *Gut* 1995;**36**:462–7.
6 Choudari CP, Palmer KR. Outcome of endoscopic injection therapy for bleeding peptic ulcer in relation to the timing of the procedure. *Eur J Gastroenterol Hepatol* 1993;**5**:591–3.
7 Swain CP, Salmon PR, Northfield TC. Does ulcer position influence presentation or prognosis of upper gastrointestinal bleeding? *Gut* 1986;**27** (1 Suppl):A632.
8 Swain CP, Storey DW, Bown SG, *et al.* Nature of the bleeding vessel in recurrently bleeding gastric ulcers. *Gastroenterology* 1986;**90**:595–608.
9 Bornman PC, Theodorou NA, Shuttleworth RD, Essel HP, Marks IN. Importance of hypovalaemic shock and endoscopic signs in predicting recurrent haemorrhage from peptic ulceration: a prospective evaluation. *BMJ* 1985;**291**:245–7.

10 Clason AE, MacLeod DAD, Elton RA. Clinical factors in the prediction of further haemorrhage or mortality in acute upper gastrointestinal haemorrhage. *Br J Surg* 1986; 73:985–7.

11 NIH Concensus Conference. Therapeutic endoscopy and bleeding ulcers. *JAMA* 1989; 262:1369–72.

12 Silverstein FE, Gilbert DA, Tedesco FJ. The National ASGE surgery on upper gastrointestinal bleeding. II. Clinical prognostic factors. *Gastrointest Endosc* 1981;27:80–93.

13 Branicki FJ, Coleman SY, Fok PJ. Bleeding peptic ulcer: a prospective evaluation of risk factors for rebleeding and mortality. *World J Surg* 1990;14:262–70.

14 Petersen WL. Clinical risk factors. *Gastrointest Endosc* 1990;36(suppl 1):S14–15.

15 Chang-Chien C, Wu C, Chen P, *et al*. Different implications of stigmata of recent haemorrhage in gastric and duodenal ulcers. *Dig Dis Sci* 1988;33:400–4.

16 Lin HJ, Perng CL, Lee SD. The predictive factors of rebleeding in peptic ulcer with non-bleeding visible vessel: a prospective observation, with emphasis on the size and colour of the vessel [abstract]. *Gastroenterology* 1992;102:A113.

17 Freeman ML, Cass OW, Peine CJ, Onstad GR. The non-bleeding visible vessel versus the sentinel clot: natural history and risk of rebleeding. *Gastrointestinal Endosc* 1993;39: 359–66.

18 Foster DN, Miloszewski KJA, Losowsky MS. Stigmata of recent haemorrhage in diagnosis and prognosis of upper gastrointestinal bleeding. *BMJ* 1978;1:1173–7.

19 Griffiths WJ, Neumann DA, Welsh JD. The visible vessel as an indicator of uncontrolled or recurrent gastrointestinal haemorrhage. *N Engl J Med* 1979;300:1411–3.

20 Storey DW, Bown SG, Swain CP, Salmon PR, Kirkham JS, Northfield TC. Endoscopic prediction of recurrent bleeding in peptic ulcers. *N Engl J Med* 1981;305:915–6.

21 Wara P. Endoscopic prediction of major rebleeding—a prospective study of stigmata of haemorrhage in bleeding ulcer. *Gastroenterology* 1985;88:1209–14.

22 Swain CP. Pathophysiology of bleeding lesions. *Gastrointest Endosc* 1990;36(suppl 1): S21–2.

23 Beckly DE, Casebow MP. Prediction of rebleeding from peptic ulcer: experience with an endoscopic doppler device. *Gut* 1986;27:96–9.

24 Kohler B, Riemann JF. The endoscopic doppler: its value in evaluating gastroduodenal ulcers after haemorrhage and as an instrument of control of endoscopic injection therapy. *Scand J Gastroenterol* 1991;26:471–6.

25 Fullarton GM, Murray WR. Prediction of rebleeding in peptic ulcers by visual stigmata and endoscopic doppler ultrasound criteria. *Endoscopy* 1990;22:68–71.

26 Rajgopal C, Palmer KR. Endoscopic injection sclerosis: effective therapy for bleeding peptic ulcer. *Gut* 1991;32:727–9.

27 Silverstein FE, Auth DC, Rubin CE, Protell RL. High power argon laser treatment via standard endoscopes. 1. A preliminary study of efficacy in control of experimental erosive bleeding. *Gastroenterology* 1976;71:558–63.

28 Swain CP, Bown SG, Storey DW, Kirkham JS, Salmon PR, Northfield TC. Controlled trial of Argon laser photocoagulation in bleeding peptic ulcer. *Lancet* 1981;ii:1313–6.

29 Vallon AG, Cotton PB, Laurence BH, Armengol-Miro JR, Saloro-Uses JC. Randomised trial of endoscopic argon laser photocoagulation in bleeding peptic ulcers. *Gut* 1981;22: 228–33.

30 Jensen D, Machicado GA, Tapia JL, Elkashoff J. Controlled trial of endoscopic argon laser for severe ulcer haemorrhage [abstract]. *Gastroenterology* 1984;86(suppl 1):1125.

31 Silverstein FE, Protell RL, Gilbert DA, *et al*. Argon vs. neodymium-Yag laser photocoagulation of experimental canine ulcers. *Gastroenterology* 1979;77:491–6.

32 Rutgeerts P, Vantrappen G, Geboes K, Brockaert L. Safety and efficacy of neodymium-Yag laser photocoagulation: an experimental study in dogs. *Gut* 1981;22:38–44.

33 Dixon JA, Berenson MM, McCloskey DW. Neodymium-Yag laser treatment of experimental canine gastric bleeding. Acture and chronic studies of photocoagulation penetration and perforation. *Gastroenterology* 1979;77:647–51.

34 Kiefhaber P, Kiefhaber V, Huber V, Nath G. Ten years' endoscopic neodymium-Yag laser coagulation in gastrointestinal haemorrhage. In: Jensen DM, Brunetand JM, eds. *Medical laser endoscopy*. Dordrecht: Kluwer Academic, 1990:109–118.

35 Swain CP, Bown SG, Salmon PR, Kirkham JS, Northfield TC. Controlled trial of Nd-Yag laser photocoagulation for bleeding peptic ulcer. *Lancet* 1986;i:1113–6.

36 Rutgeerts P, Vantrappen G, Broeckhart L. Controlled trial of YAG laser treatment of upper digestive haemorrhage. *Gastroenterology* 1982;83:410–16.

117

37 Mathewson K, Swain CP, Bland M, Kirkham JS, Bown SG, Northfield TC. Randomised comparison of Nd-Yag laser, heater probe and no endoscopic therapy for bleeding peptic ulcer. *Gastroenterology* 1990;**98**:1239–44.
38 Krejs GJ, Little KH, Westergaard H, Hamilton JK, Spady DK, Polter DE. Laser photocoagulation for the treatment of acute peptic ulcer bleeding. *N Engl J Med* 1987; **316**:1618–21.
39 MacLeod I, Mills PR, Mackenzie JF, Jolfe SN, Russell RI, Carter DC. Neodymium yttrium aluminium garnet laser photocoagulation for major haemorrhage from peptic ulcers and simple vessels. *BMJ* 1983;**286**:345–58.
40 Rohde H, Thon K, Fischer M, *et al.* Results of a defined therapeutic concept of endoscopic neodymium-Yag-laser therapy in patients with upper gastrointestinal bleeding [abstract]. *Br J Surg* 1980;**67(suppl 1)**:360.
41 Buset M, Des Marez B, Vandermeeren AA. Laser therapy for non-bleeding visible vessels in peptic ulcer haemorrhage: a prospective randomised study. *Gastrointest Endosc* 1988; **34**:173.
42 Ihre T, Johansson C, Seligson U, Torngren S. Endoscopic YAG-laser treatment in massive gastrointestinal bleeding. *Scand J Gatroenterol* 1981;**16**:633–40.
43 Escourrou J, Frexinos J, Bommelaer G. Hemorragies digestives, malformations vasculaires et laser. *Gastroenterol Clin Biol* 1981;**5**:413–16.
44 Homer AC, Powen S, Vicary FR. Is Nd-Yag laser for upper gastrointestinal bleeds of benefit in a district general hospital? *Postgrad Med J* 1985;**61**:19–22.
45 Cook DJ, Guyatt GH, Salena BJ, Laine LA. Endoscopic therapy for acute non variceal upper gastrointestinal haemorrhage: A meta-analysis. *Gastroenterology* 1992;**102**:139–48.
46 Henry DA, White I. Endoscopic coagulation for gastrointestinal bleeding. *N Engl J Med* 1988;**318**:186–7.
47 Cello JP, Grendell JH. Endoscopic laser treatment of gastrointestinal vascular ectasias. *Ann Intern Med* 1986;**104**:352–4.
48 Al-Kawas FH, O'Keefe J. Nd-Yag laser treatment of a bleeding Dieulafoy's lesion. *Gastroenterol Endosc* 1987;**33**:38–9.
49 Rutgeerts P, Geboes K, Vantrappen G. Experimental studies of injection therapy for severe non-variceal bleeding in dogs. *Gastroenterology* 1989;**97**:610–21.
50 Storey DW. Endoscopic control of peptic ulcer haemorrhage using the heater probe [abstract]. *Gut* 1983;**24(suppl 2)**:A967–8.
51 Shorvon PJ, Leung JW, Cotton PB. Preliminary experience with the heater probe at endoscopy in acute upper gastrointestinal bleeding. *Gastrointest Endosc* 1985;**31**:361–4.
52 Fullarton GM, Birnie GG, MacDonald A, Murray WR. Controlled trial of heater probe treatment in bleeding peptic ulcers. *Br J Surg* 1989;**76**:541–4.
53 Jensen DM, Machicado GA, Kovacs TOG. Controlled, randomised study of heater probe and BIPCAP for haemostasis of severe ulcer bleeding [abstract]. *Gastroenterology* 1988;**94 (suppl 1)**:A208.
54 Tekant Y, Goh P, Alexander DJA, Isaac JR, Kum CK, Ngoi SS. Combination therapy using adrenaline and heater probe to reduce bleeding in patients with peptic ulcer haemorrhage: a prospective randomised trial. *Br J Surg* 1995;**82**:223–6.
55 Johnston JH, Sones JQ, Long BCU, Leonard Posey E. Comparison of heater probe and YAG laser in endoscopic treatment of major bleeding from peptic ulcers. *Gastrointest Endosc* 1985;**31**:175–80.
56 Jensen DM, Nachicado GA, Silpa ML. Argon laser vs heater probe or BICAP for control of severe ulcer bleeding [abstract]. *Gastrointest Endosc* 1984;**30**:A134.
57 Pap JP. Heat probe versus BICAP in the treatment of upper gastrointestinal bleeding. *Am J Gastroenterol* 1987;**82**:619–21.
58 Lin HJ, Lee FY, Kang WM, Tsai YT, Lee SD, Lee CH. Heat probe thermocoagulation and pure alcohol injection in massive peptic ulcer haemorrhage: a prospective, randomised controlled trial. *Gut* 1990;**31**:753–7.
59 Chung SCS, Leung JWC, Sung K, Lok K, Li AKC. Injection or heat probe for bleeding ulcer. *Gastroenterology* 1991;**100**:33–37.
60 Choudari CP, Rajgopal C, Palmer KR. Comparison of endoscopic injection therapy versus the heater probe in major peptic ulcer haemorrhage. *Gut* 1992;**33**:1159–61.
61 Freitas D, Donato A, Monteiro JG. Controlled trial of liquid monopolar electrocoagulation in bleeding peptic ulcers. *Am J Gastroenterol* 1985;**80**:853–7.
62 Moreto M, Zaballa M, Ibanez S, Setien F, Figa M. Efficacy of monopolar electrocoagulation in the treatment of bleeding gastric ulcer: a controlled trial. *Endoscopy* 1987;**19**:54–6.

63 Papp JP. Endoscopic electrocoagulation in the management of upper gastrointestinal bleeding. *Surg Clin North Am* 1982;**62**:797–805.
64 Laine LA. Determination of the optimum technique for bipolar electrocoagulation treatment. *Gastroenterology* 1991;**100**:107–12.
65 O'Brien JD, Day SJ, Burnham WR. Controlled trial of small bipolar probe in bleeding peptic ulcers. *Lancet* 1986;**1**:464–7.
66 Brearley S, Hawker PC, Dykes PW, Keighley MRB. Perendoscopic bipolar diathermy coagulation of visible vessels using a 3·2 mm probe—a randomised clinical trial. *Endoscopy* 1987;**19**:160–3.
67 Goudie BM, Mitchell KG, Birnie GG, Mackay C. Controlled trial of endoscopic bipolar electrocoagulation in the treatment of bleeding peptic ulcer [abstract]. *Gut* 1984;**25**(**suppl 2**):A1185.
68 Kernohan RM, Anderson JR, McKelvey STD, Kennedy TL. A controlled trial of bipolar electrocoagulation in patients with upper gastrointestinal bleeding. *Br J Surg* 1984;**71**: 889–91.
69 Laine LA. Multipolar electrocoagulation of active upper gastrointestinal tract haemorrhage. A prospective controlled trial. *N Engl J Med* 1987;**316**:1613–7.
70 Laine LA. Multipolar electrocoagulation in the treatment of ulcers with non-bleeding visible vessels; a prospective controlled trial. *Ann Int Med* 1989;**110**:510–4.
71 Laine LA. Multipolar electrocoagulation vs injection therapy in the treatment of bleeding peptic ulcers: a prospective, randomised trial. *Gastroenterology* 1990;**99**:1303–6.
72 Waring JP, Sanowski RA, Sawyer RL, Woods CA, Foutch PG. A randomised comparison of multipolar electrocoagulation and injection sclerosis for the treatment of bleeding peptic ulcer. *Gastrointest Endosc* 1991;**37**:295–8.
73 Lin HJ, Perng CL, Lee FY. Endoscopic injection for the arrest of peptic ulcer haemorrhage: final results of a prospective, randomised comparative trial. *Gastrointest Endosc* 1993;**39**: 15–9.
74 Fleig WE. Solute or solvent: does water do the haemostatic job? *Endoscopy* 1994;**26**: 362–3.
75 Rajgopal C, Lessels A, Palmer KR. Mechanism of action of injection therapy for bleeding peptic ulcer. *Br J Surg* 1992;**79**:782–4.
76 Chung SCS, Leung JWC, Steele RJ, Croft TJ, Li AKC. Endoscopic injection of adrenaline for actively bleeding ulcers: a randomised trial. *BMJ* 1988;**269**:1631–3.
77 Steele RJ, Logie JR, Munro A, Nichols DM. Endoscopic haemostasis in non-variceal upper gastrointestinal haemorrhage using adrenaline injection. *J R Coll Surgeons Edin* 1989;**34**:133–6.
78 Choudari CP, Palmer KR. Endoscopic injection therapy for bleeding peptic ulcer; a comparison of adrenaline alone with adrenaline plus ethanolamine oleate. *Gut* 1994;**35**: 608–10.
79 Chung SCS, Leung JWC, Leong HT, Lo KK, Li AKC. Adding a sclerosant to endoscopic epinephrine injection in actively bleeding ulcers: randomised trial. *Gastrointest Endosc* 1993;**39**:611–5.
80 Chung SCS, Leung FW, Leung JWC. Is vasoconstriction the mechanism of haemostasis in bleeding ulcers injected with epinephrine? A study using reflectance spectrophotometry. *Gastrointest Endosc* 1988;**34**:174–5.
81 O'Brien JR. Some effects of adrenaline and anti-adrenaline compounds on platelets in vitro and vivo. *Nature* 1963;**200**:763–4.
82 Randall GM, Jensen DM, Hirabayashi K, Machicado GA. Controlled study of different sclerosing agents for coagulation of canine gut arteries. *Gastroenterology* 1989;**96**:1274–81.
83 Wordehoff D, Gros H. Endoscopic haemostasis by injection therapy in high risk patients. *Endoscopy* 1982;**14**:196–9.
84 Benedetti G, Sablich R, Lacchin T. Endoscopic injection sclerotherapy in non-variceal upper gastrointestinal bleeding. *Surg Endosc* 1991;**5**:28–30.
85 Balanzo JC, Villanueva S, Sainz JC, *et al.* Injection therapy of bleeding peptic ulcer. A prospective, randomised trial using epinephrine and thrombin. *Endoscopy* 1990;**22**:157–9.
86 Groitle H, Scheele J. Initial experience with endoscopic application of fibrin tissue adhesive in the upper gastrointestinal tract. *Surg Endosc* 1987;**1**:93–7.
87 Herold G, Preclik G, Stange F. Endoscopic injection therapy using fibrin sealant. *Hepato-Gastroenterology* 1994;**41**:116–9.
88 Panes J, Vivier J, Forne M, Garcia-Olivares E, Marco C, Garan J. Controlled trial of endoscopic sclerosis in bleeding peptic ulcer. *Lancet* 1987;**2**:1292–4.

89 Balanzo J, Sainz S, Such J. Endoscopic haemostasis by local injection of epinephrine and polidocanol in bleeding ulcer: a prospective randomised trial. *Endoscopy* 1988;**20**: 289–91.

90 Oxner RBG, Simmonds NJ, Gertner DJ, Nightingale JMD, Burnham WR. Controlled trial of endoscopic injection treatment for bleeding from peptic ulcers with visible vessels. *Lancet* 1992;**339**:966–8.

91 Loizou LA, Bown SG. Endoscopic treatment for bleeding peptic ulcer: comparison of adrenaline alone and adrenaline injection plus laser photocoagulation. *Gut* 1991;**32**: 110–3.

92 Carter R, Anderson J. Randomised trial of adrenaline injection and laser photocoagulation in the control of haemorrhage from peptic ulcer. *Br J Surg* 1994;**81**:869–71.

93 Sung JY, Sydney C, Low J, et al. Systemic absorption of adrenaline after endoscopic submucosal injection in patients with bleeding duodenal ulcer. *Gastrointest Endosc* 1993; **39**:20–2.

94 Chung SCS, Sung JY, Lai CW, Ng EKW, Chan KL, Yung MY. Epinephrine injection alone or epinephrine injection plus heat probe treatment for bleeding ulcers [abstract]. *Gastrointest Endosc* 1994;**40(suppl 1)**:A271.

95 Sohendra N, Grimm H, Stenzel M. Injection of non-variceal bleeding lesions of the upper gastrointestinal tract. *Endoscopy* 1985;**17**:129–32.

96 Kortan P, Haber G, Macron N. Endoscopic injection therapy for non-variceal lesions of the upper gastrointestinal tract. *Gastrointest Endosc* 1986;**32**:145.

97 Strohn WD, Rommele UE, Barton E, et al. Injection therapy of bleeding ulcers with fibrin or polidocanol. *Deutsche Med Wochen* 1994;**119**:249–56.

98 Rutgeerts P, Vantrappen G, Broekaert L, Coremans G, Janssens J, Hiele M. Comparison of endoscopic polidocanol injection and YAG laser therapy for bleeding peptic ulcers. *Lancet* 1989;**i**:1164–7.

99 Moreto M, Zaballa M, Suarex MJ, Ibanez S, Ojembarrena E, Castillo JM. Endoscopic local injection of ethanolamine oleate and thrombin as an effective treatment for bleeding duodenal ulcer: a controlled trial. *Gut* 1992;**33**:456–9.

100 Villaneuva C, Balanzo J, Espinos JC, et al. Endoscopic injection therapy of bleeding ulcer: a prospective and randomised comparison of adrenaline with polidocanol. *J Clin Gastroenterol* 1993;**17**:195–200.

101 Levy J, Khakoo S, Barton R, Vicary R. Fatal injection sclerotherapy of a bleeding peptic ulcer. *Lancet* 1991;**37**:504.

102 Loperfids S, Patelli G, La Torre L. Extensive necrosis of gastric mucosa following injection therapy of bleeding peptic ulcer. *Endoscopy* 1990;**22**:285–6.

103 Chester JF, Hurley PR. Gastric necrosis: a complication of endoscopic sclerosis for bleeding peptic ulcer. *Endoscopy* 1990;**22**:287.

104 Luman W, Hudson N, Choudari CP, Eastwood MA, Palmer KR. Distal biliary stricture as a complication of sclerosant injection for bleeding duodenal ulcer. *Gut* 1994;**35**: 1665–7.

105 Sugawa C, Fugita Y, Ikeda T, Walt AJ. Endoscopic haemostasis of bleeding of the upper gastrointestinal tract by local injection of ninety eight percent dehydrated ethanol. *Surg Gynaecol Obstet* 1986;**162**:159–63.

106 Pascu O, Draghici A, Acalovchi I. The effect of endoscopic haemostasis with alcohol on the mortality of non-variceal upper gastrointestinal haemorrhage: a randomised prospective study. *Endoscopy* 1989;**21**:53–5.

107 Lazo MD, Andrade R, Medina MC, Garcia-Fernandez G, Sanchex-Cantros AM, Franquelo E. Effect of injection sclerosis with alcohol on the rebleeding rate of gastroduodenal peptic ulcers with non-bleeding visible vessels: a prospective, controlled trial. *Am J Gastroenterol* 1992;**87(suppl 1)**:843–6.

108 Chiozzini G, Bortoluzzi F, Pallini P, et al. Controlled trial of absolute ethanol vs epinephrine as injection agent in gastroduodenal bleeding [abstract]. *Gastroenterology* 1989;**96**:A86.

109 Feld AD, Silverstein FE, Keegan MD. Failure of microfibrillar collagen haemostat to stop bleeding from experimental canine ulcers. *Gastrointest Endosc* 1981;**27**:132.

110 Linscheer WG, Fazio TL. Endoscopic control of upper gastrointestinal bleeding: alternate spraying of thrombin and fibrinogen. *Gastrointest Endosc* 1977;**23**:233–4.

111 Peura DA, Johnson LF, Burkhalter EJ. Use of trifluoroisopropyl cyanoacrylate polymer (MBR 4197) in patients with bleeding peptic ulcers of the stomach and duodenum: a randomised controlled study. *J Clin Gastroenterol* 1982;**4**:325–8.

112 Binmoeller KF, Thonke F, Soehendra N. Endoscopic hemoclip treatment for gastrointestinal bleeding. *Endoscopy* 1993;**25**:167–70.

113 Swain CP, Mills TN, Northfield TC. Experimental studies of new mechanical methods of endoscopic haemostasis; stitching, banding, clamping and ulcer removal [abstract]. *Gut* 1985;**26(suppl 2)**:A1151.

114 Escourrow J, Delvaux M, Buscail L, *et al.* First clinical evaluation and experimental study of a new mechanical suture device for endoscopic haemostatis. *Gastrointest Endosc* 1990;**36**:494–7.

115 Michaeltz PA, Judge D. Microwave energy compared with heater probe and BICAP in canine models of peptic ulcer haemorrhage. *Gastroenterology* 1989;**97**:676–84.

116 Panes J, Viver J, Forne M. Randomised comparison of endoscopic microwave coagulation and endoscopic sclerosis in the treatment of bleeding peptic ulcers. *Gastrointest Endosc* 1991;**37**:611–6.

117 Kalabakas AS, Porter AJ, Mule L, Birch MJ, Pollock DJ, Swain CP. Design of a microwave system for endoscopy: an experimental study of energy, tissue contact and haemostatic efficacy. *Gastroenterology* 1993;**104**:680–9.

118 Choudari CP, Rajgopal C, Elton RA, Palmer KR. Failures of endoscopic therapy for bleeding peptic ulcers; an analysis of risk factors. *Am J Gastroenterology* 1994;**89**(11): 1968–72.

119 Villanueva C, Balanzo J, Espinos JC. Prediction of therapeutic failure in patients with bleeding peptic ulcer treated with endoscopic injection. *Dig Dis Sci* 1993;**38**:2062–70.

120 Brullet E, Campo R, Bedos G, *et al.* Site and size of bleeding peptic ulcer. Is there any relation to the efficacy of haemostatic therapy? *Endoscopy* 1991;**23**:73–5.

121 Villanueva C, Balanzo J, Torras X, Soriano G, Sainz S, Vilardell F. Value of second-look endoscopy after injection therapy for bleeding peptic ulcer: a prospective and randomised trial. *Gastrointest Endosc* 1994;**40**:34–9.

122 Morris DL, Hawker PC, Brearley S, Simms M, Dykes PW, Keighley MRB. Optimal timing of operation for bleeding peptic ulcer: a prospective randomised trial. *BMJ* 1984; **288**:1277–80.

9: Radiological management of acute upper gastrointestinal bleeding

JAMES E JACKSON AND DAVID J ALLISON

In most patients who are bleeding from an upper gastrointestinal source (that is, above the ligament of Treitz), the diagnosis is made by endoscopy. Angiography is indicated only when haemorrhage continues.

Criteria for the Success of Embolisation

The success of embolisation in halting upper gastrointestinal bleeding depends upon three main factors: the ability to define the bleeding site; the source of haemorrhage; and the experience of the angiographer.

Defining the site of bleeding

The only direct angiographic sign of gastrointestinal haemorrhage is extravasation of contrast into the bowel lumen (Figures 9.1 and 9.2). This sign may be absent on initial selective angiograms, especially when the source is a small vessel (for example a branch of the retroduodenal artery), because of the intermittent nature of acute gastrointestinal bleeding. It is often necessary to rely on other "indirect" angiographic signs, such as the presence of an aneurysm (Figures 9.3 and 9.4) or the demonstration of early venous return, vascular irregularity, vascular truncation, neovascularity or varices. Occasionally no abnormality will be detected in a patient who has a proven endoscopic source of haemorrhage; in such cases "prophylactic" embolisation of the apparently normal vessels supplying the vascular territory in question may be justified.

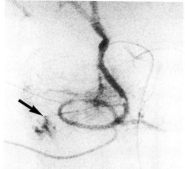

Figure 9.1

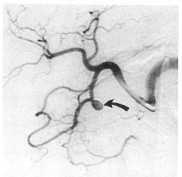

Figure 9.3

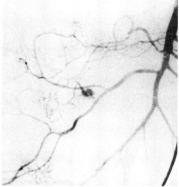

Figure 9.2

FIGURE 9.1—*Massive upper gastrointestinal bleeding following sphincterotomy: selective gastroduodenal arteriogram shows active contrast medium extravasation (arrow) from a small branch of the pancreaticoduodenal arcade supplying the second part of the duodenum.*

FIGURE 9.2—*Massive gastrointestinal haemorrhage: superior mesenteric arteriogram shows a focal area of active contrast medium extravasation in the right upper abdomen. Selective arteriograms of the right colic and inferior pancreaticoduodenal arteries were required to localise the bleeding to the duodenum from a distal branch of the latter vessel.*

FIGURE 9.3—*Pseudoaneurysm of the gastroduodenal artery secondary to chronic pancreatitis: selective common hepatic arteriogram demonstrates a small pseudoaneurysm (arrow) of the midgastroduodenal artery. Cure was effected by placing coils on either side of the abnormality, thus isolating it from the circulation.*

Digital subtraction angiography

The superior contrast resolution of digital subtraction angiography (DSA) when compared with that of conventional film will in most cases make the detection of contrast extravasation into the bowel lumen much easier, although care has to be taken to ensure that movement is kept to a minimum, to avoid the generation of confusing DSA artefacts. Bowel peristalsis is easily abolished by the use of antiperistaltic agents but respiration is more difficult to control, especially if the patient is unwell. A useful alternative is the acquisition of images during normal respiration, with multiple masks being obtained before the injection of contrast. A suitable mask will then be available for most of the images acquired after a subsequent contrast injection.

123

Subtle vascular irregularity may be missed because of the inferior spatial resolution of DSA but this is rarely a significant problem provided that magnified selective images are obtained.

DSA is almost mandatory during embolisation procedures, as it allows rapid angiography to be performed with immediate review. DSA has made embolisation considerably safer, both for this reason and because it allows the use of smaller quantities of contrast agent in patients who are often unwell. When contrast extravasation is seen, the vessel from which it originates may not be obvious on the initial study. This is particularly true when the bleeding source overlies the epigastrium, as branches of the pancreaticoduodenal arcade, the right and middle colic arteries and occasionally also the jejunal arteries may all be superimposed at this site (Figure 9.2). In such cases, superselective studies of these vessels will be required to define accurately the haemorrhaging vessel.

Source of haemorrhage

When the source of haemorrhage is a single large vessel, such as the main trunk of the gastroduodenal artery that has been directly eroded by an adjacent duodenal ulcer or a pancreatic pseudocyst (Figure 9.3), curative embolisation should be relatively straightforward, as embolisation coils (or detachable balloons) can be placed on either side of the arterial defect, thus isolating it from the circulation. When bleeding is from numerous small bleeding points, as occurs with haemorrhagic gastritis, treatment by embolisation is less likely to be successful; it may be difficult to reduce the perfusion pressure in all the vessels from which the bleeding is occurring, because of the presence of a rich collateral arterial supply to the upper gastrointestinal tract.[1]

Experience of the angiographer

The angiographer performing embolisation needs not only to be experienced in selective and superselective catheterisation but also to have a sound knowledge of the normal vascular anatomy of the territory that is being occluded. For example, a bleeding pseudoaneurysm of the gastroduodenal artery should be treated by isolating it entirely from the circulation and this may be best achieved by placing coils on either side of the neck of the aneurysm.[2] If, however, only the proximal gastroduodenal artery is occluded then the pseudoaneurysm will continue to fill, usually via the inferior pancreaticoduodenal artery arising from the superior mesenteric artery, although other sources may include the left gastroepiploic artery arising from the distal splenic artery and the transverse pancreatic artery arising from the dorsal pancreatic artery. If these potential collateral supplies are not appreciated by the angiographer then such a lesion, which is often visible only on the coeliac axis (and not the superior mesenteric) arteriogram, might be inappropriately and unsuccessfully treated by proximal occlusion of the gastroduodenal artery alone. Neglect of such simple anatomical considerations is probably the commonest cause of failure to control bleeding by embolisation.

Indications for Embolisation

Embolisation is the procedure of choice for traumatic (accidental and iatrogenic) arterial bleeding from the liver,[3-7] and also, arguably, for aneurysmal disease of the visceral arteries in the upper gastrointestinal tract.[2 8-13] The surgical treatment of many of these lesions is associated with considerable morbidity and mortality, while embolisation can be successfully performed in most patients under local anaesthesia.

Severe bleeding from benign duodenal or gastric ulcers is usually managed successfully by a combination of endoscopic methods and medical therapy, but the occasional patient will continue to bleed. The choice between embolisation or surgery in these individuals will often depend upon the expertise that is available. In most centres, however, surgical oversewing is usually performed, and embolisation is reserved for patients at high risk from a general anaesthetic and those who continue to bleed postoperatively.

Persistent, severe haemorrhage in patients with erosive or haemorrhagic gastritis is perhaps best managed by the selective infusion of vasopressin into the left gastric artery.[1] There are two main reasons for this: firstly, diffuse bleeding may be difficult to control by embolisation, because of the rich collateral supply to the stomach and duodenum; secondly, gastric infarction is a recognised risk of vasopressin therapy after failed embolisation.[14]

Contraindications to Embolisation

There are few, if any, absolute contraindications to the use of embolisation to halt acute upper gastrointestinal haemorrhage, other than those to angiography itself, such as an uncorrectable, severe bleeding diathesis or a previous history of a severe reaction to contrast medium. Particular care should be exercised, however, in those patients who have severe visceral arterial atheromatous disease, those who have undergone (failed) vasopressin therapy, and those who have a history of previous upper gastrointestinal surgery that involved the ligation of normal branches supplying the stomach. These individuals are at an increased risk of gastric infarction following embolisation.[14 15]

Technique of Embolisation

Certain general principles are common to all embolisation procedures.[16] The operator should:

- Have a thorough knowledge of the normal and variant anatomy

- Always ensure a secure catheter position before the injection of embolic material
- Always obtain good quality angiograms of the vascular territory to be embolised, so that the anatomy is fully appreciated
- Choose the right embolic agent for the lesion being embolised (see pages 127, 129 and 133)
- Always mix non-radiopaque embolic material with contrast medium before injection
- Inject embolic material in small aliquots and under continuous fluoroscopy to ensure that it is passing only into those vessels that need to be embolised
- Perform diagnostic angiograms at various times during embolisation to assess the progress of the vascular occlusion and be careful not to over-inject embolic material, otherwise it may reflux around the catheter into normal vessels
- Always stop if uncertain, and perform a check arteriogram.

More specific points of technique are perhaps best discussed by considering the approach to bleeding points in the different anatomical sites, namely the liver; the stomach and duodenum; and the pancreas.

Embolisation in the liver

Persistent, severe haemobilia, whether secondary to liver biopsy, percutaneous biliary intervention or accidental trauma, is almost always from an intrahepatic arterial source. Arteriography will often show arterial irregularity or aneurysm formation (Figure 9.4) and there may be active contrast extravasation into the biliary tree (Figure 9.5). Other angiographic signs include the presence of arterioportal shunting and, in the case of liver biopsy or biliary intervention, needle tracks may be visible as linear opacities.

Conventional surgical therapy of haemobilia consists of the ligation of extrahepatic arterial branches, and this may be successful in some individuals as it decreases perfusion pressure to the site of the arterial injury. In a significant number of patients, however, bleeding will persist because of the rapid development of an intrahepatic arterial collateral supply, and this is the principal reason why embolisation should be considered as the first-line treatment for haemobilia.[3-7]

Embolisation has a higher success rate and a lower morbidity than surgery for the control of an arterial source of haemobilia; this is because the technique allows the operator to identify and then superselectively catheterise and occlude only the abnormal intrahepatic vessel(s), while preserving the surrounding normal hepatic arterial supply. Because the hepatic arterial branches are not end arteries, the occlusion must be performed *across* the vascular abnormality (aneurysm, arterioportal communication) to prevent its continued supply from more distal intrahepatic collaterals (Figures 9.4 and 9.5). This will, in some cases, require the use of a co-axial catheter, that is, one that passes through the

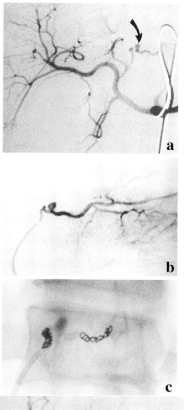

FIGURE 9.4—*Intrahepatic pseudoaneurysm treated by embolisation. The patient presented with massive haemobilia following a liver laceration secondary to trauma. (a) Coeliac axis angiogram demonstrates a small pseudoaneurysm of an intrahepatic branch of the left hepatic artery (arrow). (b) The left hepatic arterial branch has been selectively catheterised. The pseudoaneurysm is well visualised. (c) Coils have been placed on either side of the pseudoaneurysm, thus isolating it from the circulation. Note the contrast stasis within the aneurysmal sac. (d) Coeliac axis arteriogram performed after embolisation. The pseudoaneurysm is no longer opacified. The left hepatic arterial branches beyond the embolisation coils are being supplied by an accessory hepatic artery arising from the left gastric artery.*

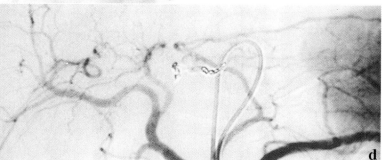

lumen of a conventional angiographic catheter, thereby allowing distal catheterisation of small vessels.

The choice of embolic agent depends partly upon operator preference and partly on the anatomy of the abnormality being occluded. A pseudoaneurysm of a small, peripheral intrahepatic artery can successfully by treated by placing metallic microcoils on either side of its neck (Figures 9.4 and 9.5). Alternatively the vessel can be "packed" with small particulate embolic material such as polyvinyl alcohol or absorbable gelatin sponge.

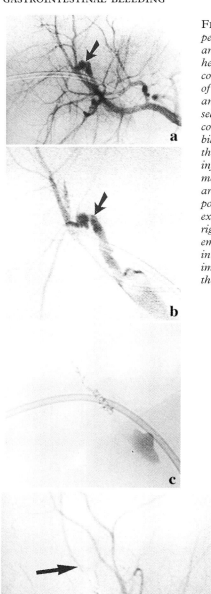

FIGURE 9.5—*Severe haemobilia after percutaneous biliary drainage treated by arterial embolisation. (a) Selective proper hepatic arteriogram demonstrates active contrast medium extravasation from a branch of the right hepatic artery (arrow). (b) The angiographic catheter has been introduced selectively into the bleeding vessel. Brisk contrast extravasation is seen into the adjacent bile duct (arrow). Note the close relationship of the biliary drainage catheter to the arterial injury. (c) Radiograph postembolisation shows metallic coils positioned on either side of the arterial injury. (d) Proper hepatic arteriogram postembolisation: the contrast medium extravasation is no longer seen. Note how the right hepatic artery branch beyond the embolisation coils (arrow) is opacified by intrahepatic collaterals; this shows the importance of isolating the arterial injury from the circulation.*

This will have the same effect as distal and proximal embolisation with coils, but is perhaps more likely to produce localised liver ischaemia and embolisation of adjacent normal hepatic arterial branches, as a result of inadvertent reflux of embolic material.

Embolisation in the stomach and duodenum

Causes of gastric and duodenal bleeding include peptic ulcers, pancreaticoduodenal arcade aneurysms (duodenem), neoplasms (usually gastric, duodenal or pancreatic in origin) and iatrogenic insults such as biopsy and surgery. While the extensive vascular supply to this portion of the bowel makes embolisation safer, it also means that the successful control of haemorrhage is more difficult; an occlusion created in one vessel supplying a bleeding point is rapidly bypassed through collateral channels, which may be difficult or impossible to catheterise. The treatment of gastric or duodenal bleeding, therefore, often requires the use of small particulate embolic material to achieve a relatively distal block.

Peptic ulceration

Persistent bleeding from a gastric or duodenal ulcer that does not respond to local endoscopic therapy often indicates erosion of the ulcer into an adjacent large artery. Operative treatment of such lesions is often successful, and in certain patients may be usefully combined with a more definitive antiulcer surgical procedure, such as highly selective vagotomy. An alternative, particularly for those patients who are poor candidates for general anaesthesia because of old age, poor lung function, or severe hypovolaemia, is angiography and embolisation.[117]

The method of embolisation used will depend upon the angiographic findings. When a defect is demonstrated within the wall of a large artery, with brisk contrast extravasation, occlusion is performed on either side of the abnormality, usually with metallic coils; this usually stops the bleeding.

More difficulty will be experienced when the source of bleeding is a small, peripheral branch of the left gastric artery (Figure 9.6) or pancreaticoduodenal arcade (Figure 9.1), or when no angiographic abnormality is visualised. In such cases an attempt should be made to reduce the perfusion pressure to this vascular territory, while avoiding the occlusion of normal visceral vessels; the superior mesenteric artery is at particular risk during occlusion of the pancreaticoduodenal arcade. Embolisation of duodenal bleeding may, therefore, involve occlusion with metal coils of the distal anterior superior pancreaticoduodenal artery, the distal retroduodenal artery and the proximal right gastroepiploic artery with metallic coils, to protect normal vessels before the injection of small particulate polyvinyl alcohol into the gastroduodenal artery.

During embolisation of a small branch of the left gastric artery, highly selective catheterisation is desirable so that small particulate emboli can be introduced directly into the bleeding vessel (Figure 9.6). If this is not done

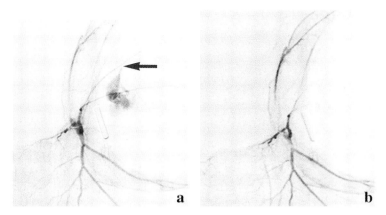

FIGURE 9.6—*Bleeding from left gastric artery due to an acute ulcer. Treatment by selective embolisation. (a) Selective left gastric arteriogram shows active contrast medium extravasation from a branch of the left gastric artery (arrow). The bleeding vessel was selectively catheterised and embolised with polyvinyl alcohol. (b) Selective left gastric arteriogram postembolisation shows complete occlusion of the bleeding vessel.*

rebleeding is not uncommon, because of collateral vessels from the short gastric arteries (which are usually extremely difficult or impossible to catheterise selectively), the right gastric artery, and the right and left gastroepiploic arteries.

Severe bleeding from a diffuse gastritis is best managed by the infusion of vasopressin selectively into the left gastric artery.[1] If this fails, or if there is recurrent bleeding when the dose of vasopressin is being reduced, then embolisation of the left gastric branches can be performed with particulate agents such as polyvinyl alcohol or absorbable gelatin sponge, in an attempt to produce a generalised decrease in perfusion pressure.

Aneurysmal disease of the pancreaticoduodenal arcade

Aneurysmal disease may be associated with acute or chronic pancreatitis, or may be secondary to atheromatous disease.[18] The combination of atheromatous disease and aneurysm formation is often associated with hypertrophy of the pancreaticoduodenal vessels, either as a result of atheromatous stenosis of the coeliac axis or, more commonly, of compression of the coeliac axis origin by the median arcuate ligament of the hemidiaphragm. The aneurysm can usually be isolated from the circulation, making embolisation the procedure of choice. When there is associated arterial hypertrophy of the pancreaticoduodenal arcade, embolisation is usually most easily performed via the inferior pancreaticoduodenal artery arising from the proximal superior mesenteric or first jejunal arteries.

Neoplastic disease

The stomach and duodenum may be involved by primary tumours (for example, carcinoma, stromal cell), by neoplasms in adjacent viscera (such as the pancreas or gall bladder) or by secondary deposits (for example, breast, melanoma). The treatment of first choice must be surgical resection but this may be neither possible nor in the patient's best interests because of tumour size or the presence of extensive metastatic disease; in such cases embolisation may be attempted. Those tumours most commonly referred for embolisation because of severe, unremitting bleeding are inoperable primary leiomyosarcomas and large, vascular pancreatic neuroendocrine tumours. A focal arterial abnormality on angiography will more often be found in patients who give a history of intermittent severe bleeds than it will in those who have a persistent slow or moderate "ooze". When a focal lesion is seen, particularly if contrast extravasation is also demonstrated, embolisation can be directed towards this abnormality even if there is a large amount of surrounding neovascularity (Figure 9.7). In many patients, however, the only angiographic abnormality visualised is that of extensive neovascularity, often with evidence of venous occlusion and resultant variceal formation. In such cases one can only aim to try and reduce perfusion pressure to the site of bleeding by occlusion of the tumour vessels. Great care has to be taken to avoid the embolisation of adjacent normal structures that may be infiltrated by the tumour.

The results of embolisation in this group of patients are not good; improvement may be obtained, but is usually short-lived.

Embolisation in the pancreas

Acute and chronic pancreatitis may be associated with severe gastrointestinal bleeding because of the involvement of adjacent vessels.[3 8–13 19–22] The splenic vein is commonly occluded, with resultant segmental portal hypertension causing splenomegaly and gastric varices. Resultant gastrointestinal bleeding can be cured by splenectomy, an operation that can often be combined with pancreatic surgery if this is indicated. A "medical splenectomy", performed by embolisation of the splenic artery, has been reported as being successful in some patients with segmental portal hypertension. This procedure is not without risk; it is associated with significant morbidity and mortality, because of the possible complications of splenic abscess formation or splenic rupture, and it might be expected that the likely subsequent growth of the spleen could cause rebleeding. If a subtotal splenic embolisation is performed, however, and some functioning splenic parenchyma left in situ, the patient's susceptibility to infection, especially by *Pneumococcus* spp, should not be increased.

Arterial erosion, either by pancreatic enzymes during an episode of acute pancreatitis, or by pressure from an adjacent pseudocyst in chronic pancreatitis (Figure 9.3), may cause life-threatening haemorrhage. This may occur into the pancreatic duct (haemosuccus pancreaticus),[8 13] in which

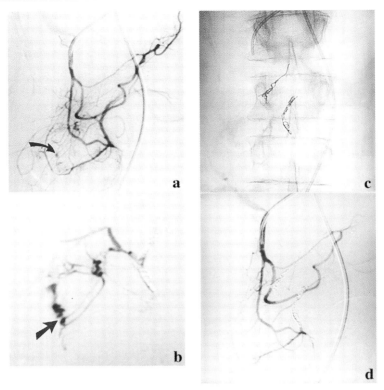

FIGURE 9.7—*Recurrent inoperable duodenal leiomyosarcoma causing episodes of severe upper gastrointestinal haemorrhage. (a) Selective gastroduodenal arteriogram shows extensive neovascularity around the second and third parts of the duodenum. A small aneurysm (arrow) is also seen. (b) During embolisation brisk contrast medium extravasation occurred from the aneurysm (arrow). (c) Radiograph postembolisation shows metallic coils within the inferior pancreaticoduodenal arteries. These have been introduced to protect the superior mesenteric artery during subsequent embolisation of the neovessels and aneurysm with polyvinyl alcohol. (d) Gastroduodenal arteriogram postembolisation shows a considerable reduction in neovascularity and occlusion of the aneurysm when compared with (a). The patient had no further large bleeds before his death 3 months later from carcinomatosis.*

case each episode of bleeding is usually associated with severe epigastric pain, or directly into the duodenum or into the retroperitoneum. The surgical treatment of acutely bleeding peripancreatic pseudoaneurysms is associated with quoted mortality rates of 16% for lesions around the pancreatic tail and up to 50% for those around the pancreatic head.[19 23 24] There are no comparable series documenting the results of embolisation in a similar group of patients, but several small series and case reports suggest that this method of treatment should be the procedure of choice, with surgery reserved for those patients in whom embolisation is not possible.[8–13]

Embolisation should, as always, be aimed at isolating the involved vessel from the circulation and this is usually possible by placing metallic coils on either side of the neck of the pseudoaneurysm. Filling the pseudoaneurysm with metallic coils should be avoided, if possible, as the cavity is likely to expand during embolisation (owing to the presence of intraluminal thrombus and the lack of a true wall), with the potential risk of rupture. On occasion, however, this method of occlusion will have to be used if the anatomy is unfavourable.

Complications of Embolisation

The possible complications of angiography and selective catheterisation include puncture site haematoma, contrast medium reaction, and arterial dissection, and there is a higher incidence of such problems in patients undergoing complex interventional procedures than in those undergoing simple diagnostic studies[25] patients requiring intervention are usually unwell, and are often not very cooperative; they may also be hypovolaemic and have abnormal clotting mechanisms as a result of repeated transfusions.

Complications specific to the embolisation procedure are those of inadvertent occlusion of a normal vascular territory (which should be avoidable), bowel infarction and persistent bleeding.

Arterial embolisation above the ligament of Treitz is associated with a low risk of ischaemic complications because of the extensive collateral vascular supply to this area. In the treatment of localised or diffuse gastric haemorrhage, occlusion of the left gastric arterial branches can be performed with fairly small calibre particulate materials with little fear of causing necrosis of the stomach, unless there has been previous surgery in the upper abdomen that might interfere with the potential collateral vascular supply (for example, gastric surgery or splenectomy), or when there is severe atheromatous disease. Similarly, small branches of the pancreaticoduodenal arcades may be safely occluded when treating duodenal haemorrhage.

Poor embolisation technique, whereby proximal arterial occlusion is performed without distal occlusion, is a common cause of recurrent bleeding. The bleeding site usually receives continued retrograde perfusion via collateral vessels, and subsequent treatment by further embolisation is then difficult or impossible because of a lack of direct vascular access to the lesion.

Conclusion

Embolisation should be the procedure of choice for arterial bleeding that occurs from the liver and for peripancreatic aneurysmal disease; results are good, provided that the embolisation technique is meticulous. Embolisation of other bleeding sites in the upper gastrointestinal tract is usually reserved for those patients who are not candidates for surgery. These patients are often in poor condition, but embolisation may prove useful, either by providing definitive treatment or by stopping bleeding for a short time and thus allowing the patient's condition to improve before later surgery.

Key points

- Extravasation of contrast is the only direct angiographic sign of gastrointestinal haemorrhage
- Use of digital subtraction angiography (DSA) is almost mandatory during embolisation procedures
- Success is most likely when the source of haemorrhage is a single large vessel
- The commonest reason for failed embolisation is probably poor understanding of vascular anatomy
- Embolisation is the procedure of choice for arterial bleeding from the liver and for peripancreatic aneurysmal disease. At other bleeding sites, it is reserved for patients unsuitable for surgery

---

References

1 Athanasoulis CA, Waltman AC, Novelline RA, Krudy AG, Sniderman KW. Angiography. Its contribution to the emergency management of gastrointestinal haemorrhage. *Radiol Clin North Am* 1976;**14**:265–80.

2 Blomley MJK, Jackson JE. Case report: a gastroduodenal artery pseudoaneurysm presenting with obstructive jaundice and treated by arterial embolisation. *Clin Radiol* 1994;**49**:715–8.

3 Fagan EA, Allison DJ, Chadwick VS, Hodgson HJF. Treatment of haemobilia by selective arterial embolisation. *Gut* 1980;**21**:541–4.

4 Kadir S, Athanasoulis CA, Ring EJ, Greenfield A. Transcatheter embolisation of intrahepatic arterial aneurysms. *Radiology* 1980;**134**:335–9.

5 Kelley CJ, Hemingway AP, McPherson GAD, Allison DJ, Blumgart LH. Non-surgical management of post-cholecystectomy haemobilia. *Br J Surg* 1983;**70**:502–4.

6 Clouse ME. Hepatic artery embolisation for bleeding and tumours. *Surg Clin North Am* 1989;**69**:419–32.

7 Dick R, Adam A, Allison DJ. Interventional techniques in the hepatobiliary system. In: Grainger RG, Allison DJ, eds. *Diagnostic radiology: an Anglo–American textbook of imaging.* 2nd ed. Edinburgh: Churchill Livingstone, 1992:1111–27.

8 Camilleri M, Hemingway AP, Chadwick VS, Blumgart LH, Hodgson HJF, Allison DJ. Embolisation of an intrapancreatic aneurysm. *Br J Radiol* 1982;**55**:685–7.

9 Mandel SR, Jaques PF, Mauro M, Sanofsky S. Nonoperative management of peripancreatic arterial aneurysms. A 10-year experience. *Ann Surg* 1987;**205**:126–8.

10 Huizinga WKJ, Kalideen JM, Bryer JV, Bell PSH, Baker LW. Control of major haemorrhage associated with pancreatic pseudocysts by transcatheter arterial embolisation. *Br J Surg* 1984;**71**:133–6.

11 Baker KS, Tisnado J, Cho S-R, Beachley MC. Splanchnic artery aneurysms and pseudoaneurysms: transcatheter embolisation. *Radiology* 1987;**163**:135–9.

12 Walker TG, Waltman AC. Angiographic management of massive haemorrhage caused by pancreatic disease. *Semin Interven Radiol* 1988;**5**:61–3.

13 Ryan CM, Benjamin IS, Allison DJ. The diagnosis and management of haemosuccus pancreaticus. *J Interven Radiol* 1989;**4**:130–4.

14 Goldman ML, Land WC, Bradley EL, Anderson J. Transcatheter therapeutic embolization in the management of massive upper gastrointestinal bleeding. *Radiology* 1976;**120**:513–21.

15 Prochaska JM, Flye MW, Johnsrude IS. Left gastric artery embolisation for control of gastric bleeding; a complication. *Radiology* 1973;**107**:521–2.
16 Allison DJ, Wallace S, Machan LS. Interventional Radiology. In: Grainger RG, Allison DJ, eds. *Diagnostic radiology: an Anglo–American textbook of imaging.* 2nd ed. Edinburgh: Churchill Livingstone, 1992:2330–90.
17 Keller FS, Barton RE, Rösch J. Angiographic diagnosis and therapy of gastrointestinal tract bleeding. In: Freeny PC, Stevenson GW, eds. *Margulis and Burhenne's alimentary tract radiology.* 5th ed. St Louis: Mosby, 1994:994–1016.
18 Granke K, Hollier LH, Bowen JC. Pancreaticoduodenal artery aneurysms: changing patterns. *Southern Med J* 1990;**83**:918–21.
19 Stanley JC, Frey CF, Miller TA, Lindenauer SM, Child CG. Major arterial haemorrhage. A complication of pancreatic pseudocysts and chronic pancreatitis. *Arch Surg* 1976;**111**: 435–40.
20 White AF, Baum S, Buranasiri S. Aneurysms secondary to pancreatitis. *Am J Roentgenol* 1976;**127**:393–6.
21 Eckhauser FE, Stanley JC, Zelenock GB, Borlaza GS, Feier DT, Lindenauer SM. Gastroduodenal and pancreaticoduodenal artery aneurysms: a complication of pancreatitis causing spontaneous gastrointestinal haemorrhage. *Surgery* 1980;**88**:335–44.
22 Bretagne J-F, Heresbach D, Darnault P, *et al.* Pseudoaneurysms and bleeding pseudocysts in chronic pancreatitis: radiological findings and contribution to diagnosis in 8 cases. *Gastrointest Radiol* 1990;**15**:9–16.
23 Kiviluoto T, Kivisaari L, Kivilaakso E, Lempinen M. Pseudocysts in chronic pancreatitis. Surgical results in 102 consecutive patients. *Arch Surg* 1989;**124**:240–3.
24 Stabile BE, Wilson SE, Debas H. Reduced mortality from bleeding pseudocysts and pseudoaneurysms caused by pancreatitis. *Arch Surg* 1983;**118**:45–51.
25 Allison DJ, Machan LS. Arteriography. In: Grainger RG, Allison DJ, eds. *Diagnostic radiology: an Anglo–America textbook of imaging.* 2nd ed. Edinburgh: Churchill Livingstone, 1992:2205–75.

Part IV
Bleeding from varices

10: Surgical management of acute upper gastrointestinal bleeding

ANDREW WU

As 70–80% of all upper gastrointestinal bleeding stops spontaneously, the small group of patients who continue to bleed remains a challenge to any clinical team. Morbidity and mortality, especially in the elderly, remain high. One response to this challenge is to set up a specialised, integrated haematemesis team, with close collaboration between physicians and surgeons, where the aim is to achieve early surgical intervention for high risk patients. This approach can reduce the mortality from 10% to 2%.[1]

Indications for Surgery

The main indications for intervening surgically in bleeding peptic ulcers relate to the age of the patient and the severity of haemorrhage. Older patients tolerate acute blood loss less well than do younger people.[2] A prospective randomised trial comparing early operation with initial expectant management and operation if necessary revealed that age was the main determinant in proceeding to surgery.[3] The policy adopted by Aintree Hospital's acute gastrointestinal bleed management team is early operative intervention after failure to obtain endoscopic control, especially in elderly patients (Figure 10.1). We operate on patients under 60 years who need eight units of blood transfused or have two rebleeds in hospital; and on patients over 60 years who need four units of blood or have one rebleed in hospital. Rarely, when a patient presents in shock after massive haemorrhage and a spurting vessel in the ulcer crater is visible on endoscopy, he or she may be rushed to the operating theatre for immediate surgery.[4]

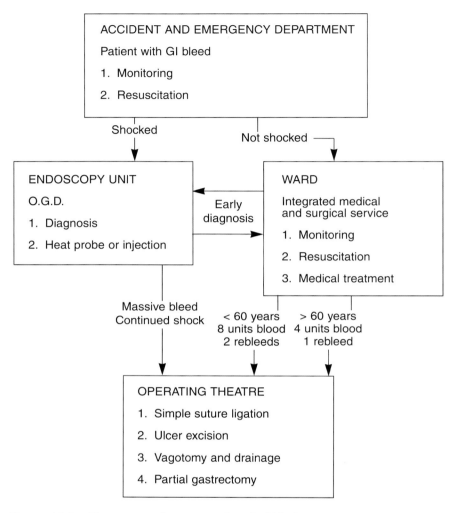

FIGURE 10.1—*Management of acute gastrointestinal bleed.*

Which Operation for Bleeding Ulcers?

An emergency operation for a bleeding peptic ulcer can be very difficult. It should not be delegated to inexperienced, junior staff, as it is clear that the experienced surgeon will produce better results. At laparotomy the stomach is usually distended with a mass of clotted blood.

Duodenal ulcer

For a duodenal ulcer, the first and second parts of the duodenum should first be mobilised (the Kocher manoeuvre) and delivered to the surface of the abdomen. A longitudinal duodenotomy passing through the pylorus will reveal the posterior ulcer crater. There is often a thrombus plug sitting on the base of the ulcer, and this should not be disturbed. The eroded vessel is then sutured and ligated with a non-absorbable material, to achieve immediate control of the bleeding. Once the danger of haemorrhage is over, then three deep, non-absorbable sutures are placed to underrun the gastroduodenal artery and, if practicable, to approximate the edges of the ulcer.

If the thrombus plug is dislodged, the resulting brisk haemorrhage can be controlled by external compression of the gastroduodenal artery from behind the duodenum, thereby lifting the ulcer forward. Similar suture ligation can then be performed. Blind suturing of a bleeding vessel should be avoided.

Gastric ulcer

To deal with a bleeding gastric ulcer a generous gastrotomy is made to quickly evacuate the clotted blood. The ulcer crater, usually situated in the lesser curve, is then sought and any active bleeding point controlled by suturing. Silk suture is best avoided because it often delays healing of the ulcer. Once the active bleeding has been arrested, then a decision must be taken as to whether a definitive procedure should be carried out.

This remains a controversial area. A multicentre randomised prospective trial compared conservative surgery (underrunning the vessel or ulcer excision) and adjuvant ranitidine with conventional surgery (vagotomy and pyloroplasty or partial gastrectomy) in 137 patients treated for bleeding peptic ulcer. The mortality was 26% after conservative surgery and 19% after conventional surgery. The only significant difference between the two groups was the incidence of fatal rebleeding, which occurred in six patients (9·6%) after conservative surgery compared with none after conventional surgery. The overall mortality was 22%.[5]

A retrospective study on 61 patients who underwent surgery for bleeding gastric ulcer reported a mortality in partial gastrectomy, undersewing of ulcer plus vagotomy and drainage, and undersewing ulcer alone of 26, 45 and 10%, respectively.[6] The mortality in another report decreased from 12 to 3·9% using an aggressive but selective management policy.[7] A selective policy tailored to meet the needs of the patient seems logical. Applying the APACHE II (Acute Physiology and Chronic Health Evaluation) scoring system for the risk factors in massive bleeding from peptic ulcers, it has been shown that non-resective procedures carry less risk of mortality when compared with gastrectomy.[8] It is my practice to manage low risk patients with conventional surgery, which is well tolerated with a low rate of rebleeding, and the high risk group with minimal surgery and adjuvant H_2 antagonist cover.

Once the bleeding from a gastric ulcer has been controlled, the surgeon may consider completely excising the ulcer and closing the healthy edges.

141

This will allow histological analysis of the ulcer, is followed by a lower rate of rebleeding, and has the advantage of being a less invasive procedure. Occasionally, poor access makes it impossible to excise the ulcer; four-quadrant biopsies should then be taken after control of the haemorrhage.

One school of thought advocates highly selective vagotomy (HSV) as a definitive procedure after control of the haemorrhage from an ulcer.[9] The procedure has a low incidence of such side effects as the dumping syndrome and intractable diarrhoea when compared with truncal vagotomy, but it is time consuming and can be associated with a ulcer recurrence rate of up to 30%.[10]

The role of the surgeon in the treatment of the upper gastrointestinal haemorrhage has changed over the past 50 years. Most patients with gastrointestinal bleeding are admitted to the care of the gastroenterologist. Although drug treatment has not appreciably affected the outcome of nonvariceal gastrointestinal bleeding, for most patients initial medical treatment, and subsequent diagnosis and endoscopic control of bleeding ulcers is successful. Only a few patients who rebleed require the services of the surgeon. However, only a closely integrated medical and surgical approach will produce optimal results, and from time to time a patient dies who could have been saved. This is usually the result of a transient lack of vigilance or a temporary breakdown in communication. Only a dedicated haematemesis management team whose performance is constantly audited and reappraised can avoid inappropriate mortality.

Management of Variceal Haemorrhage

Variceal bleeding in patients with portal hypertension continues to be a difficult clinical problem. The development of endoscopic sclerotherapy and banding has dramatically altered the management of acute variceal bleeding, and the early success rate is up to 90%. Early endoscopy can not only confirm the diagnosis but also exclude other causes of bleeding, so that injection of sclerosant into the varices can be carried out as first line treatment. This may be aided by the administration of vasopressin, propanolol or octreotide.

The Sengstaken–Blakemore tube may be required to tamponade the varices. Control of the acute bleeding may be achieved in up to 95% of patients.[11] In the acute phase sclerotherapy may be repeated once. If haemorrhage is not controlled after the second injection, further attempts will not increase the success rate and may jeopardise the patient by delaying surgical intervention. The rate of rebleeding after conservative treatment is still around 10%, and early emergency surgery is generally advocated before blood loss is excessive.

Surgical option for variceal bleeding

The most popular and least technically demanding procedure for the surgical control of variceal bleeding is oesophageal transection. This may be done using the circular stapling gun or by hand sewing. The procedure may be combined with devascularisation of the lower 5 cm of the oesophagus and the proximal two-thirds of the stomach, with or without splenectomy.[12] Oesophageal transection is successful in stopping variceal haemorrhage in 96% of patients, but the early and late rebleeding rate is as high as 60%. In patients with Child's C liver disease, the perioperative mortality rate is a massive 82%, mostly from liver failure, whereas in patients with Child's B disease, it is 16%.[13]

Emergency portasystemic shunt

The emergency portacaval shunt fell into disfavour for several reasons. Mortality was high when the procedure was carried out by non-specialists, there was an unpredictable incidence of postoperative encephalopathy and emergency sclerotherapy proved to be successful. Some dedicated groups have continued to use emergency portacaval shunting as the first treatment for variceal bleeding with admirable results, and the value of this procedure has lately been recognised again.

A non-randomised study from Italy reported on 88 patients admitted for active variceal haemorrhage over 9 years. Thirty-five underwent an emergency portacaval shunt using side-to-side anastomosis. In 31 poor risk patients with Child's B or C disease, emergency shunting controlled bleeding in all but one. There were three operative deaths. Long term endoscopic follow-up showed that the varices had disappeared in 18 patients and were substantially smaller in another 14. Chronic encephalopathy developed in 20% but was severe in only one-third.[14] Similar favourable results were published in America.[15 16]

These specialised units recommend sclerotherapy as the first treatment, and reserve portacaval shunts for patients who do not respond to two emergency injection treatments.

Side-to-side portacaval shunt

Side-to-side portacaval shunt is still not an easy operation to perform. One approach is to resect the lower part of the caudate lobe, which lies between and abuts the vena cava and the portal vein.

Distal splenorenal shunt

The distal splenorenal (Warren) shunt decompresses the oesophageal varices effectively and prevents rebleeding. Because the mesenteric vein is uninterrupted, portal circulation is maintained and patients run less risk of encephalopathy; rebleeding and operative mortality rates are comparable with those of other shunting procedures. A late complication following the Warren shunt is the development of collaterals between the splenic and the portal veins via the pancreas, which can lead to late development of hepatic encephalopathy. The technical difficulty of this operation precludes widespread adoption. However, it must be seriously considered in patients who may be suitable for subsequent liver transplantation, because it does not interfere with the portal vein.[17]

Mesocaval shunt

The mesocaval shunt can be performed relatively safely and easily by interposing a jump graft between the superior mesenteric vein and the vena cava, below the level of the third part of the duodenum.[18] A reinforced GoreTex graft of 12–16 mm diameter is ideal, and the graft must be kept as short as possible.[19] This is difficult to achieve in obese patients, but the rethrombosis rate is high if the graft is longer than a few centimetres. No randomised study has included this procedure. The operation is most suitable as an elective procedure for the treatment of ascites, portal vein thrombosis or the Budd–Chiari syndrome rather than for the acute management of variceal haemorrhage.[20]

Transjugular intrahepatic portasystemic stent (TIPS) shunt

A percutaneous technique has been developed to create a portasystemic shunt within the liver parenchyma, and this is described in Chapter 13.

Liver Transplantation

Liver transplantation is the treatment of choice in many end-stage liver diseases. The success currently achieved is mainly attributable to refinement of immunosuppression, careful patient selection and regimented postoperative care. Variceal bleeding complicating portal hypertension is not in itself an indication for liver transplantation. Because of limited donor availability and the risks associated with life-long immunosuppression, liver transplantation can be recommended only for portal hypertension associated with end-stage liver disease. Patients with good hepatic function may do quite well with another treatment modality such as a shunt. Patients who have end-stage liver disease that is secondary to primary biliary cirrhosis, cryptogenic cirrhosis, chronic non-A, non-B hepatitis or sclerosing cholangitis, and those with alcoholic cirrhosis who have reformed their drinking habits, are candidates for liver transplantation, provided that they have few or no concomitant risk factors such as advanced age or cardiopulmonary or renal disease.

For transplant candidates who present with variceal haemorrhage not controlled by sclerotherapy or other non-invasive methods, shunt surgery is advisable. The major consideration is to avoid operating in the hepatic hilum, and a distal splenorenal or mesocaval shunt is therefore to be preferred. Published figures from Pittsburgh on 302 oesophageal variceal bleeders showed survival after transplantation to be 79% at 1 year and 71% at 5 years.[21] Because the number of patients who would benefit from liver transplantation far exceeds the number of donors, a significant number of them will require definitive shunt surgery.

Acute Erosive Gastritis

The causes of acute erosive gastritis are obscure and are discussed elsewhere. Most patients present with melaena and haematemesis. Most settle with conservative measures but in a few there is torrential haemorrhage and haemodynamic shock. When the diagnosis is unclear and bleeding continues, the surgeon is under pressure to perform a laparotomy. Modern drug therapy with H_2 antagonists and proton pump inhibitors virtually eliminates gastric acid secretion, however, so an acid reducing operation such as vagotomy seems superfluous. Suturing may be tried, but is seldom fully effective. Partial gastrectomy may be possible if the proximal stomach is uninvolved. In a desperate situation, the surest way to prevent rebleeding is a total gastrectomy, which also covers the remote possibility of an occult gastrinoma.[4, 22]

Key points

- The most effective means of reducing morbidity and mortality in upper gastrointestinal haemorrhage is a specialised management team that integrates medical and surgical approaches

- Early diagnosis and surgical intervention is essential in patients in whom endoscopic treatment has failed

- Drug treatment has not appreciably affected the outcome of peptic ulcer bleeding

- Conventional surgery is preferred in bleeding ulcers when the patient is at low risk

- Minimal surgery with an adjunctive H_2 antagonist or proton pump inhibitor is indicated in high risk patients

- Variceal haemorrhage should be treated early by endoscopic sclerotherapy

- Portosystemic shunt surgery is reserved for those patients in whom sclerotherapy fails. Portacaval shunt is still the most effective way to stop variceal bleeding

- Distal splenorenal or mesocaval shunts may be preferred in patients who are strong candidates for liver transplantation

- Oesophageal transection with devascularisation may be attempted in non-specialised units

---

References

1 Holman RAE, Davis M, Gough KR, Gartnell P, Brittaon DC, Smith RB. Value of a centralised approach in the management of hematemesis and melaena. Experience in a District General Hospital. *Gut* 1990;**31**:504–8.
2 Darle N. Operative treatment in massive peptic ulcer bleeding. *Scand J Gastroenterol* 1985; **29(suppl 110)**:109–11.
3 Morris DL, Hawker PC, Brearley S. Optimal timing of operation for bleeding peptic ulcer. Prospective randomised trial. *BMJ* 1984;**228**:1277–80.

4 Steffes C, Fromm D. The current diagnosis and management of upper gastrointestinal bleeding. *Adv Surg* 1992;**25**:331–50.

5 Poxon VA, Keighly MRB, Dykes PW, Heppinstall H, Jaderberg M. Comparison of minimal and conventional surgery in patients with bleeding peptic ulcer. A multicentre trial. *Br J Surg* 1991;**78**:1344–5.

6 Rogers PN, Murray WR, Shaw R, Brar S. Surgical management of bleeding gastric ulceration. *Br J Surg* 1988;**75**:16–7.

7 Hunt PS, Korman MG, Hansky J. Bleeding duodenal ulcer. Reduction in mortality with a planned approach. *Br J Surg* 1979;**66**:633–5.

8 Schein M, Gecelter G. APACHE II score in massive upper gastrointestinal haemorrhage from peptic ulcer. Prognostic value and potential clinical application. *Br J Surg* 1989;**76**: 733–6.

9 Miedema BW, Torres PR, Farnell MB, *et al*. Proximal gastric vagotomy in the emergency treatment of bleeding of duodenal ulcers. *Am J Surg* 1991;**161**:64–7.

10 Hoffman J, Olesen A, Jensen JE. Prospective 14–18 year follow-up study after parietal cell vagotomy. *Br J Surg* 1987;**74**:1056–9.

11 Paquet KJ, Feussner H. Endoscopic sclerosis and oesophageal balloon tamponade in acute hemorrhage from esophageal varices. A prospective controlled randomised trial. *Hepatology* 1985;**5**:580–3.

12 Sugiura M, Futagawa S. Result of 636 oesophageal transections with paraoesophagostric devascularisation in the treatment of oesophageal varices. *J Vasc Surg* 1984;**1**:254–60.

13 Willson PD, Kunkler R, Blair SD, Reynolds KW. Emergency oesophageal transection for uncontrolled variceal haemorrhage. *Br J Surg* 1994;**81**:992–5.

14 Spina GP, Santambrogio R, Opocher E, *et al*. Emergency portasystemic shunts in patients with variceal bleeding. *Surg Gynecol Obstet* 1990;**171**:456–63.

15 Orloff MJ, Bell RHJ, Hyde PV, Skivolozki WP. Long term results of emergency portacaval shunts for bleeding esophageal varices in unselected patients with alcoholic cirrhosis. *Am J Surg* 1980;**192**:325–40.

16 Cello JP, Grendell JH, Crass RA, Weber TE, Trunkey DD. Endoscopic sclerotherapy versus portacaval shunts in patients with severe cirrhosis and acute variceal hemorrhage: long term follow-up. *N Engl J Med* 1987;**316**:11–15.

17 Copeland G, Shields R. Portal hypertension and oesophageal varices. *Surgery* 1991; 2342–7.

18 Cameron JL, Zuidema GD, Smith GW, *et al*. Mesocaval shunts for bleeding esophageal varices. *Surgery* 1979;**85**:257–62.

19 Henderson JM. Portal hypertension and shunt surgery. *Adv Surg* 1993;**26**:233–57.

20 Copeland GP, Shields R. Oesophageal varices and portal hypertension; is there a place for the surgeon? In: *Recent advances in surgery*. Edinburgh: Churchill Livingstone, 1992: 39–54.

21 Reyes J, Iwatsuki S. Current management of portal hypertension with liver transplantation. In: *Advances in surgery 1992*. London: Mosby, 1992:189–208.

22 Dudley HAF. Acute bleeding from upper gastrointestinal tract. In J. Wright (ed) *Hamilton Bailey's emergency surgery*. 11th ed. J Wright, 1986:301–11.

11: Variceal bleeding from the oesophagus and stomach

D PATCH AND A K BURROUGHS

Bleeding from oesophageal or gastric varices is a major complication of portal hypertension.

Natural History and Prognosis of Variceal Bleeding

The natural history and prognosis has been well studied by many groups and the following points are well accepted:

- Oesophageal and gastric varices develop in 90% of patients with alcoholic cirrhosis[1]. The same figure probably applies for other aetiologies of cirrhosis.
- In more than half of these patients, varices will enlarge over time[2]
- At least 30% of patients with varices will bleed[3]
- The risk of a first bleed is highest (70%) in the first 2 years after identification of the varices[4,5]
- Mortality from the first variceal bleed is high (25–50%) and is dependent on the severity of liver disease[1,6,7]
- Patients who have already had a variceal bleed have a high risk (70% or more) of recurrent bleeding[8,9]
- Active bleeding on endoscopy (spurting or oozing from varices) carries a poor prognosis[10]
- Early rebleeding within the first few days of hospital admission is a particular feature of variceal haemorrhage,[11,12] and is associated with an increased mortality, as in peptic ulcer bleeding
- Variceal bleeding has substantial resource implications.[13] In the UK it costs the National Health Service £6·1 million to treat 3000 acute variceal bleeding admissions per year.

Variceal bleeding is therefore a major problem with a high mortality that can be reduced only by prompt, effective resuscitation, accurate diagnosis and early treatment. The clinical problem is not only to stop bleeding as soon as possible but also to prevent early re-bleeding. Any treatment regimen should therefore be evaluated not only in terms of immediate cessation of haemorrhage, but also in terms of providing a bleed free interval of 5 days. The time of treatment or randomisation in a trial, relative to the time of admission to the first hospital to which the patient is taken, is an important variable when evaluating efficacy of treatments.[14] Clearly, the longer the time from bleeding to admission, the lower the residual risk of early rebleeding. Identification of those patients likely to rebleed early would prompt earlier, more definitive therapy (e.g. surgical shunting or TIPS).

Presentation and Diagnosis

The patient with bleeding varices can present with a single life threatening haematemesis and cardiovascular collapse, or asymptomatic anaemia.

Patients will usually present with haematemesis or melaena. Specific features to be noted in the history are: prolonged excessive alcohol intake, ingestion of non-steroidal anti-inflammatory drugs or aspirin, previous variceal haemorrhages, previously diagnosed liver disease and portal hypertension, past abdominal sepsis or surgery, or investigation of thrombocytopenia. No specific features of the haemorrhage will indicate that varices have been the source.

Examination after resuscitation must include a search for cutaneous stigmata of chronic liver disease, jaundice, hepatomegaly or splenomegaly or both, hepatic bruits, distended umbilical veins, ascites and encephalopathy. Bleeding caused by portal hypertension may also occur in the absence of specific clinical signs of chronic liver disease. Usually these patients have extrahepatic splanchnic vein thrombosis and other causes of non-cirrhotic portal hypertension.

The examination and initial investigations must include an assessment of the severity of bleeding, the severity of diseases in other systems and the severity of liver disease. The latter is still most reliably assessed by using the Child's score (Table 11.1) which is based on the bilirubin concentration, prothrombin time, albumin concentration, ascites, and the presence of portosystemic encephalopathy. The presence of portal vein thrombosis or hepatoma or both also needs to be established early on.

Upper gastrointestinal endoscopy is essential to establish an accurate diagnosis of bleeding from varices. This may need to be done under general anaesthesia just before emergency laparotomy, when the latter is being performed for exsanguinating haemorrhage. Potentially inappropriate surgery is then avoided, as balloon tamponade may arrest the bleeding.

Of patients with portal hypertension and gastrointestinal bleeding, 26–52% will have a non-variceal source,[15] such as peptic ulcers or portal hypertensive gastropathy, which highlights the need for endoscopy and a precise diagnosis. Endoscopy should be carried out as soon as resuscitation is adequate, and preferably within 6 h of admission.

148

TABLE 11.1—*Child's grading of the severity of liver disease. PBC, primary biliary cirrhosis.*

Clinical and biochemical measurement	Points scored		
	1	2	3
Encephalopathy (grade)	None	1 and 2	3 and 4
Ascites	Absent	Mild	Moderate
Bilirubin μmol/l	<34	34–50	>50
(Bilirubin for PBC)	<68	68–170	>170
Albumin (g/l)	>35	28–35	<28
Prothrombin (s prolonged)	1–4	4–6	>6
	<7	7–9	>9
	Child's A disease	Child's B disease	Child's C disease

Definitive endoscopic diagnosis during or shortly after upper gastrointestinal bleeding can be both difficult and subjective, even in the hands of the most experienced endoscopist. When the view is restricted by haemorrhage, a bleeding point cannot always be identified. The usual finding is of bright red blood around the oesophagogastric junction and, particularly in the case of gastric varices, in the gastric fundus.

A diagnosis of bleeding varices is accepted either when a venous (non-pulsatile) spurt is seen (see Figure 11.1), or there is fresh bleeding from the oesophagogastric junction in the presence of varices. In the absence of active bleeding (as in 50–70% of patients) either the presence of varices in the absence of other lesions, or a "white nipple sign"—a platelet plug on the surface of a varix[16]—suggests varices as the source of haemorrhage (see Figure 11.2).

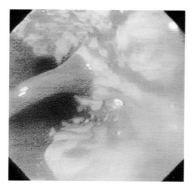

FIGURE 11.1—*A spurting varix: the clinical problem.*

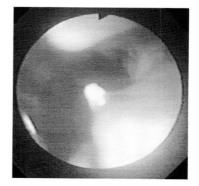

FIGURE 11.2—*A "white nipple" arising from a varix.*

When the diagnosis is in doubt (Figure 11.3), repeat endoscopy during rebleeding will reveal a variceal source in more than 75% of patients[15] and is, therefore, mandatory. Gastric varices are particularly difficult to diagnose, because of pooling of blood in the fundus. Placing the patient on his or her right side with the head up may help. If the diagnosis is still not made, splanchnic angiography will establish the presence of varices, and may display the bleeding site if the patient is actively bleeding (see Figure 11.4).

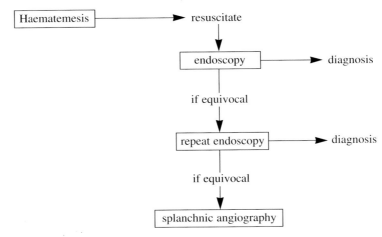

FIGURE 11.3—*Diagnostic algorithm for bleeding varices.*

In a true emergency, where the patient is exsanguinating and varices are suspected on the basis of history and examination, a Sengstaken–Blakemore tube (SBT) should be passed. If control of bleeding is obtained, varices are likely to be the source of haemorrhage. If blood continues to come up the gastric aspiration port, then varices are less likely to be the cause of blood loss (note that fundal varices are not always controlled by tamponade). Whenever this occurs, and the position of the SBT has been checked and adequate traction applied, the diagnosis of variceal bleeding should be questioned, and emergency angiography performed.

Resuscitation

The goals of resuscitation after variceal haemorrhage are to:

- Correct hypovolaemia
- Stop bleeding and prevent early rebleeding
- Prevent complications associated with bleeding
- Prevent deterioration in liver function.

Initial assessment should identify those who are at high risk of dying and require early definitive therapy. Predictive factors for early death are: severity of bleeding;[10] severity of liver disease;[7 12] presence of infection;[17] presence of renal dysfunction;[18 19] presence of cardiorespiratory disease.

The general principles of resuscitation must be followed, with attention to the "ABC" of airway; breathing; circulation. Aspiration of gastric contents

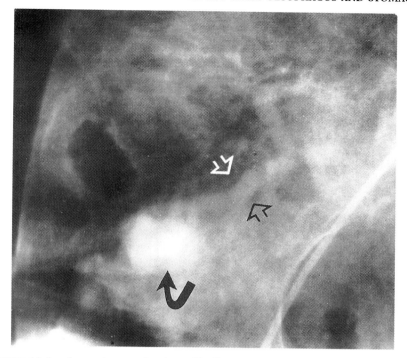

FIGURE 11.4—*An angiogram showing a bleeding ileostomy varix (outline arrows). The filled arrow shows the contrast "blush".*

and blood into the lungs is a particular danger, especially in encephalopathic patients who may have depressed pharyngeal reflexes. This risk is further exacerbated by endoscopic procedures, for which sedation may be required. If there is any concern about the safety of the airway, endotracheal intubation is mandatory.

Access to the circulation should be both peripheral and central. To achieve the latter, an internal jugular line is safer than a subclavian approach, as the carotid artery can be compressed in the case of accidental puncture, whereas the subclavian cannot. The presence of coagulopathy and thrombocytopenia is not a contraindication to central venous access.

Alcohol withdrawal syndromes are not uncommon, and can further complicate assessment of the patient's neurological state. Male patients may in particular become aggressive, removing venous lines and rendering themselves impossible to resuscitate and endoscope. In the acute situation, the endoscopy should either be delayed or the patient intubated and ventilated. If the former path is followed, 30–60 minutes of titrated intravenous chlormethiazole following an initial bolus (of up to 100 mls) may restore the patient to manageable state. It is imperative however that during the infusion these patients have continuous O_2 saturation monitoring, as well as one to one nursing. Chlormethiazole in inexperienced hands is a dangerous drug, with enormous potential for over sedation and aspiration, with no adequate reversal antidote.

Laboratory investigations

Appropriate investigations are listed in Box 11.1. Initial volume replacement should be with human albumin fraction or gelatin based colloid, as compared to dextran or hydroxyethylstarch, as these have no effect on clotting or bleeding times and less effect on platelet function.[20] Specific treatment can then be started with a vasopressor agent, when the clinical picture is suggestive of portal hypertension.

Box 11.1 Laboratory investigations required during resuscitation after variceal haemorrhage

Blood sample for:
- full blood count
- clotting screen
- cross matching (prepare 6 units of blood)
- urea and electrolytes, creatinine, glucose
- liver function tests, calcium (Ca^{2+})
- amylase, magnesium (Mg^{2+})
- blood gas
- blood culture

Ascitic tap
- diagnostic, with a request for an absolute white cell count/mm^3

Midstream urine specimen

Chest radiograph

Electrocardiogram

Meanwhile the patient should be transferred to the intensive care unit or a high dependency bed, and prepared for endoscopy. The surgical and radiological teams should be informed, and a tertiary referral centre contacted, particularly if local expertise is not available.

Cardiorespiratory monitoring

Pulse oximetry and oxygen are essential during endoscopy (see, for example, the guidelines of the British Society of Gastroenterology[21]) and there must be suitable staff to provide suction and ensure airway maintenance.

The haemodynamic consequences of haemorrhage in patients with cirrhosis may differ from those in normal individuals. These patients, particularly when decompensated, will have a reduced peripheral vasoconstrictor response because of: the established vasodilator state of cirrhosis and portal hypertension;[22][23] a disturbed baroreceptor reflex, with an attenuated response to adrenaline;[24] and an autonomic neuropathy, particularly in alcoholics. The presence of covert tissue hypoxia in decompensated cirrhosis[25] emphasises the importance of rapid restoration of circulating blood volume and oxygen-carrying capacity, to prevent critical deterioration of organ function.

None the less, the usual indications for pulmonary capillary wedge pressure measurement apply in bleeding varices: suspicion of abnormal right atrial pressures (when there is finger clubbing suggestive of hepatopulmonary syndrome); the presence of alcoholic ischaemic heart disease; and advanced age. However, it is important not to concentrate on invasive monitoring at the expense of stopping the bleeding—the endoscopy should come before the Swan–Ganz catheter.

Vasoconstrictor therapy (for example, with vasopressin) may reduce cardiac output, and increase right atrial pressure;[26] ascites also increases right atrial pressure measurements[27] and should be taken into account when assessing readings of central venous pressure.

All modes of ventilation may affect the systemic and splanchnic circulation. Positive pressure ventilation (PPV) and positive end expiratory pressure (PEEP) may cause a reduction in mean arterial pressure, cardiac output, portal venous and hepatic arterial blood flow.[28-30] These may be accompanied by deterioration in hepatic function[31], reduced cardiac output[29], and further salt and water retention, which may precipitate ascites formation. These features help to explain why mortality in patients with combined liver and respiratory failure is above 90% in intensive care units worldwide.

Transfusion of blood products

The correct volume of blood product transfusion remains controversial. Following a variceal bleed in animal models, return of arterial pressure to normal by immediate transfusion results in overshoot in portal venous pressure, with associated risk of further bleeding.[32] This effect may not be relevant in clinical practice, when volume replacement is always delayed with respect to the start of bleeding. A study in trauma patients identified a survival benefit for fluid replacement only at the time of laparotomy, perhaps because of the avoidance of clotting factor dilution beforehand.[33] How this finding relates to cirrhotic patients who already have compromised renal function, oxygen uptake and abnormal clotting is difficult to evaluate.

In clinical practice, overtransfusion should be avoided, and it is wise to aim for a haemoglobin concentration of 90–100 g/l, and right atrial pressure of 4–8 mm Hg.

The use of blood products (Box 11.2) also needs care. Large volume transfusion may worsen the haemorrhagic state, as well as causing thrombocytopenia. Many patients with cirrhosis have a tendency to fibrinolysis[34] and transfusion of more than 15 units of blood results in prolongation of the prothrombin and partial thromboplastin time.[35]

Box 11.2 Use of blood products during resuscitation after variceal haemorrhage

Initial colloid to restore volume

Blood products
- platelets if concentration $<50 \times 10^9/l$
- fresh frozen plasma if prothrombin time >20 s
- cryoprecipitate if fibrinogen $<0{\cdot}2$ g/l
- calcium gluconate, 10 ml of 10% solution for every 2 l of blood transfused

If patient is still bleeding, consider
- tranexamic acid, 1 g in 50 ml 5% dextrose, intravenously over 6 h
- desmopressin (DDAVP) $0{\cdot}3$ µg/kg, up to three doses 4 h apart

---

Transfused blood contains low concentrations of 2,3-diphosphoglycerate, with the theoretical risk that it will reduce haemoglobin-to-tissue oxygen transfer. However, there is no evidence that this is clinically significant.[36] With large volume transfusion there is a risk of citrate toxicity, although modern blood supplies contain only low concentrations. Toxicity is manifested by changes in ionized calcium levels and associated effects on the heart (prolonged QT interval, reduced cardiac output, changes in blood coagulation).[37] The associated toxicity may be enhanced by hypothermia, which also potentiates the cardiac side effects of hypocalcaemia, and further increases the affinity of haemoglobin for oxygen.

Massive transfusion has been implicated in the development of pulmonary microembolism,[38] and the use of filters is recommended for transfusions of 5 l or more in normal humans.[39] Routine use of filters in variceal haemorrhage could be considered, but they have the disadvantage of preventing rapid transfusions.

Clotting indices may be improved with fresh frozen plasma (FFP), but bleeding time is not. Often these tests look at single static points in a complex dynamic mechanism, and therefore may not be useful to assess clotting deficiencies. Nonetheless, it is reasonable to give 2 units of FFP after every 4 units of blood, and when the prothrombin time exceeds 20 s. Cryoprecipitate is indicated when the fibrinogen level is less than $0{\cdot}2$ g/l, and has the advantage of not containing fibrinolytic factors.

Platelet transfusions are necessary to improve primary haemostasis, and should be used if the baseline count is $50 \times 10^9/l$ or less, and the patient is bleeding. It is also routine to give intravenous vitamin K to patients with cirrhosis but no more than three doses of 10 mg are required. It is likely to be of little benefit except in patients with biliary-type cirrhosis.

Further measures in patients who continue to bleed despite balloon tamponade include the use of desmopressin (DDAVP)[40] and antifibrinolytic agents (Box 11.2). In stable cirrhotics the former produces a two- to fourfold increase in factor VIII and von Willebrand's factor, presumably by release from storage sites,[41] and may shorten or normalise the bleeding time.[42 43] However, in one study of variceal bleeding DDAVP in association with terlipressin was shown to be detrimental compared to terlipressin alone, and therefore its use can only be recommended when all else has failed.[44]

The use of antifibrinolytics in variceal bleeding has not been studied, although their role has been established in liver transplantation.[45 46] These agents are best used as a bridge between balloon tamponade and transjugular intrahepatic portosystemic stent (TIPS) shunting or before open surgery, when bleeding continues and preferably when increased fibrinolysis has been documented.

Prevention of Complications and Deterioration in Liver Function

Infection control and treatment

Sepsis is an important complication in patients with cirrhosis,[18 47] particularly during bleeding episodes; aspiration is then a major risk and there may be increased translocation of gut organisms.[48] Cirrhotic patients normally have defects of both humoral and cellular host defence mechanisms,[49–51] added to which is the well recognised suppression of the immune system after simple haemorrhage,[52] via impaired T lymphocyte[52] B lymphocyte[53] and macrophage[54] function. Because many of these host defences are humorally mediated, their function is further reduced by depletion in serum factors after haemorrhage and transfusion.

Sclerotherapy is associated with bacteraemia[55 56] but this does not appear to be clinically relevant. Nonetheless, even when bleeding has stopped following emergency TIPS therapy, mortality may remain at 50% because of infection.[57]

Oral selective decontamination prevents Gram negative injections after sclerotherapy[58] and gastrointestinal haemorrhage[59] but seems of little value as it takes days to decontaminate the intestine. Decontamination is not suitable for prophylaxis and it may cause the selective proliferation of resistant microorganisms. Such treatment cannot be used at the time of variceal haemorrhage, nor does it prevent infections of extradigestive or endoscopic origin.

In a study of the use of systemic antibiotics, Blaire et al.[60] recorded a significantly lower incidence of bacterial infection in 46 cirrhotic patients with gastrointestinal haemorrhage and treated with systemic orfloxacillin, compared with controls. There was a non-significant reduction in mortality. Amoxycillin with clavulanic acid was also given before endoscopy as part of the systemic antibacterial regimen. A larger prospective randomised trial, with cost analysis built in, is required. Our practice is to screen all patients for sepsis with blood, urine and ascitic cultures, plus chest radiographs. If there is a suspicion of infection (pyrexia, neutrophilia, a possible episode of aspiration), broad spectrum systemic antibiotics are used—metronidazole with third generation cephalosporin. (There is currently concern regarding possible hepatotoxic effects of amoxycillin with clavulanic acid in patients with cirrhosis.)

Spontaneous bacterial peritonitis (SBP) must be suspected in any cirrhotic patient with ascites throughout a hospital stay. Symptoms may be absent or include fever and the onset or worsening of encephalopathy or abdominal pain or both. Deterioration in renal or liver function may also herald SBP. The diagnosis is confirmed by the presence of 250 or more mononuclear cells/mm^3 on diagnostic paracentesis, or more than 500 leucocytes/mm^3.[61 62] Ascitic fluid should also be sent for culture in aerobic and anaerobic media. The antibiotic of first choice should be a third-generation cephalosporin.[63] Other agents may need to be considered depending on the clinical picture; for example, a patient who has had an indwelling percutaneous drain for ascites is likely to be colonised with Staphylococci. A high ascitic lymphocyte count should alert the clinician to the possibility of TB, a condition that appears to be increasing.

Ascites and renal management

Renal failure may be precipitated by a variceal bleed, not only because of acute tubular necrosis, but also because of the hepatorenal syndrome (HRS), which is associated with deterioration in liver function and sepsis. HRS is associated with a mortality in excess of 95%,[64] as it reflects end stage liver disease. Any iatrogenic precipitants must therefore be avoided. The intravascular volume should be maintained, initially with human albumin solution or blood. Dextrose solution is used for maintenance fluid. Catheterisation and hourly measurement of urine output is mandatory and nephrotoxic drugs should be avoided, especially aminoglycosides and non-steroidal anti-inflammatory drugs. Dopamine infusion at a renal dose (2·5 µg/kg/min) has not been shown to improve survival in clinical trials, and may actually increase gut translocation of bacterial products.[65] In the first randomised controlled trial of low dose dopamine in critically ill patients, there was no change in renal function, but a non-significant increase in cardiac death in the treatment group.[66] The use of dopamine can be recommended only when the urine output falls in the presence of satisfactory filling, and should be stopped after 24 h if no benefit is seen.

Increasing ascites may occur during the acute stage of variceal haemorrhage, but should not be the main focus of fluid and electrolyte management until bleeding has stopped and the intravascular volume is stable. If there is a rising urea and creatinine, all diuretics should be stopped, and paracentesis performed if the abdomen becomes uncomfortable; 100 ml salt poor (20%) albumin should be given for every 2 l of fluid removed. Physiological saline should be avoided as it may cause further ascites formation.

When the patient has not bled for 24 h, nasogastric feeding can be commenced with a low sodium feed. This avoids the need for maintenance fluid, removes the risk of line sepsis, as well as providing much needed nutrition.

An unexplained rise in creatinine and urea may indicate sepsis, and is an indication for antibiotic treatment.

Portosystemic encephalopathy

Factors likely to precipitate portosystemic encephalopathy include:

- Haemorrhage;
- Sepsis;
- Sedative drugs;
- Constipation;
- Dehydration;
- Electrolyte imbalance.

Hypokalaemia, hypomagnesaemia and hypoglycaemia may precipitate encephalopathy and should be aggressively corrected; for example, a patient with ascites and a serum potassium of 3·0 mmol/l is likely to require in excess of 100 mmol over 24 h.

All the above factors must be addressed in the patient with cirrhosis and variceal bleeding. As soon as the patient is taking oral fluid, lactulose 5 ml four times daily can be started. Phosphate enemas are also useful.

Nutrition

Few cirrhotics are not malnourished,[67] particularly when decompensated.[68] Most hospital diets provide a maximum of 1500 kilocalories per day, and patients with liver disease have substantially greater requirements.[69] These patients often do not want to eat, are on a "nil by mouth" regimen because of investigations, and the food itself is often unappealing. Exacerbation of malnutrition while in hospital is therefore a substantial risk.

A fine bore nasogastric feeding tube can be passed 24 h after cessation of bleeding and feeding started. Although such a tube may cause oesophageal erosion, there is no evidence that it will precipitate a variceal bleed; it allows treatment of encephalopathy in comatose patients, and makes fluid management easier. Furthermore, if liver transplantation is being considered the additional nutrition helps to get the patient in as good as condition as is possible before the operation and fluid management is simplified.[70] It is extremely rare that parenteral nutrition is required. Nutritional therapy in liver disease remains one of the most overlooked, yet one of the most important aspects of the patient's management.

Vitamin replacement

All patients with a significant history of alcohol abuse should be assumed to be folate[71 72] and thiamine[71 73] deficient, and be given at least three doses of the latter intravenously. It is easier and more practical to assume all such patients to be vitamin deficient rather than to delay treatment while awaiting a report on red cell transketolase activity.

Liver transplantation and failed sclerotherapy

Liver transplantation is discussed as a surgical option in Chapter 3. No patient, unless biologically very elderly or with concomitant diseases, should be allowed to die of liver failure without discussion with a transplant unit, even if he or she has alcoholic liver disease and is still actively drinking.

Excessive sclerotherapy is liable to cause mediastinal and oesophageal ulceration, which may complicate the post-transplant course. Thus rather than repeated emergency sclerotherapy in patients who continue to bleed, one should consider early referral for alternative treatment (such as TIPS). For example, if two sclerotherapy sessions fail to arrest bleeding, a TIPS procedure might be an appropriate alternative.

Transfer of the Patient with Bleeding Varices

A patient should not be transported to another hospital unless his or her bleeding has been controlled, either with vasopressor agents or tamponade, for 6 h. If there is any suggestion of continued blood loss, and the source is known to be variceal, then a modified Sengstaken tube with an oesophageal aspiration channel must be inserted before transfer, otherwise the risk of aspiration or hypovolaemia, particularly in the uncontrolled environment of an ambulance, is excessive.

The Sengstaken–Blakemore tube will arrest bleeding in 90% of cases.[74] Prior endotracheal intubation is necessary when there is any concern about the patient's airway; this is particularly important when the Sengstaken–Blakemore tube is being put down before transfer of the patient. Figure 11.5 shows a "Sengstaken box".

Use of balloon tamponade to control bleeding

If balloon tamponade seems to be necessary to arrest oesophageal variceal bleeding, the following procedure should be followed:

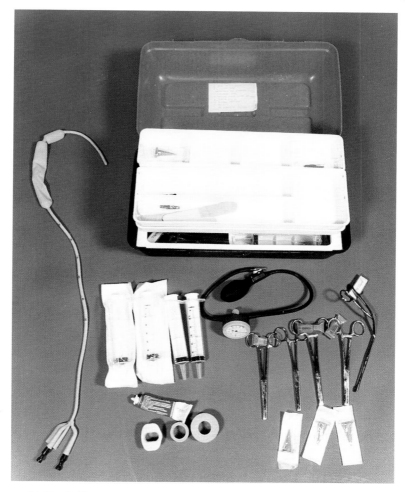

FIGURE 11.5—*A "Sengstaken box" containing a tube and manometer, and other relevant equipment, e.g. clamps, mouth pieces, KY jelly.*

1) *Prepare the area.* Ensure that good suction facilities, an oxygen saturation monitor, and oxygen supplies are all working. Two tamponade tubes should be placed in the freezer section of a fridge for at least 15 min. Three heavy duty non-serrated tubing clamps and three 60 ml bladder catheter syringes must be to hand. A modified sphygmomanometer is required to check the inflation pressure of the oesophageal balloon.

2) *Prepare the staff.* Three assistants are required, one of whom must be responsible for airway protection and suction. A gown, goggles, and gloves should be worn.

3) *Prepare the patient.* The patient is often frightened. A simple, quiet explanation, with reassurance, will help to avoid struggling. Explain that he or she must try to swallow, and that the airway will not be obstructed.

4) The patient should lie head down, in the left lateral position, with an endoscopy mouth guard and nasal oxygen prongs in place.

The assistant at the head end provides suction and maintains the airway, while keeping the mouth guard in position.

When all is ready, remove the Sengstaken–Blakemore tube from the fridge, and check balloon patency. Fully deflate both balloons, and lubricate them generously with KY jelly. Without delay, insert the tube, twisting the shaft through 180° once the balloon has passed the oropharynx; this directs the tip posteriorly towards the oesophagus. Ask the patient to swallow. If he or she gags, this is the time to advance the tube as the sphincter relaxes. Occasionally it is necessary to guide the tube into the oesophagus with the fingers—the mouth guard prevents them from being bitten.

Push the tube down at least 60 cm, and check that it is not coiled in the pharynx. Then inflate the gastric balloon with at least 250 ml of air. If inflation is difficult or the patient is in pain, deflate the balloon immediately and check that the tube is in the stomach.

Once the gastric balloon is inflated, pull the tube back until firm resistance is encountered—usually 30–40 cm depending on the patient's build. Inflate the oesophageal balloon to a pressure of 40 mm Hg.

Tape the tube securely to the side of the patient's face. Check the position of the balloons with a chest radiograph, and then organise definitive therapy.

Potential problems with this procedure and the nursing care required are listed in Box 11.3.

Box 11.3 Controlling variceal bleeding with a Sengstaken–Blakemore tube

Problems

- The tube will not go down: get another cold tube, as the original one has probably become floppy. If problems persist, get senior help
- Continued bleeding: this indicates either gastric varices, or a non-variceal source. Put the tube on traction with a 500 ml bag of saline. If bleeding continues, angiography is required.

Nursing care

- Hourly oesophageal pressure check
- Change position of tube in mouth every 6 h
- Regular oesophageal and stomach aspiration (every 15 min)
- Calming environment

Summary

All variceal bleeding episodes that do not respond to a single session of sclerotherapy should be discussed with the regional tertiary centre because of the high risk of death and the availability at the specialist centre of treatments such as TIPS and liver transplantation.

There is no evidence that vasopressor therapy for variceal bleeding improves hospital mortality, apart from two small trials of terlipressin versus placebo.[75][76] Emergency sclerotherapy does improve survival, but the mortality of variceal bleeding remains high, reflecting the importance of resuscitation and preventive measures that may specifically reduce deterioration in liver and renal function.

Key points

- Bleeding from oesophageal or gastric varices is a major complication of portal hypertension. Mortality is high and resource implications substantial

- If endoscopy fails to clarify the diagnosis, splanchnic angiography will demonstrate varices

- When the patient is exsanguinating and varices are suspected, balloon tamponade with a Sengstaken–Blakemore tube stops bleeding in 90% of cases

- An important aim of resuscitation after variceal haemorrhage is to prevent deterioration in liver and renal function

- Sepsis, renal failure and portosystemic encephalopathy may complicate bleeding episodes in patients with cirrhosis

- Many patients with cirrhosis are malnourished and benefit from nasogastric tube feeding

- Variceal bleeding must be controlled before a patient is transferred to another hospital

References

1 Christensen E, Faverhold L, Schlicthing P, et al. Aspects of the natural history of GI bleeding or coma in cirrhosis. Gastroenterology 1981;81:944–52.

2 Cales P, Desmorat H, Tinel JP, et al. Incidence of large oesophageal varices in patients with cirrhosis; application to prophylaxis of first bleeding. Gut 1990;31:1298–1302.

3 Baker LA, Smith C, Lieberman G. The natural history of oesophageal varices. Am J Med 1950;26:228–37.

4 Conn HO, Lindenmuth WW, May CJ, et al. Prophylactic portocaval anastomosis. A tale of two studies. Medicine 1972;51:27–40.

5 Resnick RH, Chairies TC, Ishihara AM, et al. A controlled study of the prophylactic portocaval shunt. A final report. Ann Intern Med 1969;70:675–88.

6 Pascal JP, Cals P, and the multicentre study group. Propranolol in the prevention of first upper GIT haemorrhage in patients with cirrhosis of the liver and oesophageal varices. N Eng J Med 1987;317:856–61.

7 Graham DY, Smith JL. The course of patients after variceal haemorrhage. Gastroenterology 1981;80:800–9.

8 Jackson FC, Perrin EB, Felix R, Smith AG. A clinical investigation of the portocaval shunt v survival analysis of the therapeutic operation. *Ann Surg* 1971;**174**:672–700.

9 Reynolds TB, Donovan AJ, Mikkelsen WP, *et al*. Results of a 12 year randomized trial of portocaval shunt in patients with alcoholic liver disease and bleeding varices. *Gastroenterology* 1981;**80**:1005–11.

10 Cardin F, Gori G, McCormick PA, Burroughs AK. A predictive model for very early rebleeding from varices [abstract]. *Gut* 1990;**31**:A1204.

11 Smith JL, Graham DY. Variceal haemorrhage, a critical evolution of survival analysis. *Gastroenterology* 1982;**82**:968–72.

12 Dedombal FT, Clarke JR, Clamp SE, Mallzia G, Kohval MR, Morgan AG. Prognostic factors in upper GI bleeding. *Endoscopy* 1986;**18(suppl)**:6–10.

13 McCormick PA, Greenslade L, Matheson L, Matsafaris M, Bosanquet N, Burroughs AK (1994). Vasoconstrictors in the management of bleeding from oesophageal varices: A clinico–economic appraisal in the UK. *Scand J Gastroenterol* 1995;**30**:377–83.

14 Burroughs AK, Mezzanotte G, Phillips A, *et al*. Cirrhotics with variceal haemorhage. The importance of the time interval between admission and the start of analysis for survival and rebleeding rates. *Hepatology* 1989;**9**:801–7.

15 Mitchell K, Theodossi A, Williams R. Endoscopy in patients with portal hypertension and upper gastrointestinal bleeding. In: Westaby D, MacDougall BRD, William R, eds. *Variceal bleeding*. London: Pitman, 1982:62–7.

16 Siringo S, McCormick PA, Mistry P, Kaye G, McIntyre N, Burroughs AK. Prognostic significance of the white nipple sign in variceal bleeding. *Gastrointest Endosc* 1991;**37**:51–5.

17 Bleichner G, Boulanger R, Squara P, *et al*. Frequency of infections in cirrhotic patients presenting with acute gastrointestinal haemorrhage, *Br J Surg* 1986;**73**:724–6.

18 Christensen E, Kreitel JJ, Meltofe Hansen S, Johansen J, *et al*. Prognosis after the first episode of gastrointestinal bleeding or coma in cirrhosis. *Scand J Gast* 1984;**24**:999–1006.

19 Garden OJ, Motyl H, Gilmour WH, *et al*. Prediction of outcome following acute variceal haemorrhage. *Br J Surg* 1985;**72**:91–5.

20 Tschirren B, Ajjoller U, Elsasser R, *et al*. Dukluische Plasmaersak mit gelatine. Zwolf jahre erjahrangen Mit 39320 Einheiten Physiogel. *Infusionstherapie* 1974;**1**:651–62.

21 BSG Guidelines. Recommendations for standards of sedation and patient monitoring during gastrointestinal endoscopy. *Gut* 1991;**32**:823–7.

22 Borizon A, Blendis L. Vascular reactivity in experimental portal hypertension. *Am J Physiol* 1987;**252**:G158–62.

23 Lunzer M, Manghani K, Newman S, *et al*. Impaired cardiovascular responsiveness in liver disease. *Lancet* 1975;**2**:382–5.

24 Moreau R, Rouleot D, Braille A, *et al*. Low dose nitroglycerin failed to improve splanchnic haemodynamics in patients with cirrhosis: evidence for an impaired cardiorespiratory baroreflex function. *Hepatology* 1989;**10**:93–7.

25 Moreau R, Lee S, Hadengue A, *et al*. Relationship between oxygen transplant and oxygen uptake in patients with cirrhosis: effect of vasoactive drugs. *Hepatology* 1989;**9**:427–32.

26 Groszman R, Kravetz D, Bosch, *et al*. Nitroglycerine improves the haemodynamic response to vasopressin in portal hypertension. *Hepatology* 1982;**2**:757–62.

27 Panos M, Moore K, Vlavlanios P, *et al*. Sequential haemodynamic changes during single total paracentesis and right atrial size in patients with tense ascites. *Hepatology* 1991;**11**:662–7.

28 Mauay J, Jashie R, Hechtrain H. Abnormalities in organ blood flow and its distribution during end expiratory pressure. *Surgery* 1979;**85**:425–32.

29 Hemmer M, Suter P. Treatment of cardiac and renal effects of PEEP with dopamine in acute respiratory failure. *Anesthesiology* 1979;**50**:399–403.

30 Aruidsson D, Lindgen S, Almquise P, *et al*. Role of the renin angiotensin system in liver blood flow reduction produced by positive and expiratory pressure ventilation. *Acta Chir Scand* 1990;**156**:353–8.

31 Johnson E, Hedley-Whyte H, Hull S. End expiratory pressures ventilation and sulphobromophthalein Na excretion in dogs. *J Appl Physiol* 1977;**45**:714–20.

32 Kravetz D, Bosch J, Ardesui M, *et al*. Haemodynamic effects of blood volume resuscitation following haemorrhage in rats with portal hypertension due to cirrhosis of the liver. Influence of the extent of portal systemic shunting. *Hepatology* 1989;**9**:808–14.

33 Bickell W, Wall M, Mattox K, *et al*. Immediate versus delayed fluid resuscitation for hypotensive patients with penetrating torso injuries. *N Engl J Med* 1994;**331**:1105–9.

34 Goodpasture EW. Fibrinolysis in chronic hepatic insufficiency. *Bulletin of Johns Hopkins Hospital* 1914;**25**:330–6.

35 Bove J. What is the factual basis, in theory and in practice, for the use of fresh frozen plasma? *Vox Sang* 1978;**35**:428.

36 Collins J. Abnormal haemoglobin–oxygen affinity and surgical haemotherapy. In: Collins J, Lumsgaard-Hansen P, eds. *Surgical haemotherapy*. Basel: Skager, 1980.

37 Bunker J, Stebas J, Coe R, *et al.* Citric acid intoxication. *JAMA* 1955;**157**:1361.

38 Solis R, Walker B. Does a relationship exist between massive blood transfusion and the adult respiratory distress syndrome. *Vox Sang* 1977;**32**:319.

39 Reul G, Beale A, Greenberg S. Protection of the pulmonary vasculature by fine screen blood filtration. *Chest* 1974;**44**:6.

40 Cattaneo N, Tenconi P, Albera I, Garcia V, Mannucci P. Subcutaneous desmopressin shortened the prolonged bleeding time in patients with liver cirrhosis. *Thromb Haemost* 1990;**64**:358–60.

41 Mannucci PM, Canciani MT, Rota L, Donovan BS. Response of factor VIII and von Willebrand's factor to DDAVP in healthy subjects and patients with haemophilia A and von Willebrand's disease. *Br J Haematol* 981;**47**:283–93.

42 Burroughs AK, Matthews K, Quadira M, *et al.* Desmopressin and bleeding time in patients with cirrhosis. *BMJ* 1985;**291**:1377–81.

43 Mannucci PM, Vicentre V, Vianello L, *et al.* Controlled trial of desmopressin in liver cirrhosis and other conditions associated with a prolonged bleeding time. *Blood* 1986;**67**: 1148–53.

44 De Franchis R, Arcidiacono PG, Andreoni B, Cestari L, Brunati S and the new Italian Endoscopic Club. Terlipressin plus desmopressin versus terlipressin alone in acute variceal haemorrhage in cirrhotics: Interim analysis of a double-blind multicenter randomized controlled trial [abstract]. *Gastroenterology* 1992;**102**:A799.

45 Smith O, Hazlehurst G, Brozovic B, *et al.* Impact of aprotonin on blood transfusions requirements in liver transplantation. *Transfusion Med* 1993;**81**:97–102.

46 Grosse H, Lobbes W, Von Broem O, Barthels M. The use of high dose aprotonin in liver transplantation; the influence on fibrinolysis and blood loss. *Thromb Res* 1991;**63**:287–97.

47 Beroff E, Grebourg T, Seriant J, Macand D, Boureille J. Epidemiology of infections in cirrhotic patients. A prospective study about 121 patients (in French). *Gastroenterol Clin Biol* 1985;**9**:10A.

48 Deitsch E, Bridges W, Baker J, *et al.* Haemorrhagic shock induced bacterial translocation is reduced by xanthine oxidase inhibition or inactivation. *Surgery* 1988;**104**:191–8.

49 Rajkovic I, Williams R. Mechanisms of abnormality in host defences against bacterial infection in liver disease. *Clin Sci* 1985;**68**:247–53.

50 Wyke R. Bacterial infections complicating liver disease. *Clin Gastroenterol* 1989;**3**:187–210.

51 Gomez F, Ruiz P, Schreiber A. Impaired function of macrophage Fcγ receptors and bacterial infection in alcoholic cirrhosis. *N Engl J Med* 1994;**331**:1122–8.

52 Stephan R, Kupper T, Geha A, *et al.* Haemorrhage without tissue trauma produces immunosuppression and enhances susceptibility to sepsis. *Surgery* 1987;**122**:62–8.

53 Stephan R, Conrad P, Janeway C, *et al.* Decreased interleukin-2 production following simple haemorrhage. *Surg Forum* 1986;**37**:73–5.

54 Ayala A, Perrin M, Chaudry I. Defective macrophage antigen presentation following haemorrhage is associated with loss of MHC class II (Ia) antigens. *Immunology* 1990;**70**: 33–9.

55 Chamara DS, Gruberg M, Barde CH, *et al.* Transient bacteria following endoscopic injection sclerotherapy of oesophageal varices. *Arch Intern Med* 1983;**143**:1350–2.

56 Cohen LB, Kaslen MA, Schol EJ, Belez ME, Fisse RD, Arons EJ. Bacteria after injection sclerosis. *Gastrointest Endosc* 1983;**29**:198–200.

57 McCormick PA, Dick R, Panagou EG, *et al.* Emergency TIPS as salvage treatment for uncontrolled variceal bleeding. *Br J Surg* 1994;**81**:1324–7.

58 Kaulhold A, Behrend W, Krausss T, Van Saene H. Selective decontamination of the digestive tract and methylene-resistant *Staphylococcus aureus*. *Lancet* 1992;**339**:1411–2.

59 Rimola A, Bory F, Teres H, Perez-Auso RM, Arroyot, Rhodes J. Oral non-absorbing antibiotics prevent infection in cirrhotics with gastrointestinal haemorrhage. *Hepatology* 1985;**5**:463–7.

60 Blaire M, Patterson D, Tranchet J, Leuachet S, Beauerand M, Purriat J. Systemic antibiotic therapy prevents bacterial infection in cirrhotic patients with gastrointestinal haemorrhage. *Hepatology* 1994;**20**:134–8.

61 Reynolds TB. Rapid presumptive diagnosis of spontaneous bacterial peritonitis. *Gastroenterology* 1986;**70**:455–7.

62 Hoefs JC, Canawati HN, Sapico FL, *et al*. Spontaneous bacterial peritonitis. *Hepatology* 1982;**2**:399–407.

63 Felisart J, Rimola A, Arroyo V, *et al*. Cefotaxime is more effective than ampicillin-tobramycin in cirrhotics with severe infections. *Hepatology* 1986;**5**:457–62.

64 Llach J, Gines P, Arroyo V, *et al*. Progostic value of arterial pressure, endogenous vasoactive systems and renal function in cirrhosis with ascites. *Gastroenterology* 1988;**94**:482–7.

65 Segal J, Phang P, Walley K. Low dose dopamine hastens the onset of gut ischaemia in a porcine model of haemorrhagic shock. *J Appl Physiol* 1992;**73**:1159–64.

66 Baldwin L, Henderson A, Hickman P. Effect of post operative low-dose dopamine on renal function after elective major vascular surgery. *Ann Intern Med* 1994;**120**:744–7.

67 Loguercio C, Sava E, Mermo R, *et al*. Malnutrition in cirrhotic patients: Anthropometric measurements as a method of assesing nutritional status. *Br J Clin Practice* 1990;**44**: 98–101.

68 Shronts EP. Nutritional assessment of adults with end stage hepatic failure. *Nutr Clin Pract* 1988;**3**:113–9.

69 Levin JA, Stanger LC, Morgan MY. Resting and post-prandial energy expenditure and fuel utilisation in patients with cirrhosis. *Hepatology* in press.

70 McCullough AJ, Tavill AS. Disordered energy and protein metabolism in liver disease. *Semin Liver Dis* 1991:305–14.

71 Leevey CM, Becker H, Tentlove W, *et al*. B-complex vitamins in liver disease of the alcoholic. *Am J Clin Nutr* 1965;**16**:339–46.

72 Wu A, Chanarin I, Levi A. Macrocytosis of chronic alcoholism. *Lancet* 1974;**2**:829–31.

73 Camilo ME, Morgan MY, Sherlock S. Red blood cell transketolase activity in alcoholic liver disease. *Scand J Gastroenterol* 1981;**16**:273–9.

74 Panes J, Teres J, Bosch J, Rhodes J. Efficacy of balloon tamponade in treatment of bleeding gastric and oesophageal varices. Results in 151 consecutive episodes. *Dig Dis Sci* 1988; **33**:454–9.

75 Freeman JG, Cobden I, Record CO. Placebo controlled trial of terlipressin (Glypressin) in the management of acute variceal bleeding. *J Clin Gastroenterol* 1989;**11**:58–60.

76 Soderlund C, Magnusson I, Torngren S, *et al*. Terlipressin (triglycyl-lysine vasopressin) controls acute bleeding oesophageal varices. A double blind randomised placebo-controlled trial. *Scand J Gastroenterol* 1990;**25**:622–30.

12: Endoscopic control of upper gastrointestinal variceal bleeding

A E S GIMSON

Haemorrhage from gastro-oesophageal varices continues to be a significant management problem despite advances in our knowledge concerning the relative roles of pharmacological and endoscopic therapy. Risk of rebleeding is related to both the severity of the liver disease (Child's grade) and portal pressure. In this chapter we shall assess the role of endoscopic therapies in the treatment of variceal haemorrhage and its primary and secondary prevention, and compare their efficacy with that of pharmacological or surgical approaches.

Prophylactic endoscopic therapy

The prophylactic use of injection sclerotherapy in both selected and unselected patients with oesophageal varices is of no proven benefit. Although a recent meta-analysis of 14 randomised trials suggested that sclerotherapy reduced the odds ratio of death to 74% (95% confidence intervals 0·60–0·93) there was significant heterogeneity in the results.[1] Pooled results with the sclerosant polidocanol were apparently significantly better than those obtained with other sclerosants. Despite these provocative results, there is no firm place for prophylactic sclerotherapy until further large trials have confirmed its value, and identified those individuals most likely to benefit.

Initial resuscitation of acute variceal haemorrhage

Irrespective of the mode of therapy to be undertaken the initial resuscitation of the patient after varix haemorrhage is of crucial importance, and discussed in detail in Chapter 11.

Endoscopic diagnosis

Upper gastrointestinal haemorrhage demands early endoscopy to confirm the diagnosis, by direct visualisation of either the bleeding site or an adherent fibrin plug. Delayed endoscopy makes it more difficult to identify the bleeding source, as up to 60% of cases stop bleeding spontaneously. Other mucosal lesions must be looked for, although in some cases it is difficult to conclude whether portal hypertensive gastropathy or varices were the source of the haemorrhage. It is also important to distinguish between bleeding from gastric and oesophageal varices as their management differs, particularly when haemorrhage is from gastric fundal varices.

Endoscopic management of active variceal haemorrhage

In most centres the initial control of oesophageal varix haemorrhage, after resuscitation, is with endoscopic techniques. The two main techniques for treating oesophageal varices have been injection sclerotherapy, using standard sclerosants, and variceal banding ligation. Injection therapy using tissue adhesives or thrombin has been predominantly used for gastric varices.

Endoscopic injection sclerotherapy (EIS)

Initially performed using a rigid oesophagoscope, endoscopic injection sclerotherapy (EIS) is now carried out with a flexible-end or oblique-viewing endoscope. In the UK ethanolamine is the most common sclerosant, but polidocanol, sodium morrhuate and absolute alcohol have all been used successfully. Injections are either intravariceal (1–5 ml per varix) or paravariceal (up to 1·5 ml per injection) starting at, or just above, the gastro-oesophageal junction. Some groups have favoured using an over-tube to isolate each varix to be injected,[23] or balloons incorporated on to the endoscope or inserted down dual-channel endoscopes to tamponade the varices,[4] but such variations have not been universally accepted. Use of the cytoprotectant sucralfate is recommended, as it may be associated with less variceal rebleeding from oesophageal ulcers.[5]

Trials have shown that emergency injection sclerotherapy is more often successful than balloon tamponade in achieving haemostasis.[6] Comparisons of EIS with surgical intervention, usually oesophageal transection, have shown lower early rebleeding rates with the more invasive techniques, but hospital mortality in such studies has not been affected.[7] Comparisons between EIS and pharmacological therapy (vasopressin, nitroglycerine, somatostatin analogue) have demonstrated that both approaches are highly effective in achieving haemostasis. Although Westaby et al.[8] achieved initial haemostasis in 88% using EIS and only 65% (p<0·05) with vasopressin and nitroglycerine, two more recent studies have found both modalities

166

equally effective, sclerotherapy achieving haemostasis in 90% and 83%, compared with 84% and 80% with pharmacological therapy.[9 10]

No one form of therapy is conclusively superior,[11] each having disadvantages. EIS requires endoscopic expertise and carries a higher complication rate than somatostatin,[9 11] whereas pharmacological therapy has the disadvantage that, if it fails, control of variceal haemorrhage with EIS becomes less effective.[8] Shemesh *et al.* demonstrated that early emergency sclerotherapy was associated with a lower in-hospital rebleeding rate (5%) than with pharmacological therapy.[12] In many centres a combined approach is favoured with initial somatostatin analogue therapy until emergency endoscopic therapy can be arranged. Pharmacological therapy can be continued for 2–5 days to prevent early rebleeding, by modifying spontaneous changes in splanchnic haemodynamics.[13]

A major problem of injection sclerotherapy has been a high complication rate in many series, including oesophageal stricture, perforation and, more commonly, sclerotherapy-induced mucosal ulceration in up to 30%.[5] Furthermore, rebleeding from such ulcers may occur in 10% of cases and such complications are more common after emergency sclerotherapy. In addition, four to six sessions of EIS may be required to eradicate all a patient's varices.

Endoscopic variceal banding ligation

Endoscopic variceal banding ligation (EVL) was introduced by van Steigmann as a means to avoid the high frequency of mucosal injury after injection sclerotherapy. The technique requires an end-viewing endoscope, a 30 cm outer sheath, and a hood attached to the endoscope tip. Prestretched elastic bands are rolled off an inner ring by pulling a trip wire up the instrument channel, to effect strangulation of a varix that has been sucked up into the outer hood. Bands are applied to varices at or just below the gastro-oesophageal junction and banding continued up the oesophagus for about 5 cm. Four to eight bands are usually required during active variceal haemorrhage, when haemostasis may be achieved either by direct ligation of the bleeding source or oesophageal spasm.

Early uncontrolled series reported primary haemostasis in 90–96% of patients, including those in whom injection sclerotherapy had failed. Three randomised controlled trials have compared EVL with injection sclerotherapy; the new technique is as effective as sclerotherapy, achieving initial haemostasis in 85–90% of cases.[14–16] These trials have also shown that EVL may have a significant advantage over sclerotherapy, in that it obliterates varices sooner and thereby reduces the rebleeding rate. In one trial EVL obliterated varices after a mean of only three sessions compared with the five needed with EIS.[15] More rapid obliteration of varices is the most likely reason for the lower rebleeding rate with EVL. Complication rates, including perforation, stricture formation, deep oesophageal ulceration and sepsis, are low[17 18] with EVL, although not all trials have found them to be significantly lower than with sclerotherapy.[15] Nevertheless despite these apparent advantages of band ligation over sclerotherapy, mortality was reduced only in van Steigmann's original trial and not in subsequent studies.

Overview of management

In clinical practice the management of acute variceal haemorrhage (Figure 12.1) depends on available expertise. If an appropriately experienced endoscopist is not available, initial therapy should be with a somatostatin analogue bolus and infusion, followed by transfer to a centre where long term management and measures for secondary prevention of variceal haemorrhage can be arranged. Where endoscopic procedures are

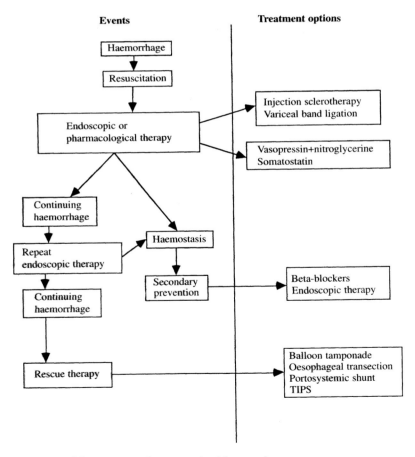

FIGURE 12.1—*Management of acute variceal haemorrhage.*

available, sclerotherapy and banding ligation are equally effective in halting the initial haemorrhage. In those 10–20% of cases who continue to bleed, or have a rebleed within 48 h, endoscopic therapy can be repeated once more but after that becomes increasingly less effective.[7 8] In these circumstances rescue therapy includes surgical procedures such as portacaval shunts (mesocaval or distal splenorenal) and oesophageal transection with or without devascularisation. The preferred option will depend on the available surgical expertise. The transjugular intrahepatic portosystemic stent (TIPS) shunt is a new technique that has generated much interest. There are no controlled trials demonstrating its improved efficacy compared with other techniques, but TIPS is associated with a low rebleeding rate.[19] Its use should be reserved for salvage therapy of continuing variceal rebleeding, in those centres with appropriate radiological expertise.

Secondary prevention of variceal haemorrhage

Initial haemostasis must be followed by secondary prevention of variceal haemorrhage. Meta-analyses have clearly demonstrated that long term endoscopic injection sclerotherapy is of benefit compared to no therapy, with a reduction in both variceal rebleeding rates and mortality irrespective of Child's grade.[20] In three recent trials comparing sclerotherapy with variceal banding ligation, the latter has been associated with a lower rebleeding rate, that presumably is related to a more rapid obliteration of varices. Early evidence therefore suggests that variceal banding ligation may become the preferred endoscopic technique for secondary prevention of variceal rebleeding.

The aim of all such therapy has been to achieve variceal obliteration, with regular review for varix recurrence, and thereby reduce rebleeding rates and mortality. Such an intensive regimen of endoscopic surveillance may not be necessary, as recent trials have suggested that similar rebleeding and mortality rates may be achieved with endoscopic therapy at the time of haemorrhage only.[21 22]

Endoscopic therapy is also at least as effective as secondary prevention with beta-blockade. In comparative trials no significant survival benefit has consistently accrued to either form of therapy, although endoscopic therapy has a higher complication rate.[23] Combination of beta-blockade with endoscopic therapy to reduce the high rate of variceal rebleeding before variceal obliteration was previously discounted,[24] but merits further consideration on the basis of a study showing a 50% reduction in rebleeding rates.[25] A meta-analysis of trials comparing sclerotherapy with distal splenorenal shunts demonstrated significantly lower rebleeding with surgical treatment, but survival benefit was equivocal because of the heterogeneity of the results.[26] No trials comparing pharmacological therapy with variceal band ligation have been reported.

Management of gastric and ectopic variceal haemorrhage

Haemorrhage from gastric varices carries a mortality higher than that associated with oesophageal varices. For lesser curve gastric varices, the results of standard injection sclerotherapy are similar to those for oesophageal varices. Sclerotherapy of fundal varices is less effective,[27] and may be associated with a high complication rate.[28] In these circumstances initial haemostasis is often best achieved with the large volume gastric balloon of the Linton–Nachlas balloon tamponade.

Other treatments that have been proposed include use of cyanoacrylate polymer injection,[29] thrombin injection,[30] endoscopic snares,[31] and TIPS. Polymer injections carry a significant complication rate[32] and TIPS procedures, although effective at initiating haemostasis, are difficult to perform during active bleeding. Thrombin injection is a relatively safe, easier and equally effective option.

Ectopic varices at sites other than the oseophagus or stomach are a source of bleeding in fewer than 3% of cases.[33] Endoscopic injection sclerotherapy has rarely been used to control haemorrhage from stomal, duodenal and anorectal varices.[33]

Key points

- Prophylactic injection sclerotherapy for oesophageal varices is of no proven benefit

- Endoscopic injection sclerotherapy (EIS) and endoscopic variceal banding ligation (EVL) are the main endoscopic techniques for treating oesophageal varices

- In achieving haemostasis, EIS is more often successful than balloon tamponade; EIS and pharmacological therapy (vasopressin, nitroglycerine, somatostatin analogue) are of similar efficacy. Many centres use a combination of pharmacological and endoscopic therapy

- EVL is as effective as EIS in initial haemostasis and the rate of rebleeding after EVL is lower; mortality, however, is not reduced

- Secondary prevention of variceal bleeding reduces mortality, and EVL is likely to become the preferred endoscopic technique for this purpose

- For gastric fundal varices, haemostasis is best achieved with large volume balloon tamponade

---

References

1 Fardy JM, Laupacis A. A meta-analysis of prophylactic endoscopic sclerotherapy for esophageal varices. *Am J Gastroenterol* 1994;**89**:1938–48.
2 Williams K, Dawson J. Fibreoptic injection of oesophageal varices. *BMJ* 1979;2:766–7.
3 Kitano S, Iwanaga T, Iso Y, *et al*. A transparent overtube for endoscopic injection sclerotherapy and results in patients with oesophageal varices. *Jpn J Surg* 1987;**17**:256–62.

4 Lewis J, Chung RS, Allison J. Sclerotherapy of oesophageal varices. *Arch Surg* 1980;**115**: 476–9.
5 Polson R, Westaby D, Gimson A, *et al.* Sucralfate for the prevention of early rebleeding following injection sclerotherapy for oesophageal varices. *Hepatology* 1989;**10**:279–82.
6 Moreto M, Zaballa M, Bernal A, *et al.* A randomised trial of tamponade or sclerotherapy as immediate therapy for bleeding oesophageal varices. *Surg Gynecol Obstet* 1988;**167**: 331–4.
7 Burroughs A, Hamilton G, Phillips A, *et al.* A comparison of sclerotherapy with staple transection of the oesophagus for emergency control of bleeding oesophageal varices. *N Engl J Med* 1986;**321**:857–62.
8 Westaby D, Hayes P, Gimson A, Polson R, Williams R. A controlled trial of injection sclerotherapy for active variceal haemorrhage. *Hepatology* 1989;**9**:274–7.
9 Planas R, Quer JC, Boix J, *et al.* A prospective randomized trial comparing somatostatin and sclerotherapy in the treatment of acute variceal bleeding. *Hepatology* 1994;**20**:370–5.
10 Sung J, Chung S, Lai C-W, *et al.* Octreotide infusion or emergency sclerotherapy for variceal haemorrhage. *Lancet* 1993;**342**:637–41.
11 Shields R, Jenkins SA, Baxter JN, *et al.* A prospective randomised controlled trial comparing the efficacy of somatostatin with injection sclerotherapy in the control of bleeding oesophageal varices. *J Hepatol* 1992;**16**:128–37.
12 Shemesh E, Czerniak A, Klein E, Pines A, Bal L. A comparison between early and delayed endoscopic sclerotherapy of bleeding oesophageal varices in non-alcoholic portal hypertension. *J Clin Gastroenterol* 1990;**12**:5–9.
13 McCormick PA, Biagini MR, Dick R, *et al.* Octreotide inhibits the meal-induced increases in the portal venous pressure of cirrhotic patients with portal hypertension: a double-blind, placebo-controlled study. *Hepatology* 1992;**16**:1180–6.
14 Stiegmann GV, Goff JS, Michaletz-Onody PA, *et al.* Endoscopic sclerotherapy as compared with endoscopic ligation for bleeding esophageal varices. *N Engl J Med* 1992;**326**:1527–32.
15 Gimson AE, Ramage JK, Panos MZ, *et al.* Randomised trial of variceal banding ligation versus injection sclerotherapy for bleeding oesophageal varices. *Lancet* 1993;**342**:391–4.
16 Laine L, el-Newihi HM, Migikovsky B, Sloane R, Garcia F. Endoscopic ligation compared with sclerotherapy for the treatment of bleeding esophageal varices. *Ann Intern Med* 1993; **119**:1–7.
17 Berner J, Gaing A, Sharma R, Almenoff P, Muhlfelder T, Korsten M. Sequelae after esophageal variceal ligation and sclerotherapy: a prospective randomised study. *Am J Gastroenterol* 1994;**89**:852–8.
18 Lo GH, Lai KH, Shen MT, Chang CF. A comparison of the incidence of transient bacteremia and infectious sequelae after sclerotherapy and rubber band ligation of bleeding esophageal varices. *Gastrointest Endosc* 1994;**40**:675–9.
19 Rossle M, Haag K, Ochs A, *et al.* The transjugular intrahepatic portosystemic stent-shunt procedure for variceal bleeding. *N Engl J Med* 1994;**330**:165–71.
20 Infante-Rivard C, Esnaola S, Villeneuve JP. Role of endoscopic variceal sclerotherapy in the long-term management of variceal bleeding: a meta-analysis. *Gastroenterology* 1989; **96**:1087–92.
21 Moreto M, Zaballa M, Ojembarrena E, *et al.* Combined (short-term plus long-term) sclerotherapy v short-term only sclerotherapy: a randomised prospective trial. *Gut* 1994; **35**:687–91.
22 Parikh SS, Desai HG. What is the aim of esophageal variceal sclerotherapy—prevention of rebleeding or complete obliteration of veins? *J Clin Gastroenterol* 1992;**15**:186–8.
23 Teres J, Bosch J, Bordas JM, *et al.* Propranolol versus sclerotherapy in preventing variceal rebleeding: a randomized controlled trial. *Gastroenterology* 1993;**105**:1508–14.
24 Vickers C, Rhodes J, Chesner I, *et al.* Prevention of rebleeding from oesophageal varices: two-year follow up of a prospective controlled trial of propranolol in addition to sclerotherapy. *J Hepatol* 1994;**21**:81–7.
25 Vinel JP, Lamouliatte H, Cales P, *et al.* Propranolol reduces the rebleeding rate during endoscopic sclerotherapy before variceal obliteration. *Gastroenterology* 1992;**102**:1760–3.
26 Spina GP, Henderson JM, Rikkers LF, *et al.* Distal spleno-renal shunt versus endoscopic sclerotherapy in the prevention of variceal rebleeding. A meta-analysis of 4 randomized clinical trials. *J Hepatol* 1992;**16**:338–45.
27 Gimson AE, Westaby D, Williams R. Endoscopic sclerotherapy in the management of gastric variceal haemorrhage. *J Hepatol* 1991;**13**:274–8.

171

28 Ng EK, Chung SC, Leong HT, Li AK. Perforation after endoscopic injection sclerotherapy for bleeding gastric varices [see comments]. *Surg Endosc* 1994;**8**:1221–2.
29 Soehendra N, Grimm H, Nam VC, *et al.* N-butyl-2-cyano-acrylate: a supplement to endoscopic sclerotherapy. *Endoscopy* 1986;**18**:25–6.
30 Williams SG, Peters RA, Westaby D. Thrombin—an effective treatment for fundal gastric varices. *Gut* 1993;**34(suppl 1)**:S48.
31 Yoshida T, Hayashi N, Suzumi N, *et al.* Endoscopic ligation of gastric varices using a detachable snare. *Endoscopy* 1994;**26**:502–5.
32 Ramond M, Valla D, Gottlib J, *et al.* Obturation endoscopique des varices oesophagogastrique par le Bucrylate. *Gastroenterol Clin Biol* 1986;**10**:575–9.
33 Rammage JK. Ectopic variceal bleeding. *Gastrointest Endosc Clin North Am* 1992;**2**:95–110.

Part V
Lower gastrointestinal haemorrhage

13: The transjugular intrahepatic portosystemic stent (TIPS) shunt

R DICK, D PATCH AND J TIBBALS

TIPS is an interventional radiological technique in which a portosystemic shunt is created entirely within the liver. It has developed because variceal bleeding in patients with portal hypertension continues to be associated with a high mortality (35–50% in all published trials) despite established surgical treatments and improvements in medical and endoscopic therapies.[1]

A percutaneous approach to producing a shunt between the portal and hepatic veins was first used in pigs by Rosch et al. in 1969.[2] Colapinto and co-workers in 1982 reported the first clinical experience in humans, though unfortunately their intrahepatic tract, dilated by an angioplasty balloon, closed early.[3] It was Richter et al. in 1990 who pioneered the use of metal stents to maintain the shunt tract and are credited with the developing popularity of this procedure.[4] More than 1000 TIPS insertions have been recorded worldwide; 50% of the procedures performed in the US are done in private clinics, despite the paucity of controlled trials confirming their efficacy.

Indications for TIPS

The indications for TIPS include established and more controversial ones.

Established indications

- Acute variceal bleeding that is unresponsive to two sessions of sclerotherapy
- As a trial of shunt surgery
- In selected patients suffering from the Budd–Chiari syndrome

Controversial/unproven indications

- Prevention of secondary variceal haemorrhage
- Reduction of ascites in patients with liver failure

- Treatment for the hepatorenal syndrome
- Interim measure while awaiting liver transplantation
- Clearance of portal vein thrombosis.

Method

TIPS may be an elective or an emergency procedure. The emergency procedure is common, the shunt being performed at short notice and "out of hours" in patients with continued variceal bleeding who have an inflated Sengstaken tube in situ. General anaesthesia is not necessary. Under local anaesthesia (10 ml lignocaine) and intravenous sedation (5 mg midazolam), the right internal jugular vein is cannulated and a French gauge 10 sheath inserted. Through this sheath the guidewires, catheter-needle assembly, balloon catheter to dilate the tract, and the metal stent assembly are introduced in turn.

The principles of the TIPS technique are shown in Figure 13.1. First the status of the portal vein is established, by superior mesenteric angiography or Doppler ultrasound. If the vein is poorly visualised, a contrast hepatic venogram performed using an occlusion balloon catheter is invaluable (Figure 13.2).

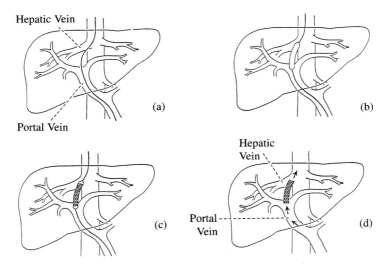

FIGURE 13.1—*Stages in the insertion of a transjugular intrahepatic stent (TIPS) shunt. (a) Guidewire bridging the hepatic and portal veins, passing through liver tissue. (b) Dilation of the liver tract by inflation of a balloon catheter. (c) Release of stent in the liver tract by means of balloon inflation. (d) Metal stent fully opened. Note that its free ends lie in the veins and the cephalad flow of the portal venous blood.*

The procedure begins with the passage of a 16 gauge modified Ross transeptal needle (or one of several commercially made needle assemblies) into the right hepatic vein. The stiff end of a 0·035 inch guidewire

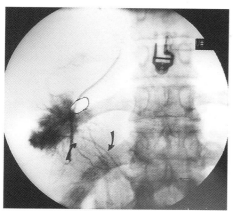

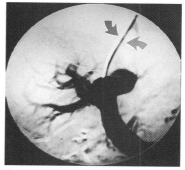

FIGURE 13.3—*Digital subtraction angiogram performed with the needle across the liver tract and in the portal vein. This image allows estimation of the length of tract to be stented. Arrows indicate puncture site through inferior wall of right hepatic vein.*

FIGURE 13.2—*Balloon occlusion hepatic venogram. Reflux into the portal system via sinusoids indicates many small veins (curved arrows) and the absence of a normal portal vein. The air-filled balloon is indicated by the straight arrow.*

(Meditech, UK) is then passed under fluoroscopic and ultrasound control through the inferior wall of the hepatic vein and advanced forcibly through the liver tract, into the confluence of the main branches of the portal vein. Once the ultrasonographer is certain that the echogenic wire tip lies within the lumen of the portal vein, the needle follows. After withdrawal of the wire, aspiration of the needle during (if necessary) its fractional retraction will yield portal venous blood. After confirmatory injection of contrast medium, the floppy tip of the heavy duty wire is advanced deeply into the superior mesenteric or splenic veins, followed by the catheter assembly (Figure 13.3). The portal pressure is measured, then an angiogram taken to assess the length of the intrahepatic tract to be stented. Next, to ensure later full expansion of the stent, the liver tract must be dilated with a 9 or 10 mm balloon catheter (French gauge 5 shaft). This manoeuvre is painful and the patient requires 25–50 mg of opiate analgesia. Once the balloon is fully deflated and removed, a stent assembly (mounted on a French gauge 7 or 9 catheter) is introduced astride the portal-hepatic vein tract and carefully deployed. Various metal stents of 10 mm diameter are available (Palmaz, Strecker, for example); the Memotherm (Angiomed) has a thermal memory and diameter of 12 mm. A definitive portal vein contrast injection is then given to confirm cephalad flow (Figure 13.4) and complete expansion can be expected. Finally pressures are recorded in the portal system and right atrium, and the catheter and introducer set removed. The patient is returned to the ward and monitored as after an angiogram. Some patients are fit for discharge within 24–48 h.

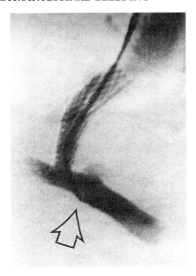

FIGURE 13.4—*Digital subtraction portogram showing upwards venous flow through a fully deployed stent. The arrow indicates the catheter tip in the portal vein. Note the division of flow between liver and stent.*

Difficulties may be experienced if the liver is small or hard, or if the hepatic vein origin is distorted. In experienced hands, TIPS takes about 2 h to perform. No significant blood loss should occur as a result of the procedure itself, and upon completion the Sengstaken balloons may safely be deflated.

Complications of TIPS

Capsular puncture

The most feared complication at the time of the procedure is capsular puncture, which may lead to rapid exsanguination and death from haemoperitoneum. It accounts for a procedural death rate of 1–2%.[5] This risk is minimised by expert ultrasound guidance showing that as the guidewire tip approaches the portal vein through the liver tract, it is at all times surrounded by hepatic tissue. Even then, accidental puncture can still occur, and this may be successfully plugged with a combination of coils, gelfoam and tissue glue. Deaths occurred in earlier studies where a combined transhepatic and transjugular approach was used to access the portal vein.

Sepsis

As with any percutaneous procedure, infection can be introduced. Patients with cirrhosis are particularly sensitive, with a markedly attenuated response to bacterial invasion. In addition to scrupulous aseptic technique, prophylactic antibiotics, including staphylococcal cover, are required.

Portosystemic encephalopathy

The true rate of portosystemic encephalopathy (PSE) is difficult to determine for several reasons; there is failure to report PSE in trials, failure to diagnose PSE, and lack of follow up. TIPS is a total shunt and one would expect TIPS placement to precipitate PSE in the same way that surgical shunts may do so; the risk factors are the same: age, diameter of the shunt, and Child's C grade liver disease. None the less, the intrahepatic position of a TIPS shunt encourages continued flow of portal blood into the liver. The rate of PSE has varied in different studies from 15 to 35%.[6,7]

TIPS-associated encephalopathy is often regarded as being easy to treat. However, the reports of this are often anecdotal and results using TIPS reduction stents appear equivocal. A paper from the Freiberg group[8] presented four patients with TIPS-induced PSE who were treated by the placement of a reducing stent (one with smaller diameter than the original stent) within the lumen of the TIPS shunt. This reduces the blood flow diversion, and should then therefore reduce the degree of encephalopathy. Two of these patients died of septicaemia at 84 and 116 days after shunt reduction. Changes were seen in serum ammonia levels, but no comment was made on electroencephalogram data. This group also looked at the use of TIPS reduction in patients who had accelerated TIPS-associated liver failure. Three out of three patients died within 6 weeks.

Haemolysis

Haemolysis is a recognised complication of TIPS and is probably related to mechanical trauma sustained by red cells as they pass through the shunt. It is usually noticeable in the first month after TIPS insertion, before endothelialisation, and may be associated with a reticulocytosis, elevation of serum bilirubin, and reduction of serum hepatoglobins with red cell fragments visible on blood film. The frequency of haemolysis was up to 35% in one reported study.[9]

Heart failure

TIPS is associated with an acute increase in right atrial pressure, pulmonary capillary wedge pressure and cardiac output. Pulmonary oedema has occurred after TIPS.[10] Compromised cardiac function is a relative contraindication to TIPS.[11]

Occlusion or stenosis

Occlusion may be acute, particularly in patients with hypercoagulable states such as Budd–Chiari. Such early occlusion will usually present with variceal bleeding, particularly when this was the original indication for the TIPS. Thrombolysis, stent dilatation, and placement of an additional stent have all been used for this type of occlusion.[12] Some workers have used plasminogen activator to dissolve acute clots, but there have been no controlled trials.[13] Use of prophylactic heparin is unproven and anticoagulation is not recommended. Prophylactic aspirin 100 mg daily did not prevent a 30% rate of occlusion or stenosis in a randomised study.[14] Factors that appear to have influenced stenosis rate are the Child's classification and prothrombin time, but not platelet count. In one study 94% of patients with Child's A disease had a significant stenosis at 1 year compared with 59% of Child's C patients.[15] Up to 50% of all patients will require reintervention at 6 months.

Accelerated liver failure and alteration of liver function tests

Most large series report 5% of patients suffering accelerated liver failure, with death as a consequence unless rescue liver transplantation is available. As with all shunts an increase in bilirubin concentration, and prothrombin time is seen after TIPS. These parameters tend to improve with time.

Results of TIPS Insertion

Uncontrolled variceal haemorrhage

Multicentre experience over a 5-year period suggests that intrahepatic stent shunts are the treatment of choice in patients with variceal bleeding who are unresponsive to medical therapy or unsuited for surgery. Bleeding gastric varices are particularly difficult to treat with sclerotherapy, and the decision to insert a shunt in these patients is more readily taken. Ninety per cent of patients with uncontrolled variceal haemorrhage will be successfully treated by TIPS; 10% of these may require two parallel shunts to achieve adequate decompression, and these patients will often need additional variceal embolisation. In this respect the TIPS shunt allows a unique access to the portal circulation.

TIPS has the advantages of shunt surgery without many of the operative risks. In most cases, the procedure does not require a general anaesthetic, thus avoiding lengthy stays on intensive care units. However, disillusion with surgical portosystemic shunts has perhaps led to over enthusiastic adoption of TIPS, particularly as there has been no randomised controlled trial comparing TIPS with another salvage therapy. Early mortality has been shown to be as high as 50% in retrospective reports of TIPS for uncontrolled variceal haemorrhage,[16 17] primarily due to overwhelming septicaemia with associated renal and liver failure. Nonetheless, in the acute bleeding situation, the results of TIPS can be very impressive, and this indication for TIPS remains the most appropriate.

Other studies have been retrospective analyses of consecutive patients who had had TIPS for uncontrolled variceal bleeding. Mortality remains at 50%; overwhelming septicaemia with associated renal failure and liver failure was usually the cause of death.[17 18]

TIPS as a trial of shunt surgery

Because of the high occlusion rate TIPS shunting should be regarded as a temporary measure, and in patients whose predominant symptoms are those of portal hypertension a TIPS may establish whether they are able to tolerate the shunt without developing uncontrolled portosystemic encephalopathy. A typical scenario is a middle aged patient who does not have progressive liver disease (for example, someone with cirrhosis who has abstained from alcohol), in whom a surgical shunt, long term, would be an alternative to liver transplantation. If the TIPS is tolerated without encephalopathy, then a surgical shunt is a reasonable alternative.

TIPS in the Budd–Chiari syndrome

There are several reports of the usefulness of TIPS in relieving the portal hypertension that is associated with the Budd–Chiari syndrome,[19 20] while the use of similar expanding metal stents to reverse the caval compression is well described.[21] Ascites may totally resolve.[22] However, in patients with grade C cirrhosis and massive ascites, early hopes that TIPS may play a major role in fluid reduction have not been realised.

Portal vein thrombosis

TIPS may be technically possible in patients with either short thromboses or recent thrombosis or both, where the clot is soft and where a wire may be passed across the obstructed segment.

TIPS for ascites

In many series of TIPS for variceal bleeding a reduction in the volume of ascites or diuretic use has been noted. Four papers have reported the use of TIPS for diuretic resistant ascites. None of these were randomised controlled studies, the obvious comparative treatment being large volume paracentesis, and they are flawed by the lack of quality of life data, particularly as this is a palliative procedure. Nonetheless, from a total of 103 patients, a complete or partial response in ascitic volume was achieved in 90%. Mortality at six months was 21%. Shunt dysfunction was heralded by reaccumulation of ascites, necessitating TIPS dilatation in 39 cases, and radiological follow up was generally intensive.[23–25 27]

Hepatorenal syndrome

Two abstracts have reported the use of TIPS for this catastrophic complication of cirrhosis. In both, the serum creatinines were generally unimpressive—the three patients with values above 300 µmol either died or had transplants. None the less, the effect of TIPS on renal blood supply is of great interest, and the demonstration of a hepatorenal reflex by the Edinburgh team, observing the effect of balloon occlusion of TIPS on renal perfusion, certainly warrants further investigation. However, as in patients with hepatic encephalopathy, the presence of the hepatorenal syndrome tends to indicate end stage liver disease. It is unlikely, therefore, that TIPS for hepatorenal syndrome will result in any significant improvement in either mortality or quality of life.

As in patients with hepatic encephalopathy, the presence of hepatorenal syndrome tends to indicate late stage liver disease. It is likely, therefore, that TIPS will not result in any significant improvement in quality of life, the complication being encephalopathy.

In liver transplantation

TIPS has been acclaimed as an optimal treatment to precede the graft of a new liver, as it removes the risk of portal hypertensive bleeding. It may reduce portal blood product requirement, and has been reported to improve nutrition.[26] However, such results have not been confirmed in a prospective study. As 5% of patients treated with TIPS will have accelerated liver failure, the procedure should be justified medically; it may not always be possible to find a suitable donor for those unpredictable few who rapidly develop acute or chronic liver failure.

Follow up

It is recommended that at 3 month intervals a patient returns for three procedures: an electroencephalogram to assess possible encephalopathy, a duplex Doppler scan to assess shunt patency and velocity (Figure 13.5) and a TIPS angiogram performed via a venous route (Figure 13.6). All of these can be safely carried out on a day stay basis. If encephalopathy develops and progresses, a "reducing stent" can be inserted (Figure 13.7).

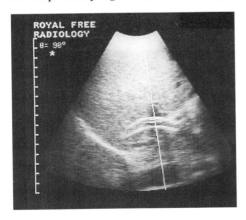

FIGURE 13.5—*Duplex Doppler ultrasound scan showing patency of TIPS stent, and a flow of 15 cm/s through the patent stent.*

Stent angiography is the most useful technique in TIPS assessment. Stent stenosis is usually heralded by ascites reaccumulation, variceal rebleeding, or

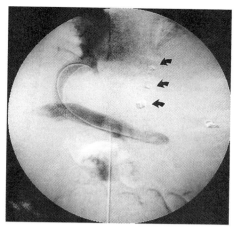

FIGURE 13.6—*Digital subtraction angiogram showing that a catheter from the femoral vein has traversed the TIPS shunt and entered the portal and then the splenic vein. The stent is patent and there is dual flow at the porta. Arrows indicate stainless steel coils in the previously embolised left gastric vein.*

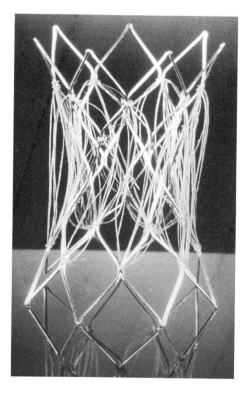

FIGURE 13.7—*A Memotherm reducing stent. After selection of a suitable internal diameter, the reducing stent is placed inside the original TIPS stent.*

a rise in the portosystemic gradient at follow up. Significant (i.e. symptomatic) stenosis will occur at six months in up to 50% of patients, hence close follow up is mandatory. Balloon dilatation of the stent is successful in the majority of cases, though intimal hyperplasia may necessitate the placement of a new stent within the lumen of the first one. A second stent is placed in parallel but this is a rare occurrence (Figure 13.8).

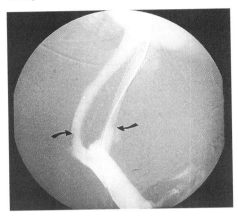

FIGURE 13.8—*Two metal stents (arrowed) were required in this patient before the portal pressure fell sufficiently to control variceal bleeding.*

Long term survival after TIPS will depend mainly on the severity of the underlying liver disease. Selectively treating portal hypertension rather than the cirrhosis is unlikely greatly to increase patient survival. Patients subsequently receiving a liver transplant are an exception; it is vital for the technical success of the transplant that the upper and lower limbs of the metal stent are not placed too deeply into the hepatic vein and portal vein respectively.

Summary

It is likely that the main indication of TIPS will remain uncontrolled variceal bleeding. The results of trials of TIPS versus other treatments are just beginning to be reported. It is expected that the indication for TIPS will narrow, and it may eventually be possible to identify a patient in whom TIPS therapy, while stopping variceal bleeding, will not prevent loss of life. Randomised controlled trials in the use of TIPS to manage ascites and to prevent secondary variceal haemorrhage are required. Because of the high stenosis rate, a TIPS shunt should be regarded as a temporary measure.

Key points

- TIPS involves the creation of a portosystemic shunt entirely within the liver
- Established indications are: acute variceal bleeding persisting after two sessions of sclerotherapy; as a trial of shunt surgery; in selected patients with the Budd–Chiari syndrome

continued

- TIPS insertion is carried out under local anaesthesia with opiate analgesia
- Capsular puncture accounts for a procedural death rate of 1–2%
- Other complications are: sepsis; portosystemic encephalopathy; haemolysis; heart failure; stent occlusion or stenosis; accelerated liver failure
- TIPS will stop uncontrolled variceal bleeding in 90% of cases; this is likely to remain its main indication
- Because of the high rate of stent occlusion, TIPS is a temporary measure; it is appropriate as a trial of shunt surgery or a bridge to liver transplantation

References

1 Burroughs AK, Mezzanote G, Phillips A, *et al.* Cirrhosis with variceal haemorrhage: the importance of the time interval between admission and the start of analysis for survival and rebleeding rates. *Hepatology* 1989;801–7.
2 Rosch J, Hanafee WN, Snow H. Transjugular portal venography and radiologic portocaval shunt: an experimental study. *Radiology* 1969;**92**:1112–4.
3 Colapinto RF, Stronell RD, Birch RL, *et al.* Creation of an intrahepatic portosystemic shunt with a Gruntzig balloon catheter. *Can Med Assoc J* 1982;**126**:267–8.
4 Richter GM, Noeldge G, Palmaz JC, *et al.* The transjugular intrahepatic portosystemic stent-shunt (TIPSS); results of a pilot study. *Cardiovasc Intervent Radiol* 1990;200–7.
5 Hayes PC, Redhead DN, Finlayson NDS. Transjugular intrahepatic portosystemic stent shunts. *Gut* 1994;**35**:445–6.
6 Sanyal AJ, Freedman AM, Schiffman ML, *et al.* Portosystemic encephalopathy following transjugular intrahepatic portosystemic shunt (TIPS): results of a prospective controlled study. *Hepatology* 1994;**20**:46–55.
7 La Berge JM, Ring EJ, Gordon RL, *et al.* Creation of transjugular intrahepatic portosystemic shunts with the Wallstent endoprosthesis; results in 100 patients. *Radiology* 1993;**187**:413–20.
8 Hauenstein KH, Haag K, Ochs A, Langer M, Rossle M. The reducing stent treatment for transjugular portosystemic shunt induced refractory hepatic encephalopathy and liver failure. *Radiology* 1995;**194**:175–9.
9 Sanyal A, Freedman A, Purdum P, Schiffman M, Luketic V. The haematologic consequences of transjugular intrahepatic portosystemic shunts. *Hepatology* 1996;**23**:32–9.
10 Wong F, Snidermann K, Liu P, Allidina Y, Sherman M, Blendis L. Transjugular intrahepatic portosystemic stent shunt: effect on haemodynamics and sodium homeostasis in cirrhosis and refractory ascites. *Ann Intern Med* 1995;**122**:816–22.
11 Azoulay D, Castaing D, Dennison A, Martino W, Eyraud D, Bismuth H. Transjugular intrahepatic portosystemic shunt worsens the hyperdynamic circulatory state of the cirrhotic patient: preliminary report of a prospective study. *Hepatology* 1994;**19**:129–32.
12 Blum U, Haag K, Rossle M, Ochs A, Gabelmann A, Boos S, *et al.* Noncavernomatous portal vein thrombosis in hepatic cirrhosis: treatment with transjugular intrahepatic portosystemic shunt and local thrombolysis. *Radiology* 1995;**195**:153–7.
13 Theilmann L, Sauer P, Roeren T, Otto G, Arnold J, Noeledge G, *et al.* Acetylsalicylic acid in the prevention of early stenosis occlusion of transjugular intrahepatic portal-systemic stent shunts: a controlled study. *Hepatology* 1994;**20**:592–7.
14 Theilmann L, Sauer P. Transjugular intrahepatic portosystemic shunt (TIPS). Results and complications. *Radiologe* 1994;**34**:174–7.
15 Sauer P, *et al.* Stent stenosis after transjugular intrahepatic portosystemic stent shunt (abstract). *Hepatology* 1994;**20(4 Pt 2)**:108A 48.
16 Jalan R, John T, Redhead D, Garden J, *et al.* A comparative study of emergency intrahepatic portocaval stent-shunt and oesophageal transection in the management of uncontrolled variceal haemorrhage. *Am J Gastroenterol* 1995;**90**:1932–7.
17 McCormick PA, Dick R, Panagou EB, *et al.* Emergency transjugular intrahepatic portosystemic stent shunting as salvage treatment for uncontrolled variceal bleeding. *Br J Surg* 1994;**81**:1324–7.

18 Barange K, et al. TIPS as an emergency procedure in actively bleeding patients with an advanced cirrhosis (abstract). *Hepatology* 1994;**20(4 Pt 2)**:104A 46.

19 Pelt M, Ring EJ, La Berge JM, et al. Treatment of Budd–Chiari syndrome with a transjugular intrahepatic portosystemic shunt. *J Vasc Intervent Radiol* 1993;**4**:263–7.

20 G A, Rossle M, Haag K, et al. TIPS for hepatorenal syndrome. *Hepatology* 1994;**20**: A:70.

21 m I, Bass N, LaBerge JM, et al. Treatment of the hepatorenal syndrome with the transjugular intrahepatic portosystemic shunt (TIPS). *Gastroenterology* 1995;**108**:A31.

22 cking CN, Sanderson AJ, Arthur MJP. Budd–Chiari syndrome (BCS)—treatment with transjugular intrahepatic portosystemic stent shunt (TIPSS). *J Intervent Radiol* 1994;**9**: 21–4.

2 Quiroga J, Sangro B, Nunez M, Bilbao I, Longo J, Garcia-Villarreal L, et al. Transjugular intrahepatic portosystemic shunt in the treatment of refractory ascites: effect on clinical, renal, humoral and haemodynamic parameters. *Hepatology* 1995;**21**:986–94.

24 Ochs A, Rossle M, Haag K, Hauenstein, et al. The transjugular intrahepatic portosystemic stent-shunt procedure for refractory ascites. *N Engl J Med* 1995;**332**:1192–7.

25 Somberg KA, Lake JR, Tomlanovich SJ, LaBerge JM, Feldstein V, Bass NM. Transjugular intrahepatic portosystemic shunts for refractory ascites: assessment of clinical and hormonal response and renal function. *Hepatology* 1995;**21**:709–16.

26 Sterneck N, et al. Intrahepatic portocaval shunts. A bridge to liver transplantation in patients with refractory variceal bleeding. *Hepatology* 1991;**15A**:801.

27 Wong F, Snidermann K, Liu P, Allidina Y, Sherman M, Blendis L. Transjugular intrahepatic portosystemic stent shunt: Effect on haemodynamics and sodium homeostasis in cirrhosis and refractory ascites. *Ann Intern Med* 1995;**122**:816–22.

14: Lower gastrointestinal haemorrhage: the scope of the problem

J N BAXTER

Lower gastrointestinal bleeding traditionally means bleeding from sites distal to the ligament of Treitz that presents as rectal bleeding. This rectal bleeding may be overt or occult, and overt bleeding can be acute massive or chronic—a useful subdivision for clinical purposes. This definition excludes from discussion those causes of lower gastrointestinal bleeding that lie in the upper gastrointestinal tract, but this artificial distinction provides a useful model for discussion of the clinical problems.

There are few data about the incidence of hospital consultations for lower gastrointestinal bleeding in adults. It has been estimated that 25–30 000 patients per year are admitted to UK hospitals with all causes of gastrointestinal bleeding, both upper and lower. In one American hospital series admissions for lower gastrointestinal bleeding accounted for about 20% of all cases of gastrointestinal bleeding.[1] If the pattern is similar in the UK, 5–6000 patients per year are admitted to hospital for investigation and treatment of lower gastrointestinal bleeding. This figure is likely to be a gross underestimate of the true incidence of lower gastrointestinal bleeding, as many patients will be admitted to hospital for definitive treatment after investigations as an outpatient. Other patients will bleed while in hospital and not be included in any data set. There is a real need for more precise data because the mortality for lower gastrointestinal bleeding is estimated to be around 11% overall and as high as 21% for acute massive bleeding.[1 2]

Most lower gastrointestinal bleeds are benign in origin, but the usual clinical approach is to suspect a neoplastic cause, particularly if the patient is over 50 years of age or has other colorectal symptoms or both. In the UK around 31 000 new cases of colorectal cancer are diagnosed annually, making the disease the second most common cause of cancer death. The prognosis is poor, with a relative survival at 5 years of 37%, because more than half the patients present with advanced disease. Rectal bleeding is a

187

common symptom of colorectal cancer and occurs in more than 66% of patients before diagnosis.[3] Bleeding is more likely to indicate an early state cancer than a late stage one.[4]

Overt chronic lower gastrointestinal bleeding

Overt chronic lower gastrointestinal bleeding is typically intermittent and usually has a benign cause in the anorectum. In a random sample of patients registered with general practitioners in the south of England, rectal bleeding noticed by the patient had an estimated 1-year prevalence of 20%.[5] Most patients who notice rectal bleeding do not consult their general practitioner, so the true cause of their rectal bleeding goes undiagnosed. Similar findings have been reported from other countries, and the reported incidence of rectal bleeding rises in the subset of the population who examine their toilet paper regularly.[6]

Rectal bleeding and colorectal cancer

There is, therefore, a high proportion of the population with symptomatic rectal bleeding who must be considered at increased risk of harbouring serious disease. However, most patients with overt chronic rectal bleeding do not have serious disease but simple, local anorectal problems and do not need full bowel investigation. So what is the positive predictive value of rectal bleeding for a colorectal neoplasm? In an important study from Australia 319 men aged over 50 years were randomly selected and asked about rectal bleeding before undergoing flexible sigmoidoscopy to at least 30 cm.[7] Of the 12 patients found to have polyps more than 10 mm in diameter, only four had admitted to rectal bleeding in the previous 6 months. Of the 271 patients who reported no rectal bleeding eight were found to have polyps, which in one case were malignant. In this study, rectal bleeding had a specificity of 86%, a sensitivity of 33% and a positive predictive value of only 8% for rectal and low sigmoid neoplasms. This means that if rectal bleeding was used as a predictor of colorectal neoplasia, then 44 of the 48 patients underwent unnecessary sigmoidoscopy. The authors therefore cautioned against any public health programme based on the use of rectal bleeding as a screening test for colorectal cancer. This was an important study, because the whole population sample was endoscoped and the true incidence of colorectal neoplasm determined. Although blood mixed with bowel motion is said to be more likely than bright red rectal bleeding to presage a polyp or cancer,[8] many patients are unable to be precise about the nature of the bleeding. However, not all workers have found that the type of bleeding is predictive for its cause. Chapius and co-workers found no differences in the positive predictive value of blood on the toilet paper, in the lavatory bowl or on the stool.[7] Related bowel symptoms have been thought to increase the diagnostic yield, but even then, because of the independent high prevalence of rectal bleeding and irritable bowel syndrome, they do not identify most cases of colorectal cancer and are highly inaccurate at determining the cause of the rectal bleeding.[9]

We lack adequate predictive criteria to identify those with rectal bleeding who need full assessment rather than limited investigation. Some patient groups are known to be at increased risk of colorectal cancer (Box 14.1) but most cases of colorectal cancer (85–90%) are sporadic and not in those perceived to be at high risk. Until molecular biologists provide us with a faecal test of higher positive predictive value, we shall continue to over investigate patients with rectal bleeding. We have to assume that all patients aged over 50 years who have chronic overt rectal bleeding may harbour a colorectal malignancy, while bearing in mind that the incidence of the condition in younger patients is 5% of all cases (Figure 14.1[13]). As most patients do not even consult their general practitioner about rectal bleeding, we have a major public health education problem, despite the fact that rectal bleeding alone is a poor predictor of serious disease. Each year an estimated 6·8 million people in the UK experience overt rectal bleeding, so there is an urgent need to devise guidelines for the identification and further investigation of those who may have colorectal cancer.

Box 14.1   Risk factors for colorectal cancer

- Previous colorectal cancer (metachronous lesion→4% at 10 years)
- Familial polyposis coli (30% are sporadic)
- Hereditary nonpolyposis colorectal cancer syndromes
  —type a, site specific (young age and right sided)
  —type b, previous cancer of breast, uterus, ovary or genitourinary system
- Family history of colorectal cancer in first degree relatives (1:17)
- Long history of ulcerative colitis
- Long history of Crohn's disease
- Previous cholecystectomy (controversial)

Role of general practice in the detection of colorectal cancer

In general practice the incidence of rectal bleeding is high but the incidence of lower gastrointestinal cancer low. In hospital practice about 10% of patients have a malignant tumour and 30% polyps.[10][11] Clearly general practice helps to define the patient population that needs full investigation. What is not clear is how efficient general practice is at detecting patients who bleed, and then either carrying out investigations or referring them for further investigation. General practitioners in the UK vary with regard to ownership of proctoscopes and sigmoidoscopes and access by direct referral for barium enema examinations and colonoscopy.[12]

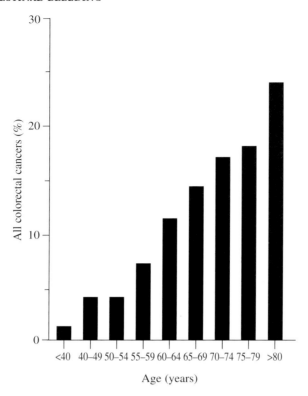

FigURE 14.1—*Incidence of colorectal cancer by age in the United Kingdom.*

It has been suggested that the minimum role for the general practitioner must be a good history and examination including anal inspection and rectal digital examination. Low risk patients (Box 14.2) can be treated conservatively, albeit still needing referral to hospital for treatment of a refractory local anorectal condition or for full bowel investigation if bleeding persists after treatment of a local anorectal problem.

Box 14.2   Patients with rectal bleeding who are at low risk of colorectal cancer

- Under 45 years of age
- No family history of colorectal cancer
- No history of other linked cancers (for example, breast cancer, or cancer of the ovary, uterus or genitourinary system)
- No associated bowel symptoms

Making best use of limited resources

An average general surgeon working in a UK district general hospital would expect to see each week four or five cases of rectal bleeding referred by a general practitioner. Assuming there are five surgeons in the hospital, this would generate about 1000 cases each year, of which up to 40% may have a significant lesion, either a polyp or cancer. Most of these patients will required further investigations and some form of treatment. The significant cost to the National Health Service of the diagnosis and treatment of these patients and of the investigation of the 60% without a significant lesion must be viewed in the context of demand for limited health care resources. However, given that early diagnosis of colorectal cancer improves outcome, the hospital must provide resources for the diagnosis and treatment of rectal bleeding despite the low positive predictive value of rectal bleeding *per se*. As in the UK 22 000 people die each year from colorectal cancer, for which the 5 year crude survival rate of all-comers is only 30%, there is a real need for an aggressive policy towards this disease. General practitioners need to have a clear algorithm for managing these patients, worked out in discussion with local hospital specialists. There needs to be debate about whether general practitioners should carry out endoscopy and about means of ensuring adequate training and quality control in those practices that do take on this role.

Bleeding haemorrhoids

Bleeding from internal haemorrhoids is responsible for most cases of overt chronic rectal bleeding, having a prevalence in one study population of around 4·4%;[4] much higher figures have also been reported. When the haemorrhoids start bleeding the patient often requests treatment. If bleeding persists despite treatment, then full bowel investigation becomes mandatory. The morbidity of bleeding haemorrhoids represents a considerable problem in health care terms; many patients do not present to their general practitioners and general practitioners not active enough in their management of the condition.

Acute massive lower gastrointestinal bleeding

Patients who present to a general practitioner with acute massive lower gastrointestinal bleeding are usually admitted urgently to hospital for investigation and treatment. However, many patients with so called "acute massive bleeding" are experiencing their first brisk bleed from a benign, self limiting anorectal condition that does not require hospital admission. Relatively few patients present with a massive bleed from significant pathology of the colorectum. Those who do may require emergency intervention, such as arteriography, emergency colonoscopy or even emergency colectomy, so they should be managed in a hospital with a full range of relevant facilities, ideally by surgeons with a special interest in coloproctology.

Occult lower gastrointestinal bleeding

Most patients with occult bleeding from the lower gastrointestinal tract are identified only when a medical practitioner suspects colonic pathology and performs a faecal occult blood test. The usual clinical scenario is that of a patient with iron deficiency anaemia where bleeding from the gastrointestinal tract is suspected, especially from the colorectum. Some patients may be identified as part of a colorectal cancer screening programme.

Most cancers of the colorectum arise in a pre-existing adenomatous polyp, but malignant change in an existing polyp is probably such a rare event that a programme of population based screening and polypectomy may be inappropriate. As 30% of the population will have a polyp by the age of 60 but the lifetime risk of malignant change is only 3%, only 10% of patients with an adenoma will develop cancer.[19] Polyps are therefore a necessary but not sufficient condition for the development of colorectal cancer.

Faecal occult blood tests

Normal faecal blood loss is around 1·2 ml/day; a loss in excess of 10 ml/day is needed to obtain a positive result from a faecal occult blood test more than 50% of the time.[15 16] The most commonly used test is a guaiac reagent test (Haemoccult), which has a 12% false positive rate.[17] The more blood in the faeces, the higher is the true positive rate.[18] The false positive rate can be reduced to around 2% with dietary restrictions.

The principal assumption underlying faecal occult blood testing is that identification of blood in the bowel motion before it becomes overt will lead to earlier diagnosis and improved outcome of colonic neoplasia—an assumption that needs proof, because it may be that early diagnosis results only in a lead time bias. Given that the diagnosis of inflammatory bowel disease is usually straightforward, most people with a positive faecal occult blood test are treated as suspects for a colonic neoplasm, either benign or malignant.

A flawed screening tool

The faecal occult blood test is not a good screening tool for colorectal cancer because most adenomas do not bleed and not all tumours bleed. The test has low sensitivity, particularly for rectal lesions. Moreover, if there is bleeding, a one-off test will not always detect it—around 40% of cancers and 80% of adenomas are missed by a single faecal occult blood screen—as the total blood lost by a patient with a tumour is often less than

2 ml/day. If testing is carried out over three days 73% of tumours can be identified, which is indicative of the episodic nature of the bleeding and the inherent sampling error.[20]

More worrying are the similar rates of adenoma among those with a positive faecal occult blood test and those with a negative test.[21 22] Also the rate of colorectal cancer in patients with a positive faecal occult blood test is the same as the expected prevalence in the general population.[23] Immunological tests for occult blood that detect human haemoglobin have a significantly lower false positive rate than that of the Haemoccult test,[24] but this is at the expense of a reduced specificity; 79% more false positives are reported, probably because of increased sensitivity for upper gastrointestinal bleeding lesions.[25]

Screening in symptomatic patients

In symptomatic patients the false positive rate with the Haemoccult test is 8·6% and the false negative rate 45·4%; a patient with a positive test should therefore be investigated, but a negative test does not exclude colorectal neoplasia.[26] It has been suggested that the real value of faecal occult blood testing is to help the general practitioner detect significant disease in patients with bowel symptoms. In a controlled study of faecal blood testing in 911 patients with bowel symptoms, 25% were subsequently shown to have colorectal neoplasia compared to 6% in the control group.[27] Unfortunately the earlier diagnosis did not result in earlier stage tumours being found, perhaps making the point that rectal bleeding, even in symptomatic patients, be it overt or occult, is not a satisfactory predictor of colorectal neoplasia.

Screening in asymptomatic patients

There is no direct evidence of the value of screening programmes in asymptomatic patients. The results of four randomised controlled trials being carried out are eagerly awaited.[28–32] Although preliminary results show that more tumours and earlier stage tumours are being diagnosed in the screened group, this lead time bias may not translate into survival advantage; the screening might select out those tumours with a relatively good prognosis. Compliance with the screening test is also a problem, and ranges from 30 to 67% in the various trials. The positive predictive values reported vary from 22 to 57% for all neoplasia to 5 to 17% for colorectal cancer.

Ahlquist has estimated (Box 14.3) that in a target population of 29 000 people aged over 50 years, around 100 colorectal cancers would be expected.[23] However, because of the many factors discussed above there is a large functional reduction in yield, so that screening such a population would achieve the prevention of only one or two cancer related deaths. Although Ahlquist's prediction is depressing, improvements could be made at the various levels that might increase the functional yield of screening.

Box 14.3   Factors affecting yield of population based screening for colorectal cancer by means of a faecal occult blood (FOB) test; after[22]

Functional reductions in yield	*Cumulative impact on salvage from 100 cancers*
● Nonparticipation in screening test (50%)	50
● FOB miss rate (70%)	15
● Poor evaluation of results (33%)	10
● Specimen too old to test (20%)	8
● Cancer too advanced to treat (25%)	6
● Lead-time bias (50%)	3
● Mortality of screening (1–2%)	1–2

When a participant in a screening programme has a positive faecal occult blood test, he or she usually has a sigmoidoscopy and barium enema examination, or preferably a colonoscopy. The cost implications of a national screening programme should be set against the loss of life and productivity that results from many patients succumbing to colorectal cancer every year. The cost per cancer detected in the UK Nottingham study has been estimated at £2700.[33] In the United States, screening costs exceed the costs avoided by diagnosing and treating the cancer.[34]

In the UK there is an urgent need to address the problem of early diagnosis of colorectal cancer, even before the patient has any rectal bleeding. It has been suggested that a better option than faecal occult blood testing would be to perform a one-off flexible colonoscopy at the age of 55, and put those patients with polyps into a follow-up programme with colonoscopy screening.

Summary

Bleeding from the lower gastrointestinal tract is a common symptom and also a common finding in asymptomatic patients. It may be the only symptom in a patient harbouring a colorectal cancer, so in all patients with rectal bleeding the possibility of this diagnosis must be considered. Whether this means a full bowel investigation requires consideration of the factors discussed. Minor anorectal conditions that give rise to rectal bleeding also need to be treated, as they are often a source of discomfort to the patient. In addition, it is desirable to ablate the rectal bleeding to avoid it confounding the diagnosis of any more significant pathology that may develop.

More data are needed about the size of the problem of lower gastrointestinal bleeding, including costs to the health service. Better predictors of neoplasia are needed than rectal bleeding, be it overt or occult. The role of general practitioners in the diagnosis and treatment of rectal bleeding needs to be clarified and algorithms developed. Acute massive bleeding from lower gastrointestinal causes should be managed by a specialised multidisciplinary team.

Key points

- Lower gastrointestinal bleeding (LGIB) is defined as bleeding from a site distal to the ligament of Treitz that presents as rectal bleeding
- Rectal bleeding may be occult or overt, and overt bleeding may be acute massive or chronic
- Of patients admitted for gastrointestinal bleeding (25–30 000 per year in the UK), about 20% have a lesion in the lower gastrointestinal tract.
- Mortality for LGIB is around 11% overall, and up to 21% for acute massive bleeding
- Most LGIB is benign, but rectal bleeding should always be considered as a possible sign of colorectal neoplasia; individual patient characteristics determine whether full bowel investigation is indicated
- Detecting rectal bleeding, whether overt or occult, is a poor means of screening for colorectal cancer. Better predictors are needed
- The role of general practitioners in the detection and management of rectal bleeding needs to be clarified

---

References

1 Forde KA. Lower gastrointestinal bleeding: the magnitude of the problem. In: Sugawa C, Schuman BM, Lucas CE, eds. *Gastrointestinal bleeding*. New York: Igaku-Shoin, 1992; 13–25.

2 Leitman IM, Paull DE, Shires GT III. Evaluation and management of massive lower gastrointestinal haemorrhage. *Ann Surg* 1989;**209**:175–80.

3 Staniland JR, Ditchburn J, de Dombal FT. Clinical presentations of diseases of the large bowel: a detailed study of 642 patients. *Gastroenterology* 1976;**70**:22–8.

4 Raftery TL, Sansom N. Carcinoma of the colon: a clinical correlation between presenting symptoms and survival. *Am Surg* 1980;**46**:600–6.

5 Jones R, Lydeard S. Irritable bowel syndrome in the general population. *BMJ* 1992;**304**: 87–90.

6 Dent OF, Goulston KJ, Zubrzycki J, Chauis PH. Bowel symptoms in an apparently well population. *Dis Colon Rectum* 1986;**29**:243–7.

7 Chapuis PH, Goulston KJ, Dent OF, Tait AD. Predictive value of rectal bleeding in screening for rectal and sigmoid polyps. *BMJ* 1985;**290**:1546–8.

8 Silman AJ, Mitchell P, Nicholls RJ, *et al*. Self reported dark red bleeding as a marker comparable with occult blood testing in screening for large bowel neoplasms. *Br J Surg* 1983;**70**:721–4.

9 Mant A, Bakey EL, Chapuis PH, *et al*. Rectal bleeding: do other symptoms aid in diagnosis? *Dis Colon Rectum* 1989;**32**:191–6.

10 Shinya H, Cwern M, Wolf G. Colonoscopic diagnosis and management of rectal bleeding. *Surg Clin North Am* 1982;**62**:897–903.

11 Goulston KJ, Cook J, Dent G. How important is rectal bleeding in the diagnosis of bowel cancer and polyps? *Lancet* 1986;**ii**:261–4.

12 Jones R, Farthing M, Leicester R. The management of rectal bleeding. *Br J Clin Pract* 1993;**47**:155–8.

13 Aitken WS, Kuzick J, Northover JMA, Whynes DK. Prevention of colorectal cancer by once only sigmoidoscopy. *Lancet* 1993;**341**:736–40.

14 Johanson JF, Sonneberg A. The prevalence of hemorrhoids and chronic constipation. An epidemiologic study. *Gastroenterology* 1990;**98**:380–6.

15 Ostrow JD, Mulvaeny CA, Hansell JR, Rhodes RS. Sensitivity and reproducibility of chemical tests for faecal occult blood with an emphasis on false-positive reactions. *Dig Dis Sci* 1973;**18**:930–40.

16 Cameron AD. Gastrointestinal blood loss measured by radioactive chromium. *Gut* 1960; **1**:177–82.

17 Morris DW, Hansell JR, Ostrow JD, Lee CS. Reliability of chemical tests for faecal occult blood in hospitalised patients. *Am J Dig Dis* 1976;**21**:845–52.

18 Stroehlein JR, Fairbanks VF, McGill BD, Go VLW. Hemoccult detection of fecal blood quantitated by radioassay. *Am J Dig Dis* 1976;**21**:841–4.

19 Williams CB, Ralbot IC, Atkin WS. Adenoma screening and colorectal cancer [letter]. *BMJ* 1991;**303**:925.

20 Macrae FA, St John DJB. Relationship between patterns of bleeding and Haemoccult sensitivity in patients with colorectal cancer or adenomas. *Gastroenterology* 1982;**82**:891–8.

21 Chapman I. Adenomatous polypi of large intestine: incidence and distribution. *Ann Surg* 1963;**157**:223–6.

22 Rickert RR, Auerbach O, Garfinkel L, Hammond EC, Frasca JM. Adenomatous lesions of the large bowel: an autopsy survey *Cancer* 1979;**43**:1847–57.

23 Ahlquist DA. Occult blood screening. *Cancer* 1992;**70Suppl** 5:1259–65.

24 Schwartz S, Ellefson M. Quantitative faecal recovery of ingested haemoglobin-heme in blood: comparisons by HemoQuant assay with ingested meat and fish. *Gastroenterology* 1985;**89**:19–26.

25 Frommer DJ, Kapparis A, Brown MK. Improved screening for colorectal cancer by immunological detection of occult blood. *BMJ* 1988;**296**:1092–4.

26 Leicester RJ, Lightfoot A, Millar J, Colin-Jones DG, Hunt RH. Accuracy and value of Haemoccult test in symptomatic patients. *BMJ* 1983;**286**:673–4.

27 Armitage NC, Hardcastle JD, Leicester R. Screening for colorectal cancer. *Practitioner* 1989;**233**:830–3.

28 Hardcastle JD, Thomas WM, Chamberlain J, *et al*. Randomised controlled trial of faecal occult blood screening for colorectal cancer: the results of the first 107 349 subjects. *Lancet* 1989;**i**:1160–4.

29 Faivre J. Preliminary results of a mass screening programme for colorectal cancer in France. In: Hardcastle JD, ed. *Screening for colorectal cancer*. Englewood, New Jersey: Normed Verlag, 1989;94–101.

30 Flehinger BJ, Herbert E, Winawer SJ, Miller DG. Screening for colorectal cancer with faecal occult blood test and sigmoidoscopy: preliminary report on the colon project of Memorial Sloan-Kettering Cancer Centre and PMI-Strang Clinic. In: Chamberlain J, Miller AB, eds. *Screening for gastrointestinal cancer*. Toronto: Huber, 1988;9–16.

31 Kewenter J, Bjork S, Haglind E, Smith L, Svanvik J, Ahren C. Screening and rescreening for colorectal cancer in 27 700 subjects. *Cancer* 1988;**62**:645–51.

32 Kronborg O, Fenger C, Sondergaard O, Pederson KM, Olsen J. Initial mass screening for colorectal cancer with faecal occult blood test. *Scand J Gastroenterol* 1987;**22**:677–86.

33 Walker A, Whynes DK, Chamberlain JO, Hardcastle JD. The cost of screening for colorectal cancer. *J Epidemiol Commun Health* 1991;**45**:220–4.

34 Byers T, Gorsky R. Estimates of costs and effects of screening for colorectal cancer in the United States. *Cancer* 1992;**70(suppl 5)**:1288–95.

15: Causes of lower gastrointestinal bleeding

J N BAXTER

Most bleeding from the lower gastrointestinal tract is of colonic origin, with some from sites in the small intestine distal to the ligament of Treitz. However, around 15–20% of episodes of lower gastrointestinal bleeding are thought to arise from more proximal parts of the small intestine or the upper gastrointestinal tract.[1] Lower gastrointestinal bleeding may present as acute massive, chronic intermittent or occult rectal bleeding. Box 15.1 lists all causes of lower gastrointestinal bleeding other than those sited in the upper gastrointestinal tract. Causes of lower gastrointestinal bleeding in children have been reviewed elsewhere[2] and are discussed also in chapter 21, so will not be dealt with here.

Box 15.1. Causes of lower gastrointestinal bleeding

Common causes
- Colonic vascular ectasias
- Diverticula
- Neoplasms
- Benign anorectal causes
  —haemorrhoids
  —fissures
  —fistula
- Inflammatory bowel disease
  —ulcerative colitis
  —Crohn's disease
- Mesenteric vascular insufficiency
- Ischaemic colitis
- Radiation colitis
- Infectious colitis

Less common causes
- Diversion colitis
- Meckel's diverticulum
- Vasculitides
- Small intestinal causes
  —vascular ectasias
  —diverticula
  —ulceration
- Intussusception
- Endometriosis
- Bleeding in runners
- Dieulafoy's lesions
- Visceral arterial aneurysm
- Brown bowel syndrome
- Cytomegalovirus colitis
- Stercoral ulcer
- Pancreatic pseudocyst
- Neoplasms
  —carcinoid
  —lymphomas
  —sarcomas
  —haemangiomas

Common Causes

Colonic vascular ectasias

During the first few decades of this century lower gastrointestinal bleeding was thought to arise largely from lower gastrointestinal neoplasms. In the 1950s diverticula were recognised as a major source, particularly in the elderly. In the 1970s, it was realised that vascular ectasias were probably a more important source of bleeding than diverticula in the elderly.[3]

Vascular ectasias have been called by a variety of names, including angiodysplasias, arteriovenous malformations, vascular dysplasias and angioectasias. They are a distinct nosological entity and can be encountered anywhere in the gastrointestinal tract. They can be distinguished from the vascular lesions of the calcinosis-Raynaud's phenomenon-sclerodactyly-telangiectasia (CRST) syndrome and hereditary haemorrhagic telangiectasia, and from haemangiomas and congenital vascular lesions.

The typical lesion is composed of ectatic thin walled veins, venules and capillaries with a deficient amount of smooth muscle in their walls.[4] Vascular ectasias occur almost entirely in the caecum and proximal ascending colon of elderly patients.[4] Boley and colleagues have hypothesised that their predominant location in the right colon is explained by Laplace's law, which states that where the diameter of a vein is greatest the wall tension is greatest, and this tension leads to obstruction of submucosal venous outflow.[4] Over time the obstruction may cause gradual dilation of submucosal veins and ultimately of capillaries and their sphincters, leading to small arteriovenous communications. Certainly this hypothesis explains the usual location of the lesions and their occurrence in older patients. They are often seen at colonoscopy in elderly patients with no history of bleeding. Vascular ectasias occur in more than 25% of people over the age of 60 as asymptomatic lesions of around 5 mm diameter, either singly or in clusters.[4] The incidence is the same in both sexes.

Only 10% of patients with vascular ectasias will bleed; the bleeding is usually chronic and recurrent, but occasionally it can be acute massive. In 90% of cases bleeding stops spontaneously,[5] but in up to 85% of patients it will recur.[6] In 10–15% of patients there is iron deficiency anaemia and stools that are intermittently positive for occult blood.[7] Cardiac disease, especially aortic stenosis, is said to be more common in these patients, and rates of up to 50% are reported.[3] However, DeMarkles and Murphy, in a review of the literature, concluded that many of the studies reporting this association were flawed; they believe that there is no evidence for an association of aortic stenosis with vascular ectasias.[1]

Diverticula

Diverticula of the bowel are thought to have become more common in parallel with a reduced consumption of fibre and longer lifespans. Diverticula arise from points of weakness in the bowel wall, where there is penetration of the nutrient blood vessels. Each diverticulum is surrounded by serosa, submucosa and mucosa, and is therefore not a true diverticulum. The surrounding blood vessels form a vascular plexus, so it is not surprising that these lesions are subject to bleeding. Diverticula are found most commonly in the distal colon, and in 90% of people are confined to the sigmoid colon.[3] In western countries the prevalence of diverticula increases with age; half of those aged over 60 years have the disorder.[8] A reduction in dietary fibre intake is thought to be largely responsible for the frequency of this condition; this cannot be the whole story, however, because vegetarians also develop diverticula, albeit with an incidence only one-third that in a control group.[9]

Bleeding is said to occur in 3–5% of those who have diverticula and is usually acute massive. Up to 70% of bleeding diverticula are found to be at the less common proximal site.[10] Bleeding usually arises from a ruptured blood vessel at the neck of the diverticulum rather than in the diverticulum itself. The cause of the bleeding is not clear but may be mechanical trauma from luminal contents; it certainly is not related to diverticulitis, which is extremely rare as a cause of bleeding.[11] The pattern of bleeding is rarely diagnostic of the site of haemorrhage, because the patient usually suddenly passes large blood clots per rectum. Bleeding is self limiting in most patients but may persist for several days.[11] Fewer than 25% have a second episode of bleeding, and most of these individuals have continuing problems.[12] It is most important never to attribute overt intermittent lower gastrointestinal bleeding to diverticular disease, because in most of these cases there is some other cause for the bleeding.[13]

Neoplasms

Neoplasms as a cause of overt or occult lower gastrointestinal bleeding are dealt with in chapter 14. Much of the diagnostic effort in lower gastrointestinal bleeding is directed to the detection of neoplasms, which must always be considered as a possible cause, especially in the older patient. A neoplasm rarely causes acute massive bleeding, and in 40–60% of patients with colonic neoplasia chronic intermittent bleeding is the primary presenting problem. Patients with a neoplastic lesion in the rectosigmoid area usually pass bright red blood; if the tumour is more proximal, the blood may be darker in colour and less obvious. Patients with a caecal carcinoma often present with a normal bowel habit and iron deficiency anaemia from chronic faecal blood loss. If investigations are negative and bleeding persists it is important ruthlessly to pursue the diagnosis of a neoplasm. In one study of 106 patients with lower gastrointestinal bleeding who had a normal barium enema, 37 patients had a neoplasm discovered on colonoscopy.[14]

Benign anorectal causes

Benign anorectal conditions are responsible for up to 80% of all minor overt rectal bleeds.[15]

The current theory as to the cause of bleeding from haemorrhoids is that they arise from a breakdown of the connective tissue and smooth muscle within the submucosal anal cushions that normally supports the vascular tissue found in these cushions.[16] The vascular tissue in the anal cushions is rich in arteriovenous anastomoses, thus explaining why the bleeding is bright red.[17] Bleeding from haemorrhoids is usually noticed on the toilet paper, in the toilet bowl or as streaks on the faeces. Rarely it can be acute massive but more usually it is chronic intermittent. Bleeding should never be accepted as coming from haemorrhoids until more serious disease has been considered and excluded.

Anal fissures are probably the most common anorectal disorder after haemorrhoids. Their pathogenesis is hotly debated, but current thought suggests that a tear develops after trauma, usually from a hard stool. If the internal sphincter responds to the tear with increasing tone then ischaemia develops, which frustrates repair.[18] Most patients with an anal fissure have anal pain and bleeding associated with defaecation.

A variety of other minor anorectal conditions can present with bleeding, for example fistula-in-ano, rectal prolapse, and severe pruritis ani.

Inflammatory bowel disease

Rectal bleeding as a significant symptom occurs in almost all patients with ulcerative colitis or non-specific colitis, and in about 24% of patients with Crohn's disease.[19 20] However, significant morbidity from lower gastrointestinal bleeding occurs in far fewer patients. Rovert and colleagues from the Mount Sinai hospital in New York reported that the incidence of severe bleeding was only 1% in all patients with inflammatory bowel disease (ulcerative colitis 1·4%, Crohn's disease 1·3%).[21] Although rare, acute massive bleeding does occur: in ulcerative colitis when the clinical situation is becoming fulminant, and occasionally in Crohn's disease affecting the colon where it is abrupt in onset. In either case severe clinical consequences are common.[22] The cause of ulcerative colitis and Crohn's disease is entirely unknown.

Mesenteric vascular insufficiency

There are many causes of vascular compromise in the lower gastrointestinal tract, but all have the final effect of rendering the bowel ischaemic. Pain is the most common symptom of mesenteric vascular insufficiency, occurring in 75–98% of patients,[23] but many patients present with rectal bleeding which in 75% is occult.[23]

In mesenteric arterial embolus, most emboli come from a fibrillating atrium or a mural thrombus. An embolism should be suspected when an elderly patient with atrial fibrillation develops acute onset bloody diarrhoea with abdominal pain. The bloody diarrhoea is a late sign, usually indicating that mucosal sloughing has already occurred.[24] In mesenteric arterial thrombosis, the thrombus usually arises from a pre-existing atheromatous lesion in a critical blood vessel. The onset of symptoms is usually more insidious than in a patient with an embolus.

Of all patients with mesenteric vascular insufficiency, 5–15% are thought to have a mesenteric venous thrombosis,[25] of which the causes are many; these include cirrhosis, congestive splenomagaly, hypercoaguable states, intraperitoneal inflammation and trauma.[26] However, around 50% of cases are idiopathic.[26] The onset of symptoms is insidious, with slowly developing venous infarction. As in arterial infarction bloody diarrhoea may occur as part of the symptom complex. In three reported series 80–100% of patients presented with either overt or occult bleeding from the lower gastrointestinal tract.[26]

Nonocclusive mesenteric ischaemia is usually secondary to a stress caused by, for example, cardiac failure or hypovolaemic shock. Bleeding per rectum is occasionally the only indication that ischaemia is developing.[27] Studies in these patients reveal that splanchnic vasoconstriction is excessive.

Ischaemic colitis is a subacute mild or transient illness with colicky abdominal pain and bloody diarrhoea, although sometimes only one of these symptoms is present. Occasionally infarction will supervene. The usual causes of ischaemic colitis are similar to those responsible for the other causes of mesenteric vascular insufficiency detailed above. Around 10% of cases are the consequence of aortic surgery. Severe bleeding is rare, but when it does occur the blood passed is plum coloured. In most patients the ischaemia is a solitary event with only 5% of individuals having recurrent episodes.[28] Damage resolves spontaneously in half the patients; of the remainder, one-third develop gangrene and a perforated bowel, one-third develop a stricture after some months, and one-third develop a colitis that is difficult to separate from ulcerative colitis except that ischaemic colitis spares the rectum, is segmental and does not respond to the usual medical therapy.[28]

Radiation colitis

Radiation induces an obliterative endarteritis in the submucosal blood vessels, which leads to ulceration and fissuring in the mucosa. Typically the patient has had radiation therapy some years beforehand. Symptoms are usually typical of those found in inflammatory bowel disease, with proctitis being especially common.[29] The appearances at endoscopy are similar to those seen in ulcerative colitis. Characteristic mucosal telangiectasia occur in up to 55% of patients.[30] Blood loss is usually chronic and may be a particular problem if the colitis becomes severe.

Infectious colitis

Infectious colitis presents like inflammatory bowel disease. Numerous parasites and bacteria may cause enteritis or colitis or both, with lower gastrointestinal bleeding. *Shigella*, *Campylobacter*, *Salmonella*, and *Yersinia* spp, *Vibrio parahaemolyticus*, and *Entamoeba histolytica* can usually be identified from stool cultures. Epidemics of *Escherichia coli 0157:H7* have been reported from nursing homes,[31] where the bacterium causes an infectious haemorrhagic colitis. Pseudomembranous colitis is a complication of antibiotic treatment where the bowel becomes infected with *Clostridium difficile*. The bloody diarrhoea with which these patients present may be difficult to distinguish from that of inflammatory bowel disease, but a stool assay for *Clostridium difficile* toxin may be diagnostic.

Less common causes of bleeding per rectum

Aortoenteric fistula

An aortoenteric fistula may arise from an aneurysm, but most develop as a result of aortic surgery, usually at the proximal site of the prosthetic graft, fistulating into the third part of the duodenum. Fistulas from iliac vessels into the ileum and colon have also been reported.[32] Pathogenesis requires the development of an adhesion between the aneurysm or graft and a loop of bowel, followed by progressive erosion through the bowel wall and secondary contamination by the intestinal flora.[33] The resultant infection is thought to aggravate the necrotic process. It is thought that the most important cause of fistula development after grafting is the failure to interpose tissue between the graft suture line and the bowel.[34] Rupture is often not immediately fatal; it is usually heralded by a small bleed that may become recurrent over hours, days or weeks before a catastrophic larger bleed occurs.[34]

Portal hypertension

Occasionally some area of the gastrointestinal tract other than the gastro-oesophageal region bears the brunt of raised portal pressure. Rarely varices occur in the colon, and can lead to a life threatening haemorrhage. Colonoscopy in patients with portal hypertension reveals vascular ectasia-like lesions in up to 70%,[35] the lesions being similar to those seen in congestive gastropathy. Anorectal varices must also be considered in these patients and not confused with haemorrhoids, which are distinct from rectal varices. No direct communication exists between the anal cushions and the portal vein. Haemorrhoids and anorectal varices can co-exist in patients with portal hypertension, among whom the incidence of haemorrhoids is the same as that in controls.[36] Anorectal varices are portal-systemic collaterals that have enlarged in an attempt to decompress the portal circulation. Massive haemorrhage from such varices has been reported but is uncommon.[37] It is interesting to consider why anorectal varices are not more common than gastro-oesophageal varices, which are present in 75% of patients with anorectal varices.[38] If an enteric stoma is surgically created, varices can occur at the mucocutaneous junction.[39]

Solitary rectal ulcer syndrome

In the solitary rectal ulcer syndrome there is often a chronic benign ulceration of the anterior rectal wall, the aetiology of which is not entirely clear. The ulcer may be large or tiny but is nearly always surrounded by hyperaemic mucosa. In around 40% of cases there is no ulcer, but instead a proliferative or flat lesion (colitis cystica profunda).[40] The cause of either lesion is probably mechanical damage from a chronic rectal prolapse. However, in some cases paradoxical contraction of puborectalis muscle may be important in aetiology.[41] The usual symptoms are similar to those of a rectal tumour, with tenesmus and the passage of small amounts of blood, but occasionally bleeding may be acute massive.

Diversion colitis

Diversion colitis is being increasingly reported as a rare complication of defunctioned colon. Endoscopically and histologically it is indistinguishable from ulcerative colitis.[42] The cause may be related to deficiency of short chain fatty acids, in the defunctioned segment of bowel.[43] Putting the defunctioned segment back into circuit cures the condition.

Meckel's diverticulum

Meckel's diverticulum, a remnant of the vitelline duct, persists in around 2% of the population and is usually sited in the ileum, about 60 cm from the ileocaecal valve. Around 50% of these diverticula contain heterotopic gastric mucosa, which may produce acid that causes ulceration in the diverticulum or adjacent ileal mucosa. Bleeding, should it occur, is more common in childhood. Occasionally the bleeding is acute massive.

Vasculitides

Vasculitides that affect the lower gastrointestinal tract include polyarteritis nodosa, Henoch–Schönlein purpura, Wegener's granulomatosis, systemic lupus erythematosis (SLE), rheumatoid arthritis, Behçet's disease, giant-cell arteritis and essential mixed cryoglobulinaemia. Histologically, most have inflammation and necrosis of blood vessels in the intestinal wall. In polyarteritis nodosa vascular involvement of large vessels can lead to intestinal ischaemia and infarction.[44] Up to 50% of patients with polyarteritis nodosa and gastrointestinal symptoms have gastrointestinal bleeding.[45] In contrast, SLE vasculitis clinically affecting the bowel is uncommon, being estimated at around 2%.[46] SLE is also associated with inflammatory bowel disease.[47] Vasculitis affecting the bowel in rheumatoid arthritis is rare, but these patients can develop lower gastrointestinal bleeding as a result of bowel ulcers, colitis and infarction.[48]

Small intestinal causes

The advent of enteroscopy has resulted in an increasing number of reports of small intestinal lesions responsible for bleeding. It has been suggested that in cases of unexplained anaemia up to 38% of patients have lesions of the small bowel, often an erosion or ulcer.[49] Consumption of non-steroidal anti-inflammatory drugs increases the likelihood of lesions in the small bowel.[49] Ulceration of the small bowel may be isolated or diffuse, and the causes are many (Box 15.2). Isolated ulceration is often secondary to another disease (Box 15.2). If an ulcer cannot be linked to a specific cause, it is labelled a non-specific or idiopathic small intestinal ulcer, 78% of which are found in the ileum.[50] Idiopathic small intestinal ulcers are very rare. Most uncomplicated isolated ulcers of the small bowel heal without surgery.

Box 15.2   Causes of small intestinal ulceration (after Miller[26])

Isolated ulcers
- Crohn's disease
- NSAIDs
- Ischaemia
- Vasculitis
- Typhoid fever
- Tuberculosis
- Lymphoma
- Ulceration of heterotopic gastric mucosa
- Jejunal ulcers associated with gastrinoma
- Cytomegalovirus infection
- Diverticulitis
- Radiation injury
- Trauma
- Carcinoma

Diffuse ulcers
- Crohn's disease
- Ischaemia
- Tuberculosis
- Fungal infections
- Bacillary dysentery
- Vasculitides
- Gastrinoma
- Coeliac sprue
- Lymphoma
- Graft versus host disease
- Idiopathic chronic ulcerative enteritis

Diffuse ulceration may also be secondary to a specific disease process (Box 15.2) or idiopathic, when it is best known as idiopathic chronic ulcerative enteritis.[26] The cause of the latter is unknown and the prognosis is poor.[26]

Diverticula other than Meckel's also occur in the small intestine. More than 50 cases of acute massive bleeding have been reported from jejunal diverticula.[26] The cause of jejunal diverticula is unknown but probably multifactorial; motility disorders and smooth muscle abnormalities may play a part.[51] The diverticula are similar to those occurring in the colon in that they contain no muscle and are found at sites of blood vessel penetration of the bowel wall. Haemorrhage results when ulceration occurs into a vessel in relation to the diverticulum.

Vascular ectasias similar to those seen in the colon are the most common cause of small intestinal bleeding, according to Lewis.[52] They can present as either acute massive haemorrhage or as occult bleeding. In a large review of vascular ectasias 2·3% were found in the dudenum, 10·5% in the jejunum and 8·5% in the ileum.[53] Some authors claim an association with Meckel's diverticulum. The theory advanced by Boley *et al.*[4] to explain the pathogenesis of vascular ectasias in the colon seems less attractive as an explanation of the origin of the lesions in the small intestine. Moreover, it is not clear why these lesions should bleed at all. Spontaneous cessation of bleeding is reported to occur in 44% of patients when followed up for a mean of 13·1 months.[54] The natural history of these lesions in the small intestine is not well described.

Telangectasias differ from vascular ectasias in that they are hereditary and associated with other skin lesions. The lesions consist of dilated blood vessels in all layers of the bowel wall. Hereditary haemorrhagic telangiectasia (Osler–Weber–Rendu syndrome) is an autosomal dominant disorder that presents with gastrointestinal bleeding in 15% of patients.[55] Turner's syndrome is also associated with telangiectasias of the small intestine, but they rarely bleed in these patients. Telangiectasias of the small bowel are also reported in the CRST syndrome (calcinosis-Raynaud's phenomenon-sclerodactyly-telangiectasia).

Haemangiomas are neoplastic tumours of blood vessels that may be single or multiple. They are usually classified as cavernous, capillary or mixed and are sometimes associated with skin lesions. They can occur in the colon as well as the small intestine.

Intussusception

Intussusception occurs most often in children, with only 5–15% of cases occurring in adults. In adults most episodes are associated with some other pathology, with only 14% being idiopathic,[56] whereas in children most are idiopathic. In the adult a neoplasm is usually the cause of a colonic intussusception, whereas only one-third of intussusceptions in the small bowel are related to small bowel neoplasms.[56 57] Intussusception in adults has been reported in patients with haemophilia, during anticoagulation therapy and after bowel surgery. Most adult patients with intussusception do not pass blood unless the colon is involved.[26]

Endometriosis

Intestinal endometriosis is estimated to be present in up to 5% of women of reproductive age, but it rarely causes bleeding.[58] In 75–90% of cases the rectum or sigmoid colon is involved, but endometriosis can be found anywhere in the lower gastrointestinal tract.[59] The mechanism by which endometrial tissue arises in these ectopic sites is not clear. The intestinal mucosa is rarely involved, the usual site being on the external wall of the bowel, the lesion may swell during menstruation and rupture the mucosa of the bowel, causing rectal bleeding.[60] Symptoms are typically hind gut in nature, with rectal bleeding that may or may not be cyclical.[61]

Lower gastrointestinal bleeding in runners

Severe bleeding per rectum in long distance runners is being increasingly reported, although low grade blood loss is much more common. Up to 23% of marathon runners have evidence of lower gastrointestinal bleeding.[62] Death has even been reported after extended running. The blood loss is usually occult and self-limiting, resolving in a few days.[63] The aetiology of the bleeding is not clear but there is clinical and experimental evidence for mesenteric ischaemia: a reduction in superior mesenteric artery blood flow of up to 30–80% has been reported after strenuous exercise.[64] Colonoscopy in marathon runners has revealed hyperaemic and eroded areas of colonic mucosa.[65]

Dieulafoy's lesions

There have been at least three reports of Dieulafoy's lesions affecting the colon.[67-69] All had appearances similar to original description of Dieulafoy's lesion of the stomach. Histologically there is a large, tortuous artery leading up to a rent in mucosa with no evidence of inflammation or other pathology.[69] The cause of these lesions is unknown. Bleeding is typically acute massive. These lesions have also been described in the small intestine, where the bleeding is also typically acute massive.[70]

Visceral artery aneurysm

Visceral arterial aneurysms and pseudoaneurysms leaking into the colon are rare; if they rupture, most will bleed into the peritoneal cavity. Most visceral arterial pseudoaneurysms are caused by pancreatitis (splenic artery), biopsies or operative trauma.[71] Whatever the aetiology of the aneurysm bleeding is usually acute massive.

Brown bowel syndrome

Brown bowel syndrome is a rare condition of vitamin E deficiency in which there is deposition of lipofuscin in the smooth muscle layer, leading to muscle atrophy.[72] In some cases it is associated with coeliac disease.[73] A case report has described the complication of massive bleeding in this condition,[74] probably resulting from weakness of the walls of blood vessels within the bowel wall. This suggests the need to treat vitamin E deficiency in malabsorption states.

Cytomegalovirus colitis

Cytomegalovirus (CMV) infection is common in recipients of heart transplants and in patients with AIDS. There have been several reports of patients with colonic lesions attributed to CMV infection, and severe lower gastrointestinal bleeding from CMV ulceration of the terminal ileum has occurred in a patient with AIDS.[75] At colonoscopy an ulcerative appearance of the mucosa is the most common finding. The ulceration may be so severe as to require emergency colon resection. The precise pathogenesis of the CMV infection is not clear, but is probably related to the immunosuppressed state. Histologically all layers of the bowel wall are involved.

Miscellaneous causes

There have been reports of erosion of a pancreatic pseudocyst and pancreatic abscess into the colon presenting with lower gastrointestinal bleeding. Patients with a severe coagulopathy from whatever cause have also been reported to present with bleeding per rectum from a generalised ooze from the bowel mucosa. In the elderly, stercoral ulcers causing lower gastrointestinal bleeding are occasionally seen. These ulcers develop in constipated patients as a result of abrasion from a hard faecal mass; the commonest site is the rectosigmoid area but the ulcers have occurred in the transverse colon[76]. Massive haemorrhage from a stercoral ulcer may occur during a manual removal of the faeces[28].

Bleeding is sometimes iatrogenic after a colonoscopic polypectomy; typically, at 1–2 weeks after the polyp excision the patient is readmitted with bleeding that is occasionally severe. The cause is thought to be from sloughing at the coagulation site, and most bleeding episodes will stop spontaneously without the need for active intervention.

Juvenile polyps are occasionally a cause of chronic intermittent bleeding in children, especially during the first decade of life.[77] These lesions are considered as hamartomas and are mainly found in the distal colon and rectum. Bleeding can occasionally be massive. Similar lesions are also found as part of the Peutz–Jeghers syndrome, where they may cause chronic blood loss.

Key points

- Most lower gastrointestinal bleeding (LGIB) is colonic in origin
- Colonic vascular ectasias and diverticula are common in elderly people and common causes of LGIB
- Bleeding from ectasias is usually chronic and recurrent, but occasionally acute massive; acute bleeding usually stops spontaneously, but rebleeding is common

continued

- Bleeding from diverticula is usually acute massive and self limiting. Overt intermittent LGIB should never be attributed to diverticular disease

- A neoplasm will rarely cause acute massive LGIB but is always a possible cause of chronic intermittent bleeding, especially in the older patient

- Most minor overt rectal bleeds are caused by benign anorectal conditions, mainly haemorrhoids or anal fissures

- Rectal bleeding is a prominent symptom in inflammatory bowel disease, but rarely associated with significant morbidity

- Many patients with mesenteric vascular insufficiency present with occult LGIB

References

1 DeMarkles MP, Murphy JR. Acute lower gastrointestinal bleeding. *Med Clin N Amer* 1993;**77**:1085–1100.
2 Vinton NE. Gastrointestinal bleeding in infancy and childhood. *Gastroent Clin N Amer* 1994;**23**:93–188.
3 Reinus JF, Brandt LJ. Vascular ectasias and diverticulosis. *Gastroent Clin N Amer* 1994; **23**:1–20.
4 Boley SJ, Sammartano RJ, Adams A, *et al*. On the nature and etiology of vascular ectasias of the colon: degenerative lesions of aging. *Gastroenterology* 1977;**72**:650–60.
5 Dickstein G, Boley SJ. Severe lower gastrointestinal bleeding in the elderly. In: Najarian JS, Delaney JP, eds. *Progress in gastrointestinal surgery*. Chicago: Year Book, 1989;525.
6 Boley SJ, Dibiase A, Brandt LJ, Sammartano R. Lower gastrointestinal bleeding in the elderly. *Am J Surg* 1979;**137**:57–64.
7 Boley SJ, Brandt LJ. Vascular ectasias of the colon. *Dig Dis Sci* 1986;**31**:S6S.
8 Painter NS, Burkitt DP. Diverticular disease of the colon: a deficiency of Western civilization. *BMJ* 1971;**2**:450–4.
9 Gear JSS, Ware A, Fursdon P. Symptomless diverticular disease and intake of dietary fibre. *Lancet* 1979;**1**:511–4.
10 Cassarella WJ, Kanter IE, Seaman WB. Right sided colonic diverticula as a cause of acute rectal haemorrhage. *N Engl J Med* 1972;**286**:450–3.
11 Gennaro AR, Rosemond GP. Colonic diverticula and haemorrhage. *Dis Colon Rectum* 1973;**16**:409–15.
12 Behringer GE, Albright NL. Diverticular disease of the colon: a frequent cause of massive rectal bleeding. *Am J Surg* 1973;**125**:419–23.
13 Everett WG. Causes of lower gastrointestinal haemorrhage [letter]. *BMJ* 1992;**305**:425.
14 Guillem JG, Forde KA, Treat MR, Neugut A, Bodian CA. The impact of colonoscopy on the early detection of colonic neoplasms in patients with rectal bleeding. *Ann Surg* 1987;**206**:606–11.
15 Lawrence MA, Hooks VH, Bowden TA. Lower gastrointestinal bleeding: a systematic approach to classification and management. *Postgrad Med J* 1989;**85**:89–100.
16 Thomson WH. The nature of haemorrhoids. *Br J Surg* 1975;**62**:542–52.
17 Stelzner F, Staubesand J, Machleidt H. Das corpus cavernosum recti: die grundlate der inneren Hamorrhoiden. *Archiv für Klinische Chirurgia* 1962;**299**:302–12.
18 Motson RW, Keck JO. Pathogenesis and treatment of anal fissure. In: *Coloproctology and the pelvic floor*. Henry MM, Swash M, eds. Butterworth-Heinemann: Oxford, 1992; 394–402.
19 Farmer RG, Hawk WA, Turnbull RB. Clinical patterns in Crohn's disease. A statistical study of 615 cases. *Gastroenterology* 1975;**70**:369–70.
20 Farmer RG. Evolution of the concept of proctosigmoiditis: clinical observation. *Med Clin N Amer* 1990;**74**:91–102.
21 Robert JH, Sachar DB, Greenstein AJ. Severe haemorrhage of the lower digestive tract in inflammatory diseases of the intestines. *Helv Chir Acta* 1989;**56**:209–10.

22 Farmer RG. Lower gastrointestinal bleeding in inflammatory bowel disease. *Gastroenterol Jap* 1991;**26(suppl 3)**:93–100.
23 Boley SJ. Early diagnosis of acute mesenteric infarction. *Hosp Pract* 1981;**16**:63–71.
24 Peters JH, Reilly PM, Merine DS, *et al*. Vascular insufficiency. In: Yamada T, Alpers DH, Owyang C, *et al*, eds. *Textbook of gastroenterology*, vol 2. Philadelphia: JB Lippincott, 1991; 2188–217.
25 Grendell JH, Ockner RK. Mesenteric venous thrombosis. *Gastroenterology* 1982;**82**:358–72.
26 Miller LS, Barbarevech C, Friedman LS. Less frequent causes of lower gastrointestinal bleeding. *Gastroent Clin N Amer* 1994;**23**:21–51.
27 Brandt LJ, Boley SJ. Nonocclusive mesenteric ischaemia. *Ann Rev Med* 1991;**42**:107–17.
28 Reinus JF, Brandt LJ. Lower intestinal bleeding in the elderly. *Clin Geriat Med* 1991;7: 301–19.
29 DeCosse JJ, Rhodes RS, Wentz WB, *et al*. The natural history and management of radiation induced injury of the gastrointestinal tract. *Ann Surg* 1969;**170**:369–84.
30 Den Hartog Jager FCA, Van Haastert M, Battermann JJ, *et al*. The endoscopic spectrum of late radiation damage of the rectosigmoid colon. *Endoscopy* 1985;**17**:214–6.
31 Griffin PM, Ostroff SM, Tauze RV, *et al*. Illnesses associated with *Escherichia coli 0157: H7* infections. *Ann Intern Med* 1988;**109**:705–12.
32 Reckless JPD, McColl I, Taylor GW. Aortoenteric fistula: an uncommon complication of abdominal aortic aneurysms. *Br J Surg* 1972;**59**:458–60.
33 Busuttil RW, Rees W, Baker JD, *et al*. Pathogenesis of aortoduodenal fistula. Experimental and clinical correlates. *Surgery* 1979;**85**:1–13.
34 Kleinman LH, Towne JB, Bernard VM. A diagnostic and therapeutic approach to aortoenteric fistulas: clinical experience with twenty patients. *Surgery* 1979;**86**:868–80.
35 Kozarek RA, Botoman VA, Bredfeldt JE, *et al*. Portal colopathy: prospective study of colonoscopy in patients with portal hypertension. *Gastroenterology* 1991;**101**:1192–7.
36 Jacobs DM, Bubpick MP, Onstand GR, Hitcock CR. The relationship of haemorrhoids to portal hypertension. *Dis Colon Rectum* 1980;**23**:567–9.
37 Johansen K, Bardin J, Orloff MJ. Massive bleeding from haemorrhoidal varices in portal hypertension. *JAMA* 1980;**244**:2084–5.
38 Hosking SW, Johnson AG. Bleeding anorectal varices—a misunderstood condition. *Surgery* 1988;**104**:70–3.
39 Graeber GM, Ratner MH, Ackerman NB. Massive haemorrhage from ileostomy and colostomy stomas due to mucocutaneous varices in patients with coexisting portal hypertension. *Surgery* 1976;**79**:107–10.
40 Martin CJ, Parks TG, Biggart JD. Solitary rectal ulcer syndrome in Northern Ireland. *Br J Surg* 1981;**68**:744–7.
41 Rutter KRP. Electromyographic changes in certain pelvic floor abnormalities. *Proc R Soc Med* 1974;**104**:525–8.
42 Bosshard RT, Abel ME. Proctitis following faecal diversion. *Dis Colon Rectum* 1984;27: 605–7.
43 Agarwal WP, Schimmel EM. Diversion colitis: a nutritional deficiency syndrome? *Nutr Rev* 1989;**47**:257–61.
44. Guillevin L, Le THD, Godeau P, *et al*. Clinical findings and prognosis of polyarteritis nodosa and Church-Strauss angiitis: a study in 165 patients. *Br J Rheumatol* 1988;27: 258–64.
45 Lopez LR, Schocket AL, Stanford RE, *et al*. Gastrointestinal involvement in leukocytoclastic vasculitis and polyarteritis nodosa. *J Rhematol* 1980;7:677–84.
46 Laing TJ. Gastrointestinal vasculitis and pneumatosis intestinalis due to systemic lupus erythematosus: successful treatment with pulse intravenous cyclophosphamide. *Am J Med* 1988;**85**:555–8.
47 Kurlander DJ, Kirsner JB. The association of chronic "non-specific" inflammatory bowel disease with lumpus erythematosus. *Ann Intern Med* 1964;**60**:799–813.
48 Chaudhuri TK, Pocak JJ. Autoradiographic studies of the distribution in the stomach of Tc-99m pertechnetate. *Radiology* 1977;**123**:223–4.
49 Morris AJ, Wasson LA, McKenzie JF. Small bowel enteroscopy in undiagnosed gastrointestinal blood loss. *Gut* 1992;**33**:887–9.
50 Boydstun JS Jr, Gaffey TA, Bartholonew LG. Clinicopathologic study of nonspecific ulcers of the small intestine. *Dig Dis Sci* 1981;**26**:911–6.
51 Krishnamurthy S, Kelly M, Rohrmann C, *et al*. Jejunal diverticulosis: a heterogeneous disorder caused by a variety of abnormalities of smooth muscle or myenteric plexus. *Gastroenterology* 1983;**85**:538–47.

52 Lewis BS. Small intestinal bleeding. *Gastroenterol Clin N Amer* 1994;**23**:67–91.
53 Meyer C, Troncale F, Galloway S, *et al.* Arteriovenous malformations of the bowel: an analysis of 22 cases and a review of the literature. *Medicine* 1981;**60**:36–48.
54 Lewis BS, Salomon P, Rivera-MacMurray S, *et al.* Does hormonal therapy have any benefit for bleeding angiodysplasia? *J Clin Gastroenterol* 1992;**15**:99–103.
55 Thompson J, Salem R, Hemingway A. Specialist investigation of obscure gastrointestinal bleeding. *Gut* 1987;**28**:47–51.
56 Nagorney DM, Sarr MG, McIlrath DC. Surgical management of intussusception in the adult. *Ann Surg* 1981;**193**:230–6.
57 Murdoch RWG, Wallace JR. Adult intussusception in Glasgow 1968–74. *Br J Surg* 1977; **74**:679–80.
58 Sampler ER, Sagle GG, Hand AM. Colonic endometriosis: its clinical spectrum. *South Med J* 1984;**77**:192–4.
59 Masson JC. Present conception of endometriosis and its treatment. *Trans West Surg Assoc* 1945;**53**:35–50.
60 Levitt MD, Hodby KJ, Van Merwyk, *et al.* Cyclical rectal bleeding in colorectal endometriosis. *Aust NZ J Surg* 1989;**59**:941–3.
61 Collin GR, Russel JC. Endometriosis of the colon: its diagnosis and management. *Am Surg* 1990;**56**:275–9.
62 Schwartz A, Vanagunas A, Kamel P. Endoscopy to evaluate gastrointestinal bleeding and marathon runners. *Annuals of Internal Medicine* 1990;**113**:632–3.
63 McMahon LF, Ryan MJ, Larson D, *et al.* Occult gastrointestinal blood loss in marathon runners. *Ann Intern Med* 1984;**100**:846–7.
64 Heer M, Repond F, Many A, *et al.* Acute ischaemic colitis in a female long distance runner. *Gut* 1987;**28**:896–9.
65 Schwartz A, Vanagunas A, Kamel P. Endoscopy to evaluate gastrointestinal bleeding in marathon runners. *Ann Intern Med* 1990;**113**:632–3.
66 Barbier P, Luder P, Triller J, *et al.* Colonic hemorrhage from a solitary minute ulcer. *Gastroenterology* 1985;**88**:1065–8.
67 Ma CK, Padda H, Pace EH, *et al.* Submucosal arterial malformation of the colon with massive hemorrhage: report of a case. *Dis Colon Rectum* 1989;**32**:149–52.
68 Richards WO, Grove-Mahoney D, Williams LF. Hemorrhage from a Dieulafoy type ulcer of the colon: a new cause for lower gastrointestinal bleeding. *Am Surg* 1988;**54**:121–4.
69 Juler GL, Labitzke HG, Lamb R, *et al.* The pathogenesis of Dieulafoy's gastric erosion. *Am J Gastroenterol* 1984;**79**:195–200.
70 Matuchansky C, Babin P, Abadie JC, *et al.* Jejunal bleeding from a solitary large submucosal artery: report of two cases. *Gastroenterology* 1978;**75**:110–113.
71 Smith JA, Macleish DG, Collier NA. Aneurysms of the visceral arteries. *Aust NZ J Surg* 1989;**59**:329–34.
72 Tosser AH, Hukill PB, Spiro HM. Brown bowel syndrome. *Ann Intern Med* 1963;**22**: 872–7.
73 Stamp GW, Evans DJ. Accumulation of ceroid in smooth muscle indicates severe malabsorption and vitamin E deficiency. *J Clin Path* 1987;**40**:798–802.
74 Hurley JP, Leary R, Connelly CE, Keeling P. Massive lower gastrointestinal bleeding in association with the brown bowel syndrome. *J Roy Soc Med* 1991;**84**:437–8.
75 Evans JD, Robertson CS, Clague MB, Snow MH, Booth H. Severe lower gastrointestinal haemorrhage from cytomegalovirus ulceration of the terminal ileum in a patient with AIDS. *Eur J Surg* 1993;**159**:373–5.
76 Reinus JF, Brandt LJ. *Clinics in Geriatric Medicine.* 1991;**7**:301–19.
77 Holgersen LO, Miller RE, Zintel HA. Juvenile polyps of the colon. *Surgery* 1971;**69**: 288–93.

Part VI
Diagnosis and management of lower intestinal haemorrhage

16: Pathophysiology of bleeding lesions in the lower gastrointestinal tract

DAVID J GALLOWAY

Bleeding from the lower gastrointestinal tract is a common and often alarming symptom in the general population. Approximately one in seven of the adult population may experience the finding of a trace of blood during self cleansing after defaecation.[1] Various attempts have been made to assess how common the problem of rectal bleeding is in the community. A study of the employees in two industrial organisations in the UK would suggest that just under 12% of the sample had noted rectal bleeding in the preceding 3 months.[2] Various attempts to obtain such prevalence data elsewhere have tended to support figures in this range.[3 4] Only a small proportion of those who admitted to such symptoms sought medical advice.

Irrespective of the pattern or severity of the lower gastrointestinal bleeding, its successful and efficient management depends on a clear understanding of the source of the bleeding and a knowledge of the underlying pathophysiology. This allows the most appropriate application of available diagnostic and therapeutic modalities.

The spectrum of pathology is influenced by several factors, including age, race, co-morbidity, lifestyle and the use of medication.

Common diagnoses

In western society the commonest causes of lower gastrointestinal bleeding in adults are:

- Internal haemorrhoids
- Diverticulosis
- Colorectal neoplasia
- Inflammatory bowel disease
- Angiodysplasia.

These five diagnoses represent distinct pathological entities, each of which is associated with a different mechanism of bleeding. Other possible causes are much less common, but should enter the differential diagnosis.[5]

213

Mechanisms of bleeding

Blood vessel damage and bleeding can follow a range of microvascular injuries, such as trauma to the vascular bed from external abrasion, especially when the tissue concerned is rendered susceptible by inflammatory change. Inflammation tends to be associated with hyperaemia or angioneogenesis, which may heighten the probability of bleeding. Abnormal vessels can also be more prone to damage from within, in that their walls may be less able to withstand the internal hydrostatic pressure and thus prone to rupture. These factors can be complicated by others, which in their own right would not necessarily result in bleeding, such as the fragility seen in colorectal mucosa damaged by radiation, ischaemia or infection.

Haemorrhoids

The nature of haemorrhoids is poorly understood by both the public and the general medical community. Within the normal anal canal there are subepithelial vascular cushions of tissue; these comprise venous dilations supported by a scaffold of connective tissue that comprises smooth muscle and fibroelastic tissue. This tissue is present from early fetal life and is unusually rich in connections with other venous plexuses (superior, middle and inferior rectal venous systems) as well as true arteriovenous communications.[6] In the upper part of the anal canal, a loose network of areolar fibrous connective tissue lies deep to the subepithelial vascular cushions, while deep to the skin of the lower part there is a much more impressive layer, composed of both muscle and fibroelastic tissue. The function of the anal cushions and changes in their functional anatomy during defaecation have been reviewed,[7] but there remains a great deal of speculation as to their exact purpose and relative importance with respect to continence control and anal sensitivity. The histological appearance of the subepithelial vascular spaces in haemorrhoidectomy specimens is essentially the same as that in tissue from the normal subject. Histological abnormalities in patients with haemorrhoids include enlargement of the capillaries in the lamina propria, fragmentation of the structural connective tissue in the layer below the epithelium, hypertrophy of the smooth muscle and a degree of oedema.[8]

The many theories about the pathogenesis of haemorrhoids include engorgement, perhaps caused by straining or the effect of a bulky faecal mass impairing venous return from the anorectal region; posture; portal hypertension; chronic inflammation or infection; vascular hyperplasia; and functional disturbances of anorectal physiology during defaecation with incomplete relaxation. The explanation currently favoured is that the anal cushions become dislocated distally, and as a result the supporting framework of fibromuscular connective tissue becomes disorganised and disrupted, so that the cushions are more likely to sustain injury.

Mechanism of bleeding

Uncomplicated haemorrhoids are not associated with erosion or ulceration and the principal mechanism resulting in bleeding seems likely to be rupture of the haemorrhoid by severe congestion, the resulting high pressure overwhelming the already compromised integrity of the anal cushion. A combination of factors is likely to be active in most episodes of haemorrhoidal bleeding, with the trauma of passing constipated stool added to the congestion and inevitable increase in pressure within the vascular spaces of the anal cushions. The pressure generated by such congestion is generally short lived, and when the rectum has emptied the prevailing tonic closure of the sphincter mechanism rapidly stops the bleeding.

Pattern of blood loss

Characteristically, haemorrhoids bleed when the bowel is active. The amount of blood lost in a typical episode is usually small (2–20 ml), but occasionally a large volume loss results in hypovolaemia and a consequent threat to life. Larger bleeds occur more often in the presence of a coagulopathy. Sometimes the bleeding that arises from the internal component of a haemorrhoid remains occult, and occurs in a retrograde fashion, making it more difficult to be confident that the haemorrhoids are responsible. The blood that accumulates in the rectum has more opportunity to become desaturated and changed in colour, thereby mimicking blood from a more proximal site. Most surgeons have encountered dramatic fresh bleeding after haemorrhoidectomy and great care should be taken with haemostasis at the time of surgery.

Diverticular disease

Diverticular disease is common in western society. The typical pseudodiverticula occur when pockets of mucosa and submucosal tissue protrude through the circular muscle coat of the bowel wall. Such protrusions occur mainly at sites of entry of tiny segmental blood vessels into the colonic wall, and while diverticula often occur between the leaves of the mesentery, they are by no means confined to that territory. The rectum, at least in its extraperitoneal course, is never affected and the sigmoid and left colon usually carry the densest concentration of diverticula.

Mechanism of bleeding

The brisk bleeding that can occur in diverticular disease may follow erosion of one of the perforating vessels that traverses the colonic wall at the site of a diverticulum, and there is evidence to support this idea.[9]

Pattern of blood loss

Bleeding in diverticular disease can be dramatic and more severe than might be expected from damage to a tiny vessel, and inflammatory change may cause additional erosive or ischaemic injury to the colorectal mucosa. In clinical practice, however, it is rare to encounter significant blood loss in a patient who presents with typical diverticulitis. While it may be tempting to blame diverticular disease for intermittent small volume blood loss, detailed colonic assessment is essential to avoid missing a lesion that may not only be the real culprit but also amenable to curative treatment. Missing a more sinsister lesion can, naturally, have dire consequences.

Colorectal neoplasia

Both benign adenomata and colorectal cancers commonly cause bleeding. The more significant lesions are generally associated with alteration in the pattern of bowel function together with the passage of mucus. There is, of course, a relationship between the type and site of the neoplasm and the symptom pattern which results. Neoplastic lesions are often associated with a degree of ulceration, although even in the absence of breaks in the mucosa the configuration and friablity of such lesions make them liable to trauma from passing bowel content. Acute, large volume blood loss is unusual, but chronic blood loss can result in haemoglobin concentrations as low as 30–50 g/l. This is more likely to occur when a developing neoplasm has the opportunity to grow and bleed for many months without causing other more distressing or obvious symptoms. Characteristically lesions in the caecum and, to a lesser extent, in the right colon present in this way. Left sided tumours almost always present with some disturbance of bowel habit, and as this tended to occur rather earlier in their natural history, there is rarely an opportunity for bleeding to lead to such low haemoglobin concentrations.

Pattern of blood loss

While patients with diverticular disease will often present in surgical practice with episodes of intermittent brisk fresh bleeding, this is unusual in cases of colorectal cancer. It is much more common for the bleeding to be a less prominent symptom (in the case of right sided colon cancer, it may not even be prominent enough to come to the notice of the patient). The key to clinical diagnosis is the associated symptoms either gastrointestinal or systemic. The rarity of certain clinical diagnoses explains why confirmation of the cause of intermittent, nonspecific lower gastrointestinal bleeding requires careful colonic assessment by colonoscopy with or without double contrast radiology.

Inflammatory bowel disease

Severe rectal bleeding in inflammatory bowel disease (ulcerative colitis and Crohn's disease) is relatively uncommon. Long term observations at the Cleveland Clinic suggest that an individual patient's symptom pattern is related to the initial location of the disease.[10 11] In those with Crohn's disease any colonic involvement was strongly linked to rectal bleeding, but the symptom occurred in fewer than 25% of all the patients studied and was somewhat unpredictable. For patients with ulcerative colitis or proctitis, bleeding is a much more consistent feature. It occurs with discharge of mucus and other colonic symptoms and its severity relates to the degree of inflammatory activity and the extent of colonic involvement. Acute severe bleeding (defined as the requirement for the transfusion of four or more units of blood in a 3 week period) occurred in 9% of the Cleveland Clinic sample with continuously active ulcerative colitis, although taking all patients together (both Crohn's disease and ulcerative colitis) it was a feature in about 1%.[12]

Crohn's disease occasionally presents with massive rectal bleeding, and this has been the subject of recent reviews.[13 14]

Angiodysplasia

The true incidence of colonic angiodysplasia is difficult to guess, but it could be responsible for about 6·0% of all cases of lower gastrointestinal bleeding.[15] The natural history of the condition is poorly understood, and the difficulty in assessing the importance and significance of a finding of angiodysplasia is compounded by the identification of synchronous lesions in up to one-third of patients. For patients who have a more proximal source of bleeding, perhaps 1·2–8·0% of cases might be accounted for by small bowel angiodysplasia. It is of interest, however, that small bowel angiodysplasia is found in 30–40% of patients who present with lower gastrointestinal bleeding of obscure causes. Lesions that cause bleeding from the colon are most commonly located in the right side (see Figure 16.1). When the upper gastrointestinal tract is the source, lesions are most often in the stomach and duodenum. The cause is not known, but the apparent age-related incidence of angiodysplasia suggests that it is an acquired vascular abnormality. Associations with other conditions, notably aortic valve disease, cirrhosis, renal insufficiency and chronic pulmonary disease, have been recorded but no alleged relationship has been well defined.[15]

Pathophysiology

It could be said that the diagnosis of angiodysplasia has come of age in the past 25–30 years. The colonic form of vascular ectasia that is now known as angiodysplasia was first demonstrated angiographically in 1960.[16] Boley has postulated that partial submucosal venous holdup leads to intermittent venous hypertension in the colonic wall and dilation of veins in the submucous plexus. With time, this process of degeneration and ectasia extends to the capillary bed in the colonic mucosa; with ultimate loss of precapillary sphincter competence an arteriovenous connection

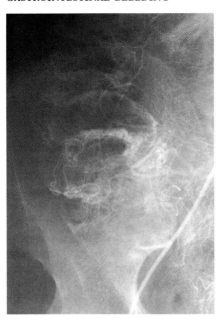

FIGURE 16.1—*A late arterial phase view showing vascular lesion in the right iliac fossa with the typical features of an abnormal aggregation of vessels together with evidence of early venous filling.*

can thus result. This theory explains the typical radiological features of angiodysplasia, that is, a tuft of submucosal vessels with early filling during the arterial phase of an angiogram, and early venous filling of larger draining veins in the locality.[17]

Mechanism of bleeding and pattern of blood loss

The pattern of bleeding varies from minor intermittent episodes to massive, life threatening loss of blood volume. It is fortunate that bleeding from an angiodysplastic lesion usually (in about 80%) stops spontaneously. The factors that trigger an angiodysplastic bleed, such as mucosal trauma or inherent vessel fragility, are a matter of speculation.[18]

A condition that shares some features of colonic angiodysplasia is portal colopathy.[19] This is associated with established portal hypertension, and patients often have other evidence of dilated portosystemic complications. A study of 20 such patients who presented with rectal bleeding indicated that the pattern was a recurring one. Colonoscopic assessment revealed multiple vascular ectasias in 14 (70%), while a smaller proportion had evidence of mild chronic colitis. While neither the severity of the portal hypertension nor the presence of stigmata of chronic liver disease were linked with the occurrence of portal colopathy, half of the patients had endoscopic evidence of congestive gastropathy.[20]

Less common diagnoses

There is of course a whole range of other conditions that characteristically present with rectal bleeding as part of the symptom complex some of which merit individual discussion.

Ischaemic colitis

Notable among the less common causes of rectal bleeding is ischaemic colitis. In presentation this condition can seem similar to colitis, with rectal bleeding, mucus and cramping abdominal pain. It can occur as a result of thrombotic or embolic occlusion of the inferior mesenteric artery, and is therefore most often seen in elderly patients with arterial disease. The mucosa of the colonic wall is the component most susceptible to ischaemic insult, and the damage can range from mild "inflammatory" changes through necrosis and ulceration (which, if it recovers spontaneously, is likely to be associated with fibrosis and luminal narrowing) to gangrenous changes in the colon that result in an abdominal catastrophe. In the less acute case of ischaemic colitis when bleeding is a feature, the cause is mucosal disintegration after hypoxic damage and subsequent oedema and attempted reconstitution of the colonic lining with granulation tissue.[21]

Infective causes

Numerous infectious conditions can result in proctitis and colitis,[22] and most can readily be distinguished by routine cultures or specific toxin measurement or both, with backup histology where appropriate. Usually the clinical differentiation of infective colitis from ulcerative colitis or Crohn's disease is not difficult, but in some circumstances diagnostic problems can arise. For example, patients who are HIV positive and immunocompromised can present particular difficulties. Widespread and fairly even inflammatory change rather suggests that ulcerative colitis is the cause. Confirmation of Crohn's disease can be more testing, because in many HIV positive patients there may be other reasons for the presence of perianal and other systemic features that often accompany the colorectal symptoms.

The prevalence of HIV infection has heightened awareness and understanding of the characteristics of intestinal infection.[23] In just under 3 years one group encountered significant gastrointestinal haemorrhage in 37 patients with AIDS. In 13 the problem lay in the upper gastrointestinal tract, while 24 patients had colorectal disease. An AIDS-associated lesion was identified as a cause of the bleeding in eight and nine, respectively, of the patients with upper and lower gastrointestinal pathology.[24] Other infectious conditions that must enter the differential diagnosis in patients presenting with diarrhoea and rectal bleeding include infection with

Clostridium difficile and *Campylobacter.* Less common causes include tuberculosis, which is much more common where this condition is endemic.[25][26]

Rare causes

Rare colorectal causes of lower gastrointestinal bleeding include the mucosal prolapse syndrome (previously known as the solitary rectal ulcer syndrome), vasculitis (associated with several different primary conditions), endometriosis, radiation induced injury and intussusception. Colonic lipomas also sometimes cause bleeding.[27] In one report most of these submucosal lesions occurred in the right colon and one-third were symptomatic. Other primary[28] and secondary tumours[29] have resulted in colonic blood loss.

Other curiosities include the rare but dramatic presentation of a vascular emergency, such as the development of an aortoenteric fistula after aortic grafting. Other vascular anomalies can also present with bleeding from the lower gut.[30]

The effect of severe or prolonged exercise on the gastrointestinal tract has been studied carefully. Gastrointestinal bleeding is not particularly common, but it is seen occasionally; it may well be the result of the relative visceral ischaemia that occurs with prolonged exercise.[31] While acute haemorrhage has been recorded, the more common outcome is that of asymptomatic blood loss that sometimes leads to microcytic anaemia.

Other extraneous influences on the colorectum should be considered. A study that set out to assess the effect of low dose warfarin or low dose aspirin, or both, found that while the use of these drugs was not associated with any major episodes of blood loss, there were more instances of rectal bleeding in men who were so treated.[32]

Noncolonic sources of rectal bleeding

An upper gastrointestinal lesion should always be considered in patients who present with massive lower gastrointestinal bleeding. Jensen and Machicado found that 11% of such patients were bleeding from an upper gastrointestinal source.[33][34]

Jejunal diverticular disease is perhaps most commonly noted as an incidental finding, but severe bleeding occasionally arises from proximal small bowel diverticula. Acquired jejunal diverticula were detected in 86 patients (27 men, 59 women, mean age 69 years) studied by a group in the south eastern United States.[35] In most cases the diagnosis was made at the time of contrast radiology to investigate abdominal symptoms (71 patients). It was made in six patients at the time of laparotomy for acute abdominal symptoms and signs, and in three during mesenteric arteriography or a radioisotope scan for massive rectal bleeding. In the remaining six the diagnosis was an incidental intraoperative finding. Surgery was indicated in 13 patients (15%), the indications being massive lower gastrointestinal bleeding in four patients, blind loop syndrome in three, small bowel obstruction in three, diverticular perforation in two, and in the remaining one, chronic abdominal pain requiring jejunal resection. In three additional patients with melaena and nine with chronic abdominal pain, jejunal diverticulosis was the only abnormality detected.

Acquired (non-Meckel's) ileal diverticular disease is even less common than the more proximal variety. Over 10 years the same group in the United States treated 21 patients (12 women, 9 men, mean age 62 years), and 13 patients had associated diverticula in another segment of the small intestine. While rectal bleeding was incidental in a few (six patients), significant rectal bleeding occurred in two.[36] Meckel's diverticulum can be associated with troublesome lower gastrointestinal bleeding, and it may be seen increasingly in patients who have immune deficiency.[37]

Small intestinal ulceration has been linked with the use of non-steroidal anti-inflammatory analgesic drugs (NSAIDs). It has long been accepted that these drugs can irritate the gastric mucosa and cause bleeding. A post-mortem study was made of 713 patients, of whom 249 had had NSAIDs prescribed during the 6 months before death. In each case the stomach, duodenum, and small intestine was carefully examined. Gastric or duodenal ulcers were found in 54 (21·7%) of the patients who used these drugs and 57 (12·3%) of those who had not—a highly significant difference (p<0·001). Small intestinal ulceration was encountered in 21 (8·4%) of the users and in three (0·6%) of the non-users (p<0·001). In three patients, all long term users of these agents, the cause of death was perforation of nonspecific ulcers of the small intestine.[38] The effects of NSAIDs on the colon are less well documented, but it is clear that patients who develop ulceration in the small intestine can present with rectal bleeding.[39]

Key points

Bleeding from haemorrhoids
The anal canal contains subepithelial vascular cushions supported by fibromuscular connective tissue. Distal dislocation of these cushions may disrupt the supportive framework. Haemorrhoidal bleeding probably occurs when high venous pressure, added to trauma from a hard stool, causes rupture of a dilated and unsupported vein. Bleeding usually is small in volume and stops after defaecation, but is occasionally major and life threatening

Diverticular disease
Diverticula, pockets of mucosa and submucosal tissue that protrude through the circular muscle coat of the bowel wall, develop mainly in the sigmoid and left colon. Brisk bleeding may occur from an eroded perforating vessel at the site of a diverticulum. Typical diverticulitis is rarely associated with significant blood loss

continued

Colorectal neoplasia
Benign adenomata and colorectal cancers often bleed. Chronic bleeding from lesions of the caecum and right colon may cause severe anaemia, while left-sided tumours usually present earlier with disturbance of bowel habit

Angiodysplasia
The colonic form of vascular ectasia is probably an acquired vascular abnormality

Ischaemic colitis
This results from thrombotic or embolic occlusion of the inferior mesenteric artery, usually in elderly patients with arterial disease. Ischaemic injury ranges from mild inflammation to catastrophic gangrene. Bleeding will follow less acute hypoxic damage to the colonic mucosa

Infective colitis
Distinguishing infective colitis from inflammatory bowel disease may be difficult in patients immunocompromised by HIV infection

1 Investigation of rectal bleeding [editorial]. *Lancet* 1989;**i**:195–7.
2 Silman AJ, Mitchell P, Nichols RJ *et al.* Self reported dark red bleeding as a marker comparable with occult blood testing in screening for large bowel neoplasms. *Br J Surg* 1983;**70**:721–4.
3 Chapuis PH, Goulston KJ, Dent OF, Tait AD. Predictive value of rectal bleeding in screening for rectal and sigmoid polyps. *Br Med J* 1985;**290**:1546–8.
4 Dent OF, Goulston KJ, Zubrzycki J, Chapius PH. Bowel symptoms in an apparently well population. *Dis Colon Rectum* 1986;**29**:243–7.
5 Miller LS, Barbarevech C, Friedman LS. Less frequent causes of lower gastrointestinal bleeding. *Gastroenterol Clin North Am* 1994;**23**:21–52.
6 Thomson WHF. The nature of haemorrhoids. *Br J Surg* 1975;**62**:542–52.
7 Loder PB, Kamm MA, Nicholls RJ, Phillips RKS. Haemorrhoids: pathology, pathophysiology and aetiology. *Br J Surg* 1994;**81**:946–54.
8 Silber G. Lower gastrointestinal bleeding. *Pediatr Rev* 1990;**12**:85–93.
9 McMahon AJ, Hansell DT. Clinical investigation of acute lower gastrointestinal haemorrhage. *Br J Clin Pract* 1989;**43**:334–8.
10 Farmer RG, Hawk WA, Turnbull RB. Clinical patterns in Crohn's disease. A statistical study of 615 cases. *Gastroenterology* 1975;**70**:369–70.
11 Farmer RG, Whelan G, Fazio VW. Long term follow up of patients with Crohn's disease: relationship between the clinical pattern and prognosis. *Gastroenterology* 1985;**88**:1818–25.
12 Farmer RG. Lower gastrointestinal bleeding in inflammatory bowel disease. *Gastroenterol Jap* 1991;**26**:93–100.
13 Ciccarelli O, Coley G. Massive rectal bleeding in Crohn's colitis. *Connecticut Med* 1986:**50**:301–2.
14 Smith-Behn J, Banez A, Brown T, Simon R, Lin P. Acute massive rectal bleeding as a presenting sign of Crohn's disease. *New York State J Med* 1988;**Oct–Nov 10**:545–6.
15 Foutch PG. Angiodysplasia of the gastrointestinal tract. *Am J Gastroenterol* 1993;**88**: 807–18.
16 Margulis AR, Heinbecker P, Bernard HR. Operative mesenteric arteriography in search of the site of bleeding in unexplained gastrointestinal haemorrhage. *Surgery* 1960;**48**: 534–9.
17 Boley SJ, Sammartano R, Brandt LJ, Sprayregen S. Vascular ectasias of the colon. *Surg Gynecol Obstet* 1979;**149**:353–9.
18 Helmrich GA, Stallworth JR, Brown JJ. Angiodysplasia: characterization, diagnosis, and advances in treatment. *South Med J* 1990;**83**:1450–3.
19 Kozarek RA, Botoman VA, Bredfeldt JE, Roach JM, Patterson DJ, Ball TJ. Portal colopathy: prospective study of colonoscopy in patients with portal hypertension. *Gastroenterology* 1991;**101**:1192–7.

20 Iredale JP, Ridings P, McGinn FP, Arthur MJ. Familial and idiopathic colonic varices: an unusual cause of lower gastrointestinal haemorrhage. *Gut* 1992;**33**:1285–8.

21 Goligher J. *Surgery of the anus, rectum and colon*, fifth ed. Eastbourne UK: Baillière Tindall 1984;1058–74.

22 Farmer RG. Infectious causes of diarrhea in the differential diagnosis of inflammatory bowel disease. *Med Clin North Am* 1990;**74**:29–38.

23 Cello JP, Wilcox CM. Evaluation and treatment of gastrointestinal tract hemorrhage in patients with AIDS. *Gastroenterol Clin North Am* 1988;**17**:639–48.

24 Evans JD, Robertson CS, Clague MB, Snow MH, Booth H. Severe lower gastrointestinal haemorrhage from cytomegalovirus ulceration of the terminal ileum in a patient with AIDS. *Eur J Surg* 1993;**159**:373–5.

25 Eboda MA, Akande B. Massive lower gastrointestinal haemorrhage from abdominal tuberculosis. *Trop Geogr Med* 1991;**43**:307–9.

26 Rais N, Plumber ST, Undre AR, Bhandarkar SD. Massive lower gastrointestinal haemorrhage as a complication of intestinal tuberculosis. *J Assn Physicians India* 1987;**35**: 647–8.

27 Hancock BJ, Vajcner A. Lipomas of the colon: a clinicopathologic review. *Can J Surg* 1988;**31**:178–81.

28 Miller GA, Borten MM. Primary carcinoid tumour of the ileum associated with massive gastrointestinal haemorrhage. *Aust NZ J Surg* 1991;**61**:645–6.

29 Gateley CA, Lewis WG, Sturdy DE. Massive lower gastrointestinal haemorrhage secondary to metastatic squamous cell carcinoma of the lung. *Br J Clin Pract* 1993;**47**:276–7.

30 Hong GS, Wong CY, Nambiar R. Massive lower gastrointestinal haemorrhage from a splenic artery pseudoaneurysm. *Br J Surg* 1992;**79**:174.

31 Moses FM. Gastrointestinal bleeding and the athlete. *Am J Gastroenterol* 1993;**88**:1157–9.

32 Meade TW. Low-dose warfarin and low-dose aspirin in the primary prevention of ischemic heart disease. *Am J Cardiol* 1990;**65**:67C–11C.

33 Jensen DM, Machicado GA. Diagnosis and treatment of severe hematochezia: the role of urgent colonoscopy after purge. *Gastroenterology* 1988;**95**:1569–74.

34 Snook JA, Holdstock GE, Bamforth J. Value of a simple biochemical ratio in distinguishing upper and lower sites of gastrointestinal haemorrhage. *Lancet* 1986;**i**:1064–5.

35 Wilcox RD, Shatney CH. Surgical implications of jejunal diverticula. *South Med J* 1988; **81**:1386–91.

36 Wilcox RD, Shatney CH. Surgical significance of acquired ileal diverticulosis. *Am Surg* 1990;**56**:222–5.

37 Patel NR, Oliva PJ, McCoy S, Soike DR, Leeper SC, Thomas E. Massive lower gastrointestinal hemorrhage in an AIDS patient: first case report of ulcerated lymphoma in a Meckel's diverticulum. *Am J Gastroenterol* 1994;**89**:133–4.

38 Allison MC, Howatson AG, Torrance CJ, Lee FD, Russell RI. Gastrointestinal damage associated with the use of nonsteroidal antiinflammatory drugs. *N Engl J Med* 1992;**327**: 749–54.

39 Varma J. Do nonsteroidal anti-inflammatory drugs cause lower gastrointestinal bleeding? A brief review. *J Am Board Fam Pract* 1989;**2**:119–22.

17: Clinical and endoscopic diagnosis of lower gastrointestinal bleeding

JOHN G LEE AND JOSEPH W LEUNG

Hemorrhage from any source along the gastrointestinal tract may present as acute lower gastrointestinal bleeding manifest by passage of bright red or maroon blood per rectum. Although such bleeding is most commonly from lesions distal to the ligament of Treitz, its cause or origin cannot be determined reliably without invasive diagnostic examinations. In 70–80% of episodes, the bleeding stops spontaneously; however, 20–25% of patients rebleed while in hospital and 50% of these patients rebleed again. Every effort must be made to determine the source of the hemorrhage before any therapeutic intervention, because the rebleeding rate, morbidity, and mortality are high after a "blind" subtotal colectomy.[1-3] Lower gastrointestinal bleeding may also present without obvious rectal bleeding or gastrointestinal symptoms; such patients complain of non-specific symptoms of chronic iron deficiency anemia. This chapter will review the clinical and endoscopic diagnosis of patients with lower gastrointestinal bleeding.

Clinical diagnosis

Blood passed per rectum may be bright red (haematochezia) or maroon, or cause melaena of varying amount and consistency. Bright red blood, especially in small amounts, usually comes from a distal colonic source, but severe haematochezia may result from a bleeding upper gastrointestinal lesion in 10–20% of patients.[4,5] Darker maroon blood or clots suggests a lesion in the more proximal colon or, rarely, small bowel. Melaena is usually seen in patients with upper gastrointestinal bleeding, but may also occur in patients with slower or intermittent lower gastrointestinal bleeding. Patients may pass more than one type of blood, because many lesions bleed intermittently and in varying intensity. It has been estimated that 80–85% of severe lower gastrointestinal bleeding is from colonic lesions,

10–15% from upper gastrointestinal lesions, and the remainder from lesions of the small bowel.[5]

Blood mixed with normal stool indicates a more proximal colonic source, while bloody diarrhoea or pyorrhoea are often associated with dysentery or inflammatory bowel disease. Typically, anorectal lesions produce haematochezia free of stool, at the end of the bowel movement, and associated with straining; often blood is noticed dripping into the toilet bowl or on the toilet paper. Patients with external haemorrhoids, fissures, or ulcers experience painful defaecation while those with internal haemorrhoids have painless bowel movements. Bleeding rectal lesions may also produce normal looking stool covered with red blood or clots. With the exception of anorectal varices, it is unusual to have heavy or prolonged bleeding, bleeding not associated with bowel movements, dark maroon blood, or melaena solely from anorectal sources. Severe lower gastrointestinal bleeding should not be attributed to anorectal sources without first examining the proximal colon and the upper gastrointestinal tract. The differing presentations of acute lower gastrointestinal bleeding are summarised in Box 17.1.

Box 17.1   Most patients with acute lower gastrointestinal bleeding seek medical attention because of rectal bleeding

- Bright red rectal bleeding (haematochezia) is usually from the distal colon or, if severe, from the upper gastrointestinal tract
- Passage of maroon blood or clots suggests a lesion in the more proximal colon, or, rarely, the small bowel
- Melaena usually indicates upper gastrointestinal bleeding, but may occur with slow or intermittent lower gastrointestinal bleeding
- Blood mixed with normal stool indicates a more proximal bleeding site
- Bloody diarrhoea or pyorrhoea suggests dysentery or inflammatory bowel disease
- Anorectal lesions typically produce haematochezia free of stool

---

Because patients with lower gastrointestinal bleeding tend to be older than those with upper gastrointestinal bleeding, its clinical presentation is more varied and complex; occult bleeding may be especially insidious, with most symptoms being related to iron deficiency anaemia. Besides fatigue, malaise, pallor, and tachycardia, pronounced iron deficiency may produce koilonychia, glossitis, and cheilitis; others complain of angina or worsening cardiac symptoms.

Gastrointestinal malignancies and angiodysplasia cause most occult bleeding, although acute, haemodynamically significant bleeding can also occur from both types of lesions. The presence of risk factors, such as a positive family history or previous colonic polyps, or symptoms such as weight loss and recent change in bowel habits or stool calibre, suggest colorectal cancer. In patients with constricting colon cancer (i.e. an "apple core" lesion) the predominent complaint may be chronic diarrhoea from stool leakage. Haematochezia is more common with distal colorectal cancers than with right sided lesions, which tend to produce occult bleeding.

In younger patients, vascular lesions are usually found as part of hereditary or congenital disorders such as the Osler–Weber–Rendu syndrome; in the elderly, most vascular lesions are a degenerative type of angiodysplasia. Angiodysplasia should be strongly suspected in patients with previous episodes of undiagnosed lower gastrointestinal bleeding. Although patients may have recurrent bleeding from multiple angiodysplasia lesions, not all episodes are clinically significant.

The presence of pain may help to determine the cause of bleeding. Patients with diverticulitis, angiodysplasia, carcinoma, or colonic ulcer usually report sudden onset of painless haematochezia, whilst those with ischaemic colitis, inflammatory bowel disease, or infectious diarrhoea generally experience some degree of abdominal pain and systemic signs such as fever. Severe abdominal pain, especially in the presence of fever, leukocytosis, tachycardia, and abdominal distention, suggests toxic megacolon or perforation and is a contraindication to colonoscopy.

Patients with colitis may present with rectal bleeding accompanied by diarrhoea or pyorrhoea. Inflammatory bowel disease should be suspected in patients with extracolonic symptoms such as arthritis or skin lesions. Colonic involvement occurs in 25% of patients with Crohn's disease. Pseudomembranous colitis should be considered in patients who have taken antibiotic drugs or had previous bouts of pseudomembranous colitis, as well as in those with underlying systemic disease such as inflammatory bowel disease and malignancy. Risk factors for ischaemic colitis include recent vascular surgery, hypotension, and cardiovascular disease. Patients with lower gastrointestinal bleeding from ischaemic colitis typically report mild to moderate, crampy abdominal discomfort 12–24 h before haematochezia.

Perhaps the only cause of lower gastrointestinal bleeding that can be diagnosed confidently from the history is postpolypectomy bleeding. Immediate bleeding results from failed haemostasis after snare polypectomy, while delayed bleeding occurs from ulceration that develop 7–10 days after snare cautery or hot biopsy. Use of non-steroidal anti-inflammatory drugs increases the risk of delayed postpolypectomy bleeding.

Every patient with lower gastrointestinal bleeding should be asked about upper gastrointestinal symptoms such as heartburn and dyspepsia, as 10–20% of lower gastrointestinal bleeding results from lesions proximal to the ligament of Treitz. Recent use of non-steroidal anti-inflammatory drugs is significantly more common in patients with either upper or lower gastrointestinal bleeding than it is in control patients.[6]

Physical examination

Physical examination is helpful for assessing the extent of bleeding but any findings are too non-specific to determine the cause. Patients who lose 15–20% of their blood volume will present with orthostatic hypotension; shock occurs after 25–35% blood loss. Patients with chronic blood loss may not show orthostatic changes, but often have signs of anemia such as pallor. The skin should be carefully inspected for stigmata of liver disease as well as presence of telangiectasia. The abdomen should be assessed for organomegaly, masses, and tenderness. Presence of rebound tenderness or guarding are relative contraindications to colonoscopy. The pitch and frequency of bowel sounds as well as any bruit should be noted. The perianal area should be inspected for fissures, haemorrhoids, masses, and fistula. Digital examination of the anorectum should be directed at identifying masses and strictures; in addition any material on the gloved examining finger should be assessed for colour, amount, consistency, presence of stool, and tested for occult blood unless obvious. Routine blood tests are not helpful in determining the cause of lower gastrointestinal bleeding, but the plasma urea/creatinine ratio can be used to separate upper from lower gastrointestinal bleeding.[7 8] In one prospective study, the plasma urea/creatinine ratio was always less than 110 in patients with lower gastrointestinal bleeding.[8]

We recommend anoscopy in every patient with lower gastrointestinal bleeding because it may yield valuable diagnostic information and can be performed easily and quickly. Internal haemorrhoids are best visualised with the patient on his or her side and performing a Valsalva manoeuvre. Presence of blood proximal to the anoscope does not preclude an anorectal source and warrants further investigation. Most patients with severe haemorrhage should have a complete examination of the colon before the bleeding is attributed to an anorectal lesion.

A nasogastric lavage must be performed in every patient with severe rectal bleeding because the consequences of missing an upper gastrointestinal tract lesion may be catastrophic. Patients in whom there is strong clinical suspicion of upper gastrointestinal bleeding should be evaluated endoscopically rather than by nasogastric lavage.

Diagnostic examinations in lower gastrointestinal bleeding

Diagnostic modalities appropriate for investigation of patients with lower gastrointestinal bleeding include radionuclide scanning, angiography, and colonoscopy. Choice of method is dictated largely by the biases of the clinician and the availability of expertise, as no one technique has been shown to be superior to another in all cases. Radionuclide scanning is best suited for patients with intermittent bleeding, because such episodes may be diagnosed by repeated scanning after the initial injection. It should be reserved for stable patients, because it cannot be performed at the bedside and has no therapeutic capabilities.

Patients with acute, hemodynamically significant bleeding should undergo either angiography or colonoscopy. Although angiography does not require colonic lavage, preparation of the angiography suite and personnel can be equally time consuming; in one study the average delay was 6 h.[9]

Bias in published studies on lower gastrointestinal bleeding

There are few well designed and executed studies on lower gastrointestinal bleeding; to our knowledge radionuclide scanning, angiography, and colonoscopy have not been compared prospectively in a scientific fashion. Most studies are selected, retrospective case series with sparse clinical follow up; some do not distinguish between haemorrhage and trivial rectal bleeding. Most data are analysed in an unblinded fashion and often such results are not verified independently. Although most studies interpret negative results as true negatives (that is, the patient stopped bleeding), this analysis may not always be correct. Consequently, it is difficult to calculate the exact sensitivity, specificity, and positive predictive value of radionuclide scanning, angiography, or colonoscopy in the diagnosis of lower gastrointestinal bleeding.

Colonoscopic diagnosis

Procedure

Emergency colonoscopy is technically successful in most patients with acute bleeding, but requires colonic lavage for optimal visualisation. Commercially available electrolyte polyethylene glycol solutions (Golytely or Colyte) are inexpensive, safe, and effective purgatives for patients with acute bleeding. We find it convenient to use the nasogastric tube (passed for lavage to rule out an upper gastrointestinal tract source) to administer the Golytely solution until the effluent is clear of gross blood and clots; further lavage delays the colonoscopy and may decrease its diagnostic sensitivity. This process is well tolerated by most patients and requires minimal nursing or patient participation. Most patients clear after 4 l of Golytely and we find that enemas are rarely necessary. Unprepared colonoscopy is rarely diagnostic and may be dangerous; we do not recommend it. The time required for colonic lavage is not significantly longer in patients with severe lower gastrointestinal bleeding and may even be shorter, because of the cathartic action of blood on the gastrointestinal tract. In our experience, some of the cleanest preparations have been in patients with severe bleeding.

Use of a large channel therapeutic colonoscope or a double channel colonoscope facilitates the endoscopic procedure. A water pik (a device which can be used for irrigation during endoscopy) is helpful in cases with active hemorrhage. Equipment for haemostasis by injection, thermocoagulation or laser photocoagulation should be readily available.

Hot biopsy may also be effective, but the unpredictable depth of injury with monopolar electrocoagulation limits its utility for haemostasis of bleeding lesions.

The colonoscopy procedure is no different from standard colonoscopy if colonic lavage has been performed properly. In patients with brisk bleeding or who have been poorly prepared, it may be necessary to turn the patient to visualise the colonic lumen. Because mucosal trauma and suction marks can mimic colonic lesions, it is advisable to note any abnormalities during the insertion of the colonoscope (Figure 17.1).

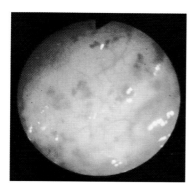 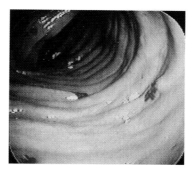

FIGURE 17.1—*(left). Clusters of non-bleeding telangiectasia were noticed in the left colon of a patient with cavernous hemangioma of the liver.*

FIGURE 17.2—*(right). Multiple, small angiodysplasia in the jejunum, observed using push enteroscopy.*

If standard colonoscopy or angiography or both fail to clarify the diagnosis and the patient continues to bleed, intraoperative colonoscopy may localise the bleeding site. An experienced gastrointestinal surgeon should first mobilise the colon and insert a catheter into the appendix for colonic irrigation. When the effluent is clear, the colonoscope is inserted into the rectum and advanced proximally under manual guidance. The ileum is cross clamped to prevent excessive small bowel insufflation. Transillumination of the colonic wall in a darkened operating room facilitates visualisation of tumours and angiodysplasia. If there is still no diagnosis, intraoperative small bowel endoscopy can be performed using a colonoscope or, preferably, an enteroscope (Figure 17.2) Both antegrade and retrograde endoscopy is possible under manual guidance.

Colonoscopic bleeding pattern

Most lesions responsible for lower gastrointestinal bleeding are easily recognised if actively bleeding during the colonoscopy, or if associated with stigmata of recent haemorrhage such as visible vessel or clot. In all other cases, only a presumptive diagnosis can be made on the basis of the colonoscopic findings. Colonoscopic investigation probably overestimates diverticulosis and angiodysplasia as causes of lower gastrointestinal bleeding because they are so common.

Active arterial bleeding may be seen with ulcers (caused by cancer, colitis, ischemia or infection), diverticulosis, and postpolypectomy bleeding. The appearance of a bleeding colonic ulcer is similar to that of upper gastrointestinal lesions. In diverticular bleeding, the bleeding vessel is usually found in the edge of the diverticulum and less often at the base. Patients with colorectal cancer (Figure 17.3), colitis (Figure 17.4), and angiodysplasia tend to have diffuse oozing without a localised bleeding point; active arterial bleeding is uncommon in absence of ulceration in such patients.

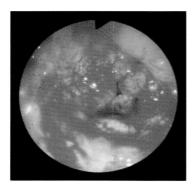 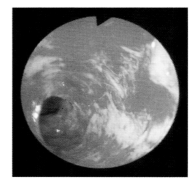

FIGURE 17.3—*(left). A concentric, stenotic colon cancer that was extremely friable and bled easily on contact. No focal bleeding point was identified.*

FIGURE 17.4—*(right). The colonic lumen appeared stenotic in this patient with lower gastrointestinal bleeding caused by ischaemic colitis. Some patients with ischaemic colitis develop colonic strictures after resolution of the acute bleeding lesion.*

Colonoscopic appearance of bleeding lesions

Anorectal lesions are uncommon causes of severe lower gastrointestinal bleeding. Anal fissures may be difficult to appreciate when using colonoscopy, but rectal pain experienced on insertion of the colonoscope is a strong indicator of anorectal disease. Anal fissures are best seen using an anoscope. Internal hemorrhoids and rectal varices can be missed during colonoscopy, unless careful examination is performed during retroflexion.

Diverticula Although more than 90% of diverticula are found in the sigmoid colon, most bleeding diverticula are right sided; approximately one-third of patients with diverticulosis have proximal colonic diverticulosis. Diverticula usually occur in clusters but multiple bleeding lesions are uncommon, as is haemorrhage in the setting of acute diverticulitis. Blood from other sources may collect in diverticula in the dependent portion of the colon, so the presence of blood alone does not establish a diagnosis of diverticular bleeding.

Angiodysplasia is characterised by a complex, frond like network of submucosal vessels with a prominent draining vein. Small lesions may be confused with trauma or suction marks and vice versa, but the presence of vascular details serves to distinguish angiodysplasia (Figure 17.5). Many patients with angiodysplasia have multiple lesions, so it is difficult to be sure of the bleeding lesion unless active haemorrhage is observed; presence of a clot is a less reliable indicator, because angiodysplasia lesions are fragile and easily traumatised.

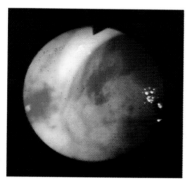 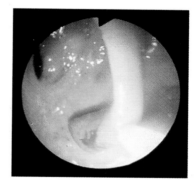

FIGURE 17.5—*(left). Two large angiodysplasia in the right colon. Notice the distinctive appearance of the fine submucosal vessels.*

FIGURE 17.6—*(right). A pedunculated polyp with slight bleeding. Severe bleeding is rare from non-malignant polyps.*

Tumours Significant bleeding (either acute or occult) from non-malignant tumours is uncommon (Figures 17.6, 17.7). Most patients with colorectal cancer experience intermittent but recurrent bleeding (Figure 17.8).

Colitis The anatomical pattern may be helpful in distinguishing between different types of colitis. Rectal disease is almost always seen in patients with ulcerative colitis, pseudomembranous colitis, and radiation colitis; in these cases a definitive diagnosis can be established without performing a complete colonoscopy. There is often a sharp demarcation between diseased and normal mucosa in patients with ischaemic colitis and ulcerative colitis, while the margin is blurred in those with other forms of colitis. Crohn's disease is characterised by skip areas of aphthous ulceration and "cobblestone" appearance.

Different forms of colitis may appear similarly endoscopically, with oedema, erythema, friability, and in severe cases purulent exudate and ulceration; however, the presence of small raised, yellowish pseudomembranes is diagnostic of pseudomembranous colitis, and that of aphthous ulcers of Crohn's disease. The absence of typical lesions does not exclude the diagnosis of pseudomembranous colitis or Crohn's disease.

231

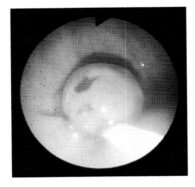 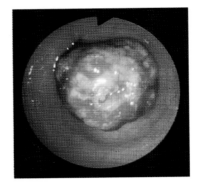

FIGURE 17.7—*(left). An adenomatous polyp with no stalk and bleeding from ulceration. Snare polypectomy successfully controlled the lower gastrointestinal bleeding.*

FIGURE 17.8—*(right). A large malignant polyp with ulceration and bleeding.*

Mucosal abnormality in radiation colitis is related to the distribution and accumulated dosage of radiation. Mucosal changes including cyanosis and oedema are often seen during radiation therapy, but significant bleeding is unusual at this time. Most bleeding occurs 6–18 months after therapy, from radiation-induced telangiectasia. In radiation colitis, unlike other forms, the mucosa appears normal except for the presence of multiple telangiectasias, most commonly in the rectum. The bleeding pattern is related to the amount of bowel irradiated as well as the accumulated dosage.

Results of colonoscopy

Caos *et al.* performed colonoscopy after Golytely preparation in 35 consecutive patients with lower gastrointestinal bleeding.[10] They found that the volume of Golytely required, the amount of residual solution in the colon, time for preparation, and the time taken to reach the caecum in patients with acute lower gastrointestinal bleeding were not significantly different from those in patients undergoing elective colonoscopy. Except for one patient with colonic stricture, all patients had satisfactory colonic lavage and underwent complete colonoscopy. Of 24 patients with an established colonoscopic diagnosis, 19 had active bleeding. Colonoscopy identified the bleeding lesion in 13 of 16 patients with severe bleeding and thermocoagulation controlled the bleeding successfully in 11 of 12 patients. Rossini *et al.* reported that carcinoma, diverticular disease, and ulcerative colitis accounted for half of all bleeding pathologies found in 311 of 409 patients with massive lower gastrointestinal haemorrhage who underwent emergency colonoscopy.[11] Jensen and Machicado studied 80 patients with severe haematochezia, initially using saline then sulphate purges.[4] Upper gastrointestinal lesions were responsible for haematochezia in 11% of cases and small bowel lesions in 9%. Although all patients were thought to have active bleeding at the time of colonoscopy, only 6 of 13 patients diagnosed with a diverticular source had active bleeding. Both colonoscopy and angiography were performed in 22 patients (order not stated); the yield of angiography was 14% with a 9% complication rate compared with 86% and 4%, respectively, for colonoscopy. Thirty nine per cent of subjects underwent endoscopic therapy but the long term success rate was not presented. A retrospective review of 58 colonoscopies performed in patients with lower gastrointestinal bleeding (25 during active haemorrhage) by Colacchio et al. showed 28 positive findings, of which 22 (85%) were in patients with active bleeding.[12] Similar to the data of Jensen and Machicado, colonoscopy was more sensitive (57% v 18%) than angiography in diagnosing the cause of bleeding among the 28 patients who underwent both examinations.

Recommendation

We believe that patients with evidence of active lower gastrointestinal bleeding (haemodynamic instability unresponsive to resuscitation, ongoing rectal bleeding, continued transfusion requirement) are best investigated using emergency colonoscopy or angiography. Radionuclide scanning is more suitable for the examination of patients with intermittent bleeding. According to available data, colonoscopy is more sensitive for identifying the bleeding lesion. Radionuclide scanning has 40–50% sensitivity in identifying ongoing bleeding, but it may not correctly localise the bleeding site. We prefer colonoscopy as the initial diagnostic approach, because it is more sensitive than angiography, it can be performed at the bedside, active bleeding is not required for a positive diagnosis (that is, stigmata of recent haemorrhage, such as visible vessel or clot), and effective haemostasis is possible with less morbidity and mortality than is associated with angiography.

Key points

- Most patients with acute lower gastrointestinal bleeding (LGIB) present with rectal bleeding
- Occult LGIB, usually caused by malignancy or angiodysplasia, often presents as iron deficiency anaemia
- LGIB accompanied by mild to moderate abdominal pain with or without fever suggests ischaemic colitis, inflammatory bowel disease, or infectious diarrhoea. Severe pain suggests toxic megacolon or perforation, and is a contraindication to colonoscopy
- Acute, haemodynamically significant LGIB warrants angiography or colonoscopy. Radionuclide scanning is best suited to stable patients with intermittent bleeding
- Unprepared colonoscopy is rarely diagnostic and may be dangerous. Colonic lavage is effective and enemas rarely necessary

---

References

1 Drapanas T, Pennington G, Kappelman M, Lindsey E. Emergency subtotal colectomy: preferred approach to management of massively bleeding diverticular disease. *Ann Surg* 1973;**177**:19–26.

2 McGuire H, Haynes B. Massive hemorrhage from diverticulosis of the colon: guidelines for therapy based on bleeding patterns observed in fifty cases. *Ann Surg* 1972;**175**:847–53.

3 Wright H, Pelliccia O, Higgins E, Sreenivas V, Gupta A. Controlled, semielective, segmental resection for massive colonic hemorrhage. *Am J Surg* 1980;**139**:535–7.

4 Jensen D, Machicado G. Diagnosis of severe hematochezia. The role of urgent colonoscopy after purge. *Gastroenterology* 1988;**95**:1569–74.

5 Levinson S, Powell D, Callahan W, *et al.* A current approach to rectal bleeding. *J Clin Gastroenterol* 1981;**3**:9–16.

6 Lanas A, Sekar M, Hirschowitz B. Objective evidence of aspirin use in both ulcer and nonulcer upper and lower gastrointestinal bleeding. *Gastroenterology* 1992;**103**:862–9.

7 Olsen L, Andreassen K. Stools containing altered blood—plasma urea:creatinine ratio as a simple test for the source of bleeding. *Br J Surg* 1991;**78**:71–3.

8 Snook J, Holdstock G, Bamforth J. Value of a simple biochemical ratio in distinguishing upper and lower sites of gastrointestinal haemorrhage. *Lancet* 1986;**1**:1064–5.

9 Browder W, Cerise E, Litwin M. Impact of emergency angiography in massive lower gastrointestinal bleeding. *Ann Surg* 1986;**204**:530–6.

10 Caos A, Benner K, Manier J, *et al.* Colonoscopy after Golytely preparation in acute rectal bleeding. *J Clin Gastroenterol* 1986;**8**:46–9.

11 Rossini F, Ferrari A, Spandre M, *et al.* Emergency colonoscopy. *World J Surg* 1989;**13**:190–2.

12 Colacchio T, Forde K, Patsos T, Nunez D. Impact of modern diagnostic methods on the management of active rectal bleeding. *Am J Surg* 1982;**143**:607–10.

18: Radiological investigation and management of lower gastrointestinal haemorrhage

JAMES E JACKSON AND DAVID J ALLISON

The choice of radiological investigation in a patient with lower gastrointestinal haemorrhage (i.e., that occurs beyond the ligament of Treitz or duodenojejunal flexure) depends upon the rate of blood loss. When bleeding is acute and life threatening, and endoscopy has failed to detect the responsible site, the patient should be referred for immediate angiography. Radiolabelled red blood cell scanning may occasionally be useful in this group of patients, but the inability of this investigation accurately to define the source of haemorrhage in most individuals means that it should generally be reserved for those in whom angiography has failed to localise the bleeding site. Barium studies have no place in the investigation of acute gastrointestinal haemorrhage. Not only are they unlikely to detect the source of bleeding but the barium within the bowel loops will seriously compromise the efficacy of any subsequent diagnostic or therapeutic procedure entailing angiography.

The approach to chronic or occult lower gastrointestinal bleeding is different. If upper and lower gastrointestinal endoscopy have failed to detect a source of bleeding then barium studies should be carried out. A barium enema will often be performed first, especially if there is a suspicion that the entire colon was not imaged at colonoscopy. The small bowel should then be investigated with an intubated study (small bowel enema). Isotope scans have little place in the investigation of this group of patients, except perhaps for the young patient in whom a Meckel's diverticulum is a more likely cause of bleeding.

Cross-sectional imaging techniques such as ultrasound and computed tomography are rarely useful in the investigation of chronic gastrointestinal bleeding. It is perhaps worthwhile performing an abdominal ultrasound study, however, before proceeding to angiography when less invasive investigations have failed to locate the source of haemorrhage. Occasionally unsuspected but relevant abnormalities will be detected (for example, liver metastases from undetected bowel primary tumour; portal, splenic or superior mesenteric venous occlusion with resultant varices; hydronephrosis caused by a desmoplastic reaction surrounding a carcinoid tumour that extends down to the root of the mesentery and involves the ureter).

The cause of gastrointestinal haemorrhage will be detected by endoscopy and these non-invasive radiological investigations in most patients with chronic blood loss. Angiography will, therefore, be required in only relatively few patients.

Diagnosis of acute bleeding

Massive haemorrhage from the lower gastrointestinal tract is most common in patients who are more than 50 years old.[1] Listed in Box 18.1 are a variety of possible causes many of which are more likely to present with chronic blood loss (for example, neoplasms of the small and large bowel, inflammatory bowel disease) but may occasionally present with an acute, life threatening bleed.

Box 18.1   Causes of massive lower gastrointestinal haemorrhage

- Diverticular disease
- Colonic angiodysplasia*
- Small bowel angiodysplasia*
- Postradiotherapy telangiectasia*
- Inflammatory bowel disease*
- Ischaemic colitis
- Infectious colitis
- Small or large bowel varices
- Colonic neoplasms*
- Small bowel neoplasms*
- Meckel's diverticulum
- Anastomotic ulcers
- Recent surgery (anastomosis or biopsy)
- Solitary rectal ulcer
- Vasculitis (e.g. Polyarteritis nodosa)
- Colorectal haemangioma
- Recent colonic polypectomy

*More commonly cause chronic blood loss

Scintigraphy

While it is our opinion (and that of others[2]) that scintigraphy is of limited value in the investigation of patients with acute lower gastrointestinal bleeding, in those centres where angiography is not available it may provide useful information to the surgeon before laparotomy.[3]

Two different scintigraphic agents are available for the investigation of patients with massive lower gastrointestinal bleeding: technetium-labelled sulphur colloid and technetium-labelled red blood cells ($^{99}Tc^m$-RBC).

Sulphur colloid

After intravenous injection, sulphur colloid is rapidly cleared from the intravascular compartment by the reticuloendothelial system; the circulation half-time in patients with normal liver function is 2·5–3·5 min.[4] Active haemorrhage (with a rate of bleeding as low as 0·05–0·1 ml/min[5]) is seen as a focus of activity away from the background uptake by the liver and spleen. Unfortunately the short circulation half-time of this agent means that detectable activity disappears from the circulation within 5–10 min of injection. Unless the patient is actively bleeding at, or soon after, the time of injection of the radioisotope, the study will be negative. Furthermore, the high background activity in the liver and spleen may obscure extravasated sulphur colloid in the right and left upper quadrants. For these reasons, scintigraphy with $^{99}Tc^m$-labelled red blood cells (RBC) is the preferred technique.[6]

$^{99}Tc^m$-RBC

After intravenous injection of the radiolabelled red blood cells, images are acquired continuously over the first 60–90 min. If there is no evidence of bleeding after this time, the patient can be re-imaged at any time over the next 24 h when active bleeding is thought to be occurring. A positive scan is seen as a focus of activity corresponding to a portion of the gastrointestinal tract, which either increases in intensity or changes in location within the gut (Figure 18.1).

Unfortunately, although this technique is more sensitive than sulphur colloid in detecting active gastrointestinal bleeding it is poor at accurately localising the source of haemorrhage, particularly if this is in the small bowel,[2] because:

- Many of the small bowel loops are superimposed, and it is often impossible to tell whether the extravasation occurred from proximal or distal loops.
- The rate of transit of intestinal contents, particularly within the jejunum, is extremely rapid. Small amounts of extravasated radioisotope from a jejunal bleeding point will often become apparent only when they have migrated to the more distal small bowel, thus giving a false impression that the bleeding occurred from this more distal site.

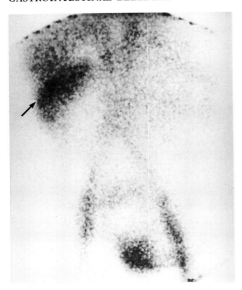

FIGURE. 18.1—$^{99}Tc^m$-labelled red blood cell scan. At 20 min after injection of the isotope the scan demonstrates a large area of increased activity overlying the hepatic flexure (arrow) indicating a diverticular bleed.

For these reasons it is our policy to proceed directly to angiography in a patient with acute gastrointestinal haemorrhage, and reserve scintigraphy for those patients in whom an angiogram has been negative. If the isotope scan demonstrates active bleeding the patient is immediately transferred to the angiography suite for a repeat arteriogram to localise the site of bleeding. Occasionally the site of bleeding will be obvious on the $^{99}Tc^m$-RBC scan, and in such cases the patient may proceed directly to surgery without a further arteriographic study.

Arteriography

The angiographic localisation of gastrointestinal bleeding relies on the detection of contrast extravasation into the bowel lumen. This is seen only in about 50–70% of patients, even when there is clinical evidence of recent active bleeding, because of the intermittent nature of blood loss. During each arteriogram the injected contrast medium will be present only for a few seconds within the vessel from which the bleeding has occurred; if there is no active bleeding during that short period, contrast extravasation will not be seen. In many patients, therefore, the angiographer has to rely on other angiographic abnormalities, which may be subtle. The most useful secondary sign is that of early venous return; this finding should prompt a more detailed study with superselective catheterisation and magnified images. Introduction of a catheter into a more selective position may provoke bleeding and contrast extravasation will then be seen.

Digital subtraction angiography is helpful, because its increased contrast resolution when compared with conventional film will make small amounts of contrast extravasation more apparent. The problems of movement artefact caused by bowel peristalsis and patient respiration may be overcome in most cases (see chapter 9).

It is difficult to determine the likely source of acute gastrointestinal bleeding on the clinical history and endoscopic findings alone. The upper gastrointestinal tract is the source of haemorrhage in up to 10% of patients with severe rectal bleeding.[7] Blood may clear rapidly from the stomach and duodenum into the more distal bowel, and a normal upper gastrointestinal endoscopy does not, therefore, exclude a bleeding point in this portion of the gut. Similarly, haematemesis may rarely occur from a bleeding point beyond the ligament of Treitz. Finally, blood from a bleeding source in the descending colon or the rectum can reflux back into the more proximal bowel and may, therefore, be seen in the right sided colon and even the terminal ileum on colonoscopy. The message for the angiographer is that a full study of all of the vessels supplying the gastrointestinal tract (inferior mesenteric artery, superior mesenteric artery, coeliac axis) is mandatory in most cases regardless of the history and endoscopic findings. Having said this, bleeding is statistically most likely to arise from a branch of the superior mesenteric artery, and it is common to study this vessel first. If no angiographic abnormality is seen the inferior mesenteric artery should be catheterised, and then the coeliac axis and its branches.

Finding a bleeding site should not stop the angiographer from completing a full "three vessel" study. The reasons for this are twofold: firstly, there may rarely be more than one source of haemorrhage; secondly, abnormalities in other vascular territories may provide clues to the cause of the gastrointestinal bleeding. For example, the findings of small intrahepatic aneurysms on the coeliac axis arteriogram in a patient with contrast extravasation from a small bowel vessel will suggest the diagnosis of polyarteritis nodosa. Similarly the finding of numerous vascular liver lesions will suggest the presence of malignant disease.

Active contrast extravasation will not be seen in up to half of patients who have had a recent acute gastrointestinal haemorrhage; nor will many of these have any other angiographic signs suggesting the likely source of bleeding. It can be useful in some of these individuals to try to provoke rebleeding by the use of a vasodilator, heparin or a thrombolytic agent injected directly into the artery (usually the superior mesenteric artery) thought most likely to be the source of haemorrhage. This "provocation" technique should not be entered into lightly as there is a risk of producing catastrophic bleeding, but it has proved useful in some patients with a history of several life threatening bleeds in whom the source of haemorrhage has not been found at previous angiography or laparotomy.[8-10] Facilities to resuscitate patients must be available if this technique is used.

Diverticular disease

In elderly patients diverticular disease is the most common cause of acute massive lower gastrointestinal haemorrhage.[11] The disease itself is characteristically worse in the left colon, but about 50% of diverticular bleeds are from the ascending colon.[12] In 80–90% of patients, the bleeding stops spontaneously, although it will recur in approximately 25%.[13] At arteriography the characteristic findings are those of contrast medium extravasation directly into the diverticulum itself, with subsequent spilling into the gut lumen (Figure 18.2).

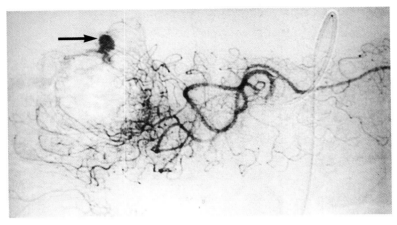

FIGURE. 18.2.—*Arteriogram of active diverticular bleeding. This selective arteriogram of the right colic/middle colic trunk demonstrates active extravasation of contrast medium into a diverticulum at the hepatic flexure (arrow).*

Angiodysplasia

Since the 1970s, colonic angiodysplasia has been recognised as a common cause of gastrointestinal bleeding.[14–18] The aetiology of this vascular abnormality is unknown, although it has been suggested that repeated intermittent, low grade obstruction to submucosal veins in the bowel wall, caused by transient elevations of intraluminal pressure, may be responsible. It has been suggested that there is an association with valvular heart disease, especially aortic stenosis.[19 20]

Angiodysplasia may be diagnosed angiographically or endoscopically. The characteristic angiographic findings (Figure 18.3) are:

- Prominent, tortuous arterial branches supplying the antimesenteric border of the caecum or the ascending colon or both
- Vascular lakes, usually lying on the antimesenteric border of the bowel
- Early, prominent and persistent venous drainage.

Identifying a site of angiodysplasia at arteriography does not (unless contrast extravasation is demonstrated, which is unusual) prove that it is the source of haemorrhage, and a full angiographic study is mandatory to exclude other disease.

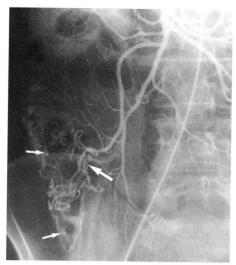

FIGURE 18.3.—*Arteriogram of caecal angiodysplasia. This superior mesenteric arteriogram shows enlarged vessels supplying the antimesenteric border of the caecum, vascular lakes (small arrows) and very early venous return (large arrow) in a florid case of angiodysplasia.*

If the patient comes to surgery, specialised injection techniques of the resected specimen can localise the angiodysplastic lesions for the histologist.[21]

Small bowel angiodysplastic lesions are less common but most are probably also acquired, as they are unusual below the age of 40 years. They are often more subtle on angiography than the colonic lesions, but are often detected because of the finding of a focal area of early venous return.

Therapy of acute bleeding

In most individuals angiography is used to localise the source of gastrointestinal haemorrhage and treatment is then surgical. A major reason for this is that the finding of contrast extravasation on angiography is non-specific and the underlying cause for the bleeding is often not apparent. Thus an acutely bleeding small bowel angiodysplastic lesion may have the same appearance as an actively bleeding avascular small bowel tumour or an area of ulceration caused by a vasculitis or inflammatory bowel disease. In some patients, however, the use of arterial embolisation or the localised infusion of vasopressin may be useful, either as a definitive treatment in cases where there is a confident diagnosis, or as a means of stabilising the patient before surgery (Figure 18.4).

Embolisation

While embolisation in the upper gastrointestinal tract is generally safe,[1 11 22–27] beyond the ligament of Treitz there is a moderately high risk

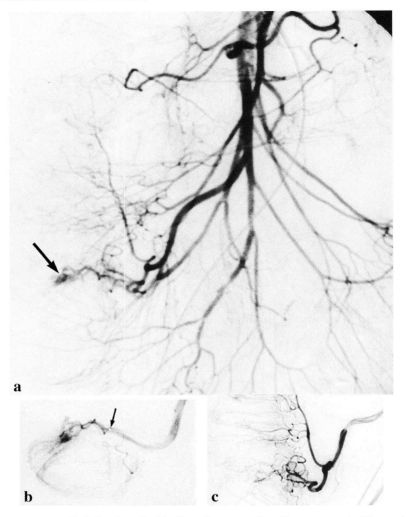

FIGURE 18.4.—*Embolisation of a bleeding ulcer at an ileocolic anastomosis. The patient had previously undergone a caecectomy.*
(a) Superior mesenteric arteriogram shows a focal area of increased vascularity (arrow) at the ileocolic anastomosis supplied by distal branches of the ileocolic artery.
(b) A coaxial 3-French catheter (which passes down the lumen of the conventional angiographic catheter) has been introduced into a distal branch of the ileocolic artery supplying the area of abnormal vascularity. The tip of the coaxial catheter is arrowed.
(c) Selective arteriogram after embolisation shows that the abnormal vascular blush has been occluded (compare with (a)). (Reproduced courtesy of Churchill Livingstone.)

of gut infarction because of the presence of a poor collateral circulation. The aim of embolisation should be to reduce the perfusion pressure to the area of contrast extravasation, thus allowing haemostasis while preserving the collateral circulation to the gut wall. Occlusion of the vasa rectae must, therefore, be avoided as these vessels do not anastomose with one another and gut infarction is likely to ensue. Embolisation may be performed with particulate agents such as polyvinyl alcohol and absorbable gelatin sponge or metallic coils (see Figure 18.4).

Vasopressin

The use of intra-arterial vasopressin to halt acute upper or lower gastrointestinal haemorrhage gained widespread acceptance in the United States in the 1970s and 1980s[11] but was never as popular in the UK and Europe. Vasopressin will often successfully control haemorrhage during the infusion itself, but rebleeding is common when the agent is discontinued and there are several serious side effects associated with its use. For example, cardiovascular complications include arrhythmia, bradycardia, hypertension, cardiac arrest, myocardial infarction, visceral infarction[28 29] and vascular occlusion at the puncture site; all have been reported and may occur in up to 43% of patients.[30] A further problem is maintaining the selective catheter position during the infusion. For these reasons the use of vasopressin has fallen out of favour in many centres. In our institution, if the patient is not a surgical candidate, intra-arterial vasopressin is no longer used and embolisation is the procedure of first choice.

Peroperative localisation of bleeding site

When a source of haemorrhage is localised to the small bowel at arteriography, the angiographer can inform the surgeon from which jejunal or ileal artery the bleeding is arising. Even so, the site of bleeding may be extremely difficult to find at surgery, despite the use of on-table enteroscopy and small bowel transillumination. It is our practice to localise the abnormality for the surgeon by introducing an angiographic catheter into the vessel supplying this area before transferring the patient to theatre. The abnormal segment of bowel is then easily delineated at the time of surgery by injecting methylene blue or fluorescein via the catheter.[31]

Investigations for chronic bleeding

Scintigraphy

Meckel's scan ($^{99}Tc^m$ pertechnetate)

While acute bleeding from a Meckel's diverticulum most commonly occurs in early childhood, presentation may be delayed until early adult life. In the young adult, therefore, who presents with acute or chronic gastrointestinal blood loss, a Meckel's scan should be performed after normal upper and lower gastrointestinal endoscopy. However, this study is not very sensitive in the adult population and detects perhaps just more than half the Meckel's diverticula. This is presumably because only 67%

of diverticula in adults who present with bleeding contain ectopic gastric mucosa,[32] compared with 95% in the paediatric population.[33] A negative scintigram should not, therefore, exclude the diagnosis.

White cell scanning

When there is a strong suspicion that the cause of chronic gastrointestinal blood loss is inflammatory or infectious bowel disease, a scan using white cells labelled with indium or technetium may be useful for determining the nature, extent and activity of the disease.[34 35]

Barium studies

Barium enema

Colonoscopy and the barium enema are complementary examinations and the choice of which to perform first will depend upon the resources available. If the entire colon is visualised at endoscopy (and the endoscopist must be confident that the caecum was reached), then the barium enema does not need to be performed. Similarly, if a good quality barium enema has been obtained in a well prepared bowel, then one can probably proceed with a small bowel study.

Abnormalities commonly detected on barium enema examination include diverticula, pedunculated or sessile polyps, carcinomas and evidence of inflammatory bowel disease.

Small bowel enema

Several studies have documented the increased sensitivity of the intubated small bowel enema, when compared with the barium follow through, for the detection of small bowel disease. This is particularly so for Meckel's diverticula,[36-38] tumours of the small bowel (leiomyomas, carcinoid tumours[39]) and inflammatory bowel disease.[40] Many relevant abnormalities may be missed on a conventional follow through examination, and the intubated small bowel study should, therefore, be the investigation of choice in the patient with chronic gastrointestinal blood loss after a normal endoscopy. We shall describe the radiological findings in a few of the more common causes of gastrointestinal bleeding.

Meckel's diverticulum[36-38] is seen radiologically as a blind-ending sac arising from the antimesenteric border of the ileum; it can vary in length from about 0·5 cm to more than 20 cm. The diverticulum may fill only transiently and it is important to use compression to separate adjacent bowel loops. A triradiate pattern of mucosal folds or a triangular plateau is sometimes present at the base of the diverticulum, and sometimes a gastric rugal pattern is seen within the diverticulum itself. Occasionally the diverticulum will become inverted and will be seen as a filling defect within the bowel lumen.

Carcinoid tumours[39] characteristically involve the terminal ileum and are often small and easily missed on a conventional small bowel follow through. On the small bowel enema they are seen as single or multiple, intramural or intraluminal filling defects. There may be stricturing of the bowel lumen and there is often acute angulation of bowel loops and valvulae and bowel wall thickening, because of a surrounding desmoplastic reaction.

Leiomyomas[41]　An intraluminal leiomyoma is seen on barium studies as a round, smooth intraluminal filling defect (Figure 18.5). It may occasionally form the apex of an intussusception (Figure 18.6). A serosal leiomyoma is seen as a mass indenting the lumen of the bowel and displacing the adjacent barium-filled bowel loops.

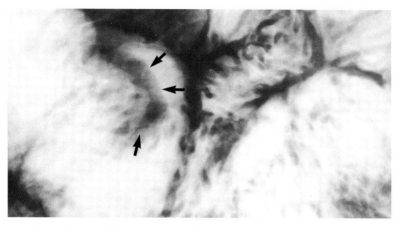

FIGURE 18.5.—*Jejunal leiomyoma on a barium examination of the small bowel. The smooth, rounded filling defect (arrows) is seen in a distal jejunal loop.*

Inflammatory bowel disease[40 42]　Crohn's disease is by far the commonest condition to involve the small bowel in industrialised countries in the northern hemisphere. The radiological signs on barium studies are many, and include ulceration with sinus and fistula formation, thickening of the bowel wall and valvulae conniventes, strictures and skip lesions.

Arteriography[21]

If scintigraphy and barium studies are negative, angiography should be performed. Contrast extravasation will not be seen in this group of patients with chronic bleeding, because of the slow rate of blood loss. The radiologist has to rely, therefore, on other angiographic abnormalities that may be subtle. These include focal areas of early venous return, areas of increased vascularity, neovascularity, vascular irregularity and aneurysm formation. Needless to say, the acquisition and interpretation of the angiographic images requires a great deal of experience and this group of patients should

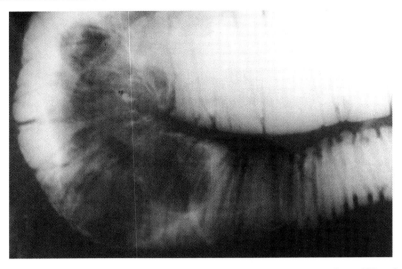

FIGURE 18.6.—*Intussuscepting leiomyoma. Small bowel enema shows a large filling defect in the distal jejunum consistent with an intussusception. This was confirmed at operation. A leiomyoma 1 cm in diameter formed the apex of the intussusceptum.*

not be investigated by the "occasional" angiographer. It is not enough, in most patients, to perform a conventional "three vessel" visceral arteriogram, in which only the inferior mesenteric artery, superior mesenteric artery and coeliac axis are selectively catheterised and studied. Superselective studies of some or all of the following arteries—jejunal, ileal, ileocolic, right colic, middle colic, splenic, common hepatic, left gastric and gastroduodenal—will be necessary in many individuals if subtle abnormalities are to be detected.

Images will be of sufficiently good quality using a digital subtraction angiographic (DSA) technique in most individuals, but this is one of the few groups of patients in which the improved spatial resolution of conventional film may be necessary to detect vascular abnormalities.

Unlike acute gastrointestinal haemorrhage, where the finding of contrast extravasation can be caused by several different pathologies, a specific diagnosis can often be suggested from the angiographic findings in chronic gastrointestinal bleeding.

Meckel's diverticulum

Most Meckel's diverticula[43–45] are supplied by a persistent vitellointestinal artery that is visualised as a long, often non-branching, vessel arising from a distal ileal artery (Figure 18.7). In some cases this vessel may be obvious on the selective superior mesenteric arteriogram, but superselective studies of the distal ileal vessels are often necessary, with oblique views, to "open up" overlapping bowel loops. Occasionally there is an area of increased vascularity within the Meckel's diverticulum itself or in the ileal loop at the base of the diverticulum, which presumably represents ectopic gastric mucosa or ulceration.

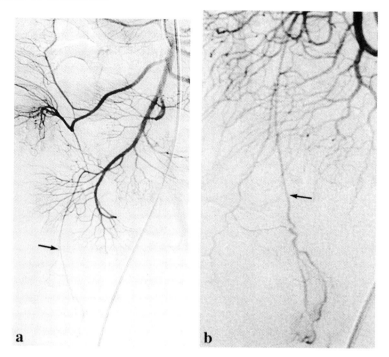

FIGURE 18.7.—*Meckel's diverticulum diagnosed by arteriography. (a) Selective superior mesenteric arteriogram demonstrates a long vessel arising from a distal ileal artery, consistent with a persistent vitellointestinal artery (arrow). (b) Superselective arteriogram with the catheter in the distal superior mesenteric artery better shows the vitellointestinal artery supplying the Meckel's diverticulum (arrow) (Reproduced courtesy of Churchill Livingstone.)*

Carcinoid tumours

Carcinoid tumours[39] have a characteristic angiographic appearance. The primary tumour itself is often hypervascular and the surrounding vessels irregular, with a "corkscrew" pattern resulting from the surrounding desmoplastic reaction. Many of the arteries may be occluded, and there is almost always occlusion of the draining veins with some resultant variceal formation. There may be vascular liver metastases.

Leiomyomas

Leiomyomas[46] are almost always hypervascular and exhibit early venous drainage. Most are well defined and rounded, although this is not invariable (Figure 18.8), and do not show the vascular irregularity and venous occlusions seen in carcinoid tumours.

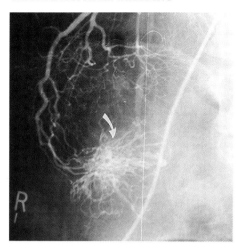

FIGURE 18.8.—*Leiomyoma in the distal ileum diagnosed by arteriography. Localised view of a superior mesenteric arteriogram shows a very vascular tumour involving the distal ileum (arrow), proven at subsequent operation to be a leiomyoma. The tumour is less well defined than is usual for these tumours.*

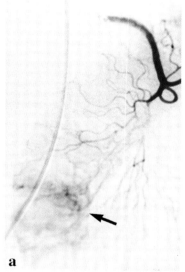

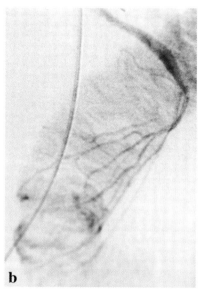

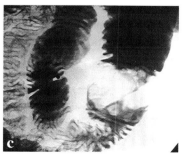

FIGURE 18.9.—*Jejunal adenocarcinoma. (a) Selective jejunal arteriogram shows an area of patchy hypervascularity within the proximal jejunum (arrow). (b) Prominent early venous return is seen from this lesion. (c) Small bowel enema shows the typical "apple-core" appearance of an adenocarcinoma in the proximal jejunum.*

Adenocarcinomas

Adenocarcinomas are usually hypovascular with areas of patchy increased tumour staining, although occasionally there is marked generalised hypervascularity. Areas of neovascularity are usually present, with vascular irregularity, but these changes may be subtle (Figure 18.9).

Conclusion

The investigation of the patient with acute or chronic lower gastrointestinal bleeding requires close liaison between physician, surgeon and radiologist. In patients with gastrointestinal haemorrhage, there should be early referral for angiography after normal endoscopy. Embolisation may be life-saving in some individuals.

Chronic gastrointestinal bleeding should be investigated initially by endoscopy and then by barium studies, Meckel's scintigraphy in children and young adults, and finally by angiography.

Key points

- If endoscopy fails to diagnose acute, life-threatening bleeding, immediate angiography is indicated

- Scintigraphy, using sulphur colloid or $^{99}Tc^m$-labelled red blood cells, can provide useful preoperative information about massive bleeding where angiography is unavailable

- For acute haemorrhage, angiography is a full "three vessel study" including the superior mesenteric artery, where bleeding is most likely, then the inferior mesenteric artery and the coeliac axis

- Angiographic localisation of acute bleeding depends on the detection of contrast extravasation into the bowel lumen. Arterial embolisation may be life saving

- If upper and lower gastrointestinal endoscopy fail to diagnose chronic or occult bleeding, barium studies should be carried out

- A barium enema commonly detects diverticula, pedunculated or sessile polyps, carcinoma and signs of inflammatory bowel disease

- Arteriography of chronic bleeding requires the detection and interpretation of subtle abnormalities and is not for the "occasional" arteriographer

---

References

1 Zuckerman DA, Bocchini TP, Birnbaum EH. Massive haemorrhage in the lower gastrointestinal tract in adults: diagnostic imaging and intervention. *Am J Roentgenol* 1993; **161**:703–11.
2 Hunter JM, Pezim ME. Limited value of technetium 99m-labelled red cell scintigraphy in localization of lower gastrointestinal bleeding. *Am J Surg* 1990;**159**:504–7.

3 Smith R, Copely DJ, Bolen FH. ^{99m}Tc RBC scintigraphy: correlation of gastrointestinal bleeding rates with scintigraphic findings. *Am J Roentgenol* 1987;**148**:869–74.

4 Alavi A. Detection of gastrointestinal bleeding with ^{99m}Tc-sulphur colloid. *Semin Nucl Med* 1982;**12**:126–38.

5 Alavi A, Dann R, Baum S, Biery DN. Scintigraphic detection of acute gastrointestinal bleeding. *Radiology* 1977;**124**:753–6.

6 Bunker SR, Lull RJ, Tanasescu DE, et al. Scintigraphy of gastrointestinal haemorrhage: superiority of ^{99m}Tc red blood cells over ^{99m}Tc sulphur colloid. *Am J Roentgenol* 1984;**143**: 543–8.

7 Boley SJ, Brandt LJ. Vascular ectasias of the colon. *Dig Dis Sci* 1986;**31**:265–425.

8 Rösch J, Keller FS, Wawrukiewicz AS, Krippaehne WW, Dotter CT. Pharmacoangiography in the diagnosis of recurrent massive lower gastrointestinal bleeding. *Radiology* 1982;**145**: 615–9.

9 Koval G, Benner KG, Rösch J, Kozak BE. Aggressive angiographic diagnosis in acute lower gastrointestinal haemorrhage. *Dig Dis Sci* 1987;**32**:248–53.

10 Glickerman DJ, Kowdley KV, Rösch J. Urokinase in gastrointestinal tract bleeding. *Radiology* 1988;**168**:375–6.

11 Athanasoulis CA, Waltman AC, Novelline RA, Krudy AG, Sniderman KW. Angiography. Its contribution to the emergency management of gastrointestinal haemorrhage. *Radiol Clin North Am* 1976;**14**:265–80.

12 Boley SJ, Brandt LJ, Frank MS. Severe lower intestinal bleeding; diagnosis and treatment. *Baillière's Clin Gastroenterol* 1981;**10**:65–91.

13 Boley SJ, Bibiase A, Brandt LJ, Sammartano R. Lower intestinal bleeding in the elderly. *Am J Surg* 1979;**137**:57–64

14 Baum S, Athanasoulis CA, Waltman AC, et al. Angiodysplasia of the right colon, a cause of gastrointestinal bleeding. *Am J Roentgenol* 1977;**129**:789–94.

15 Boley SJ, Sammartano R, Adams A, DiBiase A, Keinhaus S, Sprayregen S. On the nature and aetiology of vascular ectasias of the colon (degenerative lesions of ageing). *Gastroenterology* 1977;**72**:650–60.

16 Allison DJ. Gastrointestinal bleeding: radiological diagnosis. *Br J Hosp Med* 1980;**23**: 358–65.

17 Allison DJ, Hemingway AP, Cunningham DA. Angiography in gastrointestinal bleeding. *Lancet* 1982;**ii**:30–3.

18 Allison DJ, Hemingway AP. Colonic angiodysplasia: radiology. In: Bennett JR, Hunt RH, eds. *Therapeutic endoscopy and radiology of the gut*, 2nd ed. London: Chapman and Hall, 1990;190–8.

19 Galloway SJ, Casarela WK, Shimkin PM. Vascular malformations of the right colon as a cause of bleeding in patients with aortic stenosis. *Radiology* 1974;**113**:11–5.

20 Boss EG, Rosenbaum GM. Bleeding from the right colon associated with aortic stenosis. *Am J Dig Dis* 1971;**16**:269–75.

21 Allison DJ. Gastrointestinal angiography. In: Grainger RG, Allison DJ, eds. *Diagnostic radiology: an anglo-american textbook of imaging*, 2nd ed. Edinburgh: Churchill Livingstone, 1992;977–93.

22 Reuter SR. Embolization of gastrointestinal haemorrhage. *Am J Roentgenol* 1979;**133**: 557–8.

23 Chuang VP, Wallace S, Zornoza J, Davis LJ. Transcatheter arterial occlusion in the management of rectosigmoid bleeding. *Radiology* 1979;**133**:605–9.

24 Walker WJ, Goldin AR, Shaff MI, Allibone GW. Percatheter control of haemorrhage from the superior and inferior mesenteric arteries. *Clin Radiol* 1980;**31**:71–80.

25 Rosenkrantz H, Bookstein JJ, Rosen RJ, Goff WB, Healy JF. Postembolic colonic infarction. *Radiology* 1982;**142**:47–51.

26 Palmaz JC, Walter JF, Cho KJ. Therapeutic embolization of the small-bowel arteries. *Radiology* 1984;**152**:377–82.

27 Gomes AS, Lois JF, McCoy RD. Angiographic treatment of gastrointestinal haemorrhage: comparison of vasopressin infusion and embolization. *Am J Roentgenol* 1986;**146**:1031–7.

28 Berardi RS. Vascular complications of superior mesenteric artery infusion with pitressin in treatment of bleeding oesophageal varices. *Am J Surg* 1974;**127**:757–61.

29 Roberts C, Maddison FE. Partial mesenteric arterial occlusion with subsequent ischaemic bowel damage due to pitressin infusion. *Am J Roentgenol* 1976;**126**:829–31.

30 Conn HO, Ramsby GR, Storer EH, et al. Intra-arterial vasopressin in the treatment of upper gastrointestinal haemorrhage: a prospective, controlled clinical trial. *Gastroenterology* 1975;**68**:211–21.

31 Ohri SK, Jackson JE, Desa LA, Spencer J. The intraoperative localisation of the obscure bleeding site using fluorescein. *J Clin Gastroenterol* 1992;**14**:331–4.

32 Dixon PM, Nolan DJ. The diagnosis of Meckel's diverticulum: a continuing challenge. *Clin Radiol* 1987;**38**:615–9.

33 Rutherford RB, Akers DA. Meckel's diverticulum: a review of 148 paediatric patients, with special reference to the pattern of bleeding and to mesodiverticular vascular bands. *Surgery* 1966;**59**:618–26.

34 Roddie ME, Peters AM, Danpure HJ, *et al.* Imaging inflammation with Tc-99m HMPAO labelled leukocytes. *Radiology* 1988;**166**:767–72.

35 Peters AM, Roddie ME, Danpure HJ, *et al.* Tc-99m HMPAO labelled leucocytes: comparison with In-111 tropolonate labelled granulocytes. *Nucl Med Comm* 1988;**9**: 449–63.

36 Maglinte DDT, Elmore MF, Isenberg M, Dolan PA. Meckell's diverticulum: radiologic demonstration by enteroclysis. *Am J Roentgenol* 1980;**134**:925–32.

37 Bartram CI, Amess JA. The diagnosis of Meckel's diverticulum by small bowel enema in the investigation of obscure intestinal bleeding. *Br J Surg* 1980;**67**:417–8.

38 Salomonowitz E, Wittich G, Hajek P, Jantsch H, Czembirek H. Detection of intestinal diverticula by double-contrast small bowel enema: differentiation from other intestinal diverticula. *Gastrointest Radiol* 1983;**8**:271–8.

39 Jeffree MA, Barter SJ, Hemingway AP, Nolan DJ. Primary carcinoid tumours of the ileum: the radiological appearances. *Clin Radiol* 1984;**35**:451–5.

40 Nolan DJ, Gourtsoyiannis NC. Crohn's disease of the small intestine: a review of the radiological appearances in 100 consecutive patients examined by a barium infusion technique. *Clin Radiol* 1980;**30**:597–603.

41 Miller RE, Lehman G. Gastrointestinal haemorrhage from ileal leiomyoma. Utility of the complete reflux small bowel examination. *Gastrointest Radiol* 1978;**2**:367–9.

42 Nolan DJ. The small intestine. In: Grainger RG, Allison DJ, eds. *Diagnostic radiology: an anglo-american textbook of imaging*, 2nd ed. Edinburgh: Churchill Livingstone, 1992; 883–908.

43 Oglevie SB, Smith DC, Gardiner GA. Angiographic demonstration of bleeding in an unusually located Meckel's diverticulum simulating colonic bleeding. *Cardiovasc Intervent Radiol* 1989;**12**:210–2.

44 Routh WD, Lawdahl RB, Lund E, Garcia JH, Keller FS. Meckel's diverticula: angiographic diagnosis in patients with non-acute haemorrhage and negative scintigraphy. *Pediatr Radiol* 1990;**20**:152–6.

45 Okazaki M, Higashihara H, Saida Y, *et al.* Angiographic findings of Meckel's diverticulum: the characteristic appearance of the vitelline artery. *Abdom Imaging* 1993;**18**:15–19

46 Valls C, Sancho C, Bechini J, Dominguez J, Montana X. Intestinal leiomyomas: angiographic imaging. *Gastrointest Radiol* 1992;**17**:220–2.

19: Endoscopic haemostasis in the lower gastrointestinal tract

MICHAEL J BOURKE AND NORMAN E MARCON

The focus of this chapter will be the therapeutic approach to haemorrhage arising within the colon and rectum, with an emphasis on endoscopic modalities. Most patients with lower gastrointestinal bleeding present with either subacute or chronic rectal bleeding unaccompanied by haemodynamic compromise, or anaemia without overt gastrointestinal blood loss. These patients usually do not require admission to hospital, and can be investigated electively. The small group of patients with life threatening haematochezia accompanied by hypovolaemia require hospital admission and urgent investigation. It is upon this group that our discussion will initially centre.

The mortality rate for lower gastrointestinal haemorrhage has significantly improved over the past two decades,[1] in contrast to that of upper gastrointestinal haemorrhage which has remained static at 6–10%.[2–4] This improvement is largely attributable to new diagnostic techniques, in particular angiography, radionuclide scanning and endoscopy[1] that have allowed more effective localisation of the bleeding point[1 5 6] and obviated the need for poorly targeted empirical surgical therapy. The latter approach with a rebleeding rate of 30% and a mortality rate of 20–40%.[7–9] With the success of endoscopic haemostatis within the upper gastrointestinal tract, the challenge that now confronts the physician who deals with gastrointestinal haemorrhage is the routine provision of safe and effective endoscopic haemostasis within the lower digestive tract.

Approach to the Patient with Severe Haematochezia

Patients with severe haematochezia associated with haemodynamic compromise are most appropriately cared for in an intensive care setting. These patients are often elderly: in a series of studies involving a total of 150 patients with severe haematochezia, the mean age was 59–64·5 years.[6 10 11] Coexistent major medical and surgical illnesses are therefore common.[10] Resuscitation should proceed along the usual lines (see Chapter 6). Accurate assessment of blood loss can be confounded by the colon acting as a reservoir.[1] Fragile patients with a history of cardiopulmonary disease may require central venous monitoring, with or without measurement of pulmonary capillary wedge pressure.[12]

A detailed history and physical examination are essential, although often the site and cause of the bleeding cannot be confidently predicted from this data.[13] This is in contrast to less acute presentations of lower gastrointestinal blood loss, in which a careful history may provide a substantive clue to the location of the pathology.[14] An appreciation of the differential diagnosis pertinent to each facilitates a positive diagnosis and a provisional decision about suitable endoscopic therapy. If there is suspicion of upper gastrointestinal haemorrhage,[10 15] upper endoscopy should be performed.

Sigmoidoscopy should be performed after adequate resuscitation,[16 17] and should be regarded as a routine part of the primary assessment. Actively bleeding lesions within the rectum or anus may be identified and visualisation of the rectal mucosa may detect colitis and obviate the need for further investigation. When a bleeding lesion is present in the rectum and the sigmoidoscope can be passed above the bleeding site to where no blood is seen, the distal localisation of the bleeding site is highly accurate.[18]

Urgent colonoscopy after purge: the evidence

The choice of initial investigation in a patient with massive lower gastrointestinal haemorrhage is a matter of controversy.[16-21] The debate is compounded by the lack of a clear definition of the condition, and the wide variability of diagnostic success reported with particular techniques.[6 10 20-24] Excellent results in large series of patients have been reported with different approaches.[6 10 25 26] However, the wide variation in the severity of bleeding between various studies means that their results are not directly comparable. Consequently, published studies should be interpreted with caution. Clearly the critical factor in obtaining a good outcome is rapid and accurate localisation of the bleeding point. The choice of initial investigation rests between angiography or colonoscopy after purge, and these two investigations should be regarded as complementary rather than competitive.

Colonoscopy in severe lower gastrointestinal haemorrhage has been reported by several workers.[6 10 11 27-32] Jensen and Machicado reported their experience with 80 patients with severe haematochezia who had received a mean of 6·5 units of blood and had negative anoscopy, rigid sigmoidoscopy and nasogastric aspiration before evaluation.[10] These patients underwent emergency panendoscopy, followed by purge and colonoscopy within the intensive care unit. Using this regimen, a diagnosis was established in 94% of cases (74% colonic; 11% upper gastrointestinal; 9% small bowel—fresh blood seen emanating from the ileocaecal valve). Seventeen patients underwent both urgent angiography and emergency colonoscopy with a diagnostic yield of 12 and 82% respectively. Sixty-four percent of patients required intervention for control of bleeding. Thirty-nine percent received therapeutic endoscopy and 24% surgery. Three patients had rectal lesions diagnosed by retroflexion in the rectum; these had been missed by rigid sigmoidoscopy and anoscopy. Four patients had significant fluid overload (in three cases after saline purge); all responded promptly to medical therapy without sequelae. All of these patients had successful urgent colonoscopy, and no other complications among these 80 patients were reported. Angiography was attended by a 9% complication rate.

Caos *et al.* have reported their experience with 35 patients who presented with acute rectal bleeding and had received a mean of 4·8 units of blood before purgation with Golytely and colonoscopy.[6] A diagnosis was established in 77%, with 11 of 12 patients receiving successful endoscopic haemostasis. The mean volume of Golytely ingested for the rectum effluent to clear, the residual volume aspirated during colonoscopy, the time taken to achieve a clear effluent and the time taken to reach the caecum were compared with the same parameters in a randomly selected group of 35 patients undergoing elective colonoscopy. No significant differences were noted.

The results of other series support those discussed above, with diagnostic efficacy ranging from 70 to 90%.[11 27–30 32] There are no randomised prospective trials comparing angiography with colonoscopy after purge in the diagnosis and management of severe lower gastrointestinal haemorrhage. Cussons and Berry have reported a comparison between angiography and intraoperative colonoscopy.[33] One of the nine patients had a bleeding site localised by angiography with a mean time of 90 min for the procedure. Intraoperative colonoscopy with lavage via a caecostomy tube placed at laparotomy revealed the bleeding point in seven of these nine patients, with a mean operative time of 3 h.

Clearly, the success of emergency colonoscopy after purge or urgent angiography in severe lower gastrointestinal haemorrhage is highly dependent on the skill of the operator. However, an experienced colonoscopist should have no difficulty in intubating the caecum in well over 90% of such patients.[6 10] Endoscopic haemostasis is possible in up to 40% of patients in this setting. In the studies referred to, no attempts were made to arrest diverticular bleeding.[6 10 11 29 32] Colonoscopy equipment is portable and the procedure can be performed at the patient's bedside within the intensive care unit.[10] Colonoscopy is not limited by bleeding rates; stigmata of haemorrhage or lesions likely to be responsible for bleeding can be detected even if bleeding has ceased. In contrast, angiography requires transfer to the angiography suite and achieving a diagnosis is highly dependent on the presence of continuing active haemorrhage. A minimum bleeding rate of 0·5 ml/min is often quoted, although this figure is derived from animal studies and may not be applicable in the clinical arena.[16] We believe urgent colonoscopy after purge to be the investigation of first choice in severe lower gastrointestinal haemorrhage. Angiography should be reserved for those patients in whom colonoscopy fails to detect the source or is impossible because of truly massive haemorrhage.

Endoscopic therapy

We shall discuss the application of endoscopic therapy to diverticular bleeding, angiodysplasia and postpolypectomy haemorrhage.

Diverticular bleeding

Reports of angiographic studies suggest that most diverticular haemorrhage originates in the right colon,[3 22 23] whereas endoscopic studies have found[34 35] an approximate equal frequency of cases involving right or left colonic diverticula.[36–39]

The natural history of diverticular haemorrhage is well understood. Bleeding stops spontaneously in 75–85% of patients.[1 7 17 38] Of these patients, 20–25% will bleed again during the initial hospital admission or subsequently.[1 7 17] Unfortunately, no clinical or endoscopic factors predictive of rebleeding or continued haemorrhage have been identified. This, associated with the benign course for most of these patients, has made it difficult to adopt an aggressive interventional approach. It is clear, however, that a transfusion requirement exceeding 1500 ml in the first 24 h is associated with the need for surgical intervention.[17 41]

In several studies, each involving more than 30 patients with severe haematochezia and using colonoscopy after purge, diverticula have been positively identified as the bleeding source (on the basis of active bleeding or adherent fresh clot resistant to washing) in about 20% of all cases.[6 10 11] In these series a precise diagnosis of the bleeding site was made by emergency endoscopy in more than 75% of cases.[6 10 11] Endoscopic haemostasis was not attempted for diverticular haemorrhage in these studies, because of a lack of information about the natural history of actively bleeding colonic diverticula, and concern about possible complications from endoscopic therapy.[39] However, 25–50% of these patients required surgery for continuing haemorrhage.

The numerous small studies of endoscopic haemostasis for bleeding colonic diverticula started with Johnson and Sones in 1986.[40] Four patients, all suboptimal surgical candidates, of whom three had actively bleeding diverticula and one a "sentinel clot" at the base of a diverticulum, were treated with heater probe coagulation using a mean energy of 173 J and "modest appositional force (sufficient to tamponade bleeding)". Since then endoscopic haemostasis for diverticular haemorrhage has been reported using:

- Injection of adrenaline[37 42 43] in three patients using 1:10 000, with volumes ranging up to 16 ml,[37] and a standard sclerotherapy needle (Figure 19.1)
- Injection of fibrin sealant into a visible vessel in one patient requiring retreatment the following day, with successful haemostasis; 2 ml fibrin sealant (Tissucol) was injected on each occasion[38]
- Endoscopic haemoclip in one patient[44]

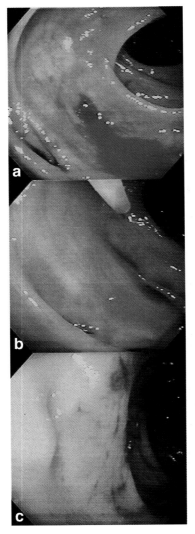

FIGURE 19.1—*(a) Active haemorrhage from a diverticulum in the hepatic flexure; (b) treated with injection of adrenalin 1 in 10 000; (c) after successful treatment.*

- Bipolar electrocoagulation in three patients, all of whom had rebled and had visible vessels at the edge of right colonic diverticula.[39] Savides and Jensen used the large, 3·2 mm gold probe with a setting of 3 or 4 on a 50 W bipolar generator, and 1–2 s pulses to achieve flattening of the visible vessel. The gold probe was preferred to other thermal devices because of its better safety profile.[39]

All case reports reveal 100% efficacy in the endoscopic control of diverticular haemorrhage.[37-39 42-44] The cumulative experience is small, however, and it is difficult to draw any firm conclusions. Thermal means of haemostasis are probably not suitable for bleeding emanating from within a diverticulum, because of the risk of perforation of the thin walled diverticular dome. Injection of adrenalin would be a safer alternative in this situation. Radiologists using aspiration biopsy techniques have revealed the safety of transgressing the colonic wall with fine needles,[45] even in the unprepared colon; although such perforation is not the goal of injection therapy, it should not be associated with serious sequelae should it occur. Injection has the advantage of being inexpensive, using highly portable equipment, unassociated with tissue damage and requiring less precision in targeting.[46] Bipolar electrocoagulation is feasible for visible vessels on the edge of diverticula.[39] Endoscopic haemoclip treatment is appealing as it is not tissue destructive.[44]

Prospective studies of the clinical parameters and endoscopic stigmata of diverticular haemorrhage are required, to clarify which patients are at an increased risk of rebleeding or continued haemorrhage necessitating surgery, and so identify which patients are likely to benefit from endoscopic haemostasis.

Angiodysplasia

Angiodysplasia or vascular ectasia of the colon were first demonstrated arteriographically in 1960.[47] In the 1970s, with the advent of selective angiography and increasing use of colonoscopy, it became apparent that angiodysplasia of the colon was as important a cause of acute lower gastrointestinal bleeding as diverticular disease.[48-51] It is now widely accepted that these two lesions account for most episodes of severe lower gastrointestinal haemorrhage.[16 17 52 53]

Angiodysplasia is a common incidental finding at colonoscopy performed for reasons unrelated to bleeding in patients over 60 years of age. The pathophysiological trigger of haemorrhage remains unknown. Haemorrhage from colonic angiodysplasia ceases spontaneously in more than 90% of cases,[52] although as most patients have recurrent bleeding and anaemia, definitive therapy to eliminate the offending lesion(s) is indicated. Colonic angiodysplasia has been identified as the source of bleeding in 10–30% of patients with severe haematochezia who received colonoscopy after purge.[6 10 11] The latter figure most likely reflects the true prevalence of this lesion in patients presenting in this manner. The patients studied by Des Marez et al.[11] were not all routinely subjected to bowel preparation, and colonic preparation must be optimal to maximise the diagnostic yield of angiodysplasia.

Endoscopic treatment of colonic angiodysplasia has been reported using various techniques including argon or Nd:YAG laser[59] monopolar[58 60-64] or multipolar[56 64] electrocoagulation and the heater probe.[56]

Laser photocoagulation

Cello and Grendell reported their experience with argon laser photocoagulation in a total of 43 patients with gastrointestinal bleeding and "vascular ectasias" in various locations, including 25 patients with lesions limited to the colon.[57] A setting of 5–7·5 W was chosen, 90% of patients required only one treatment session, and 17 of the 25 had no further bleeding during a mean follow up of 392 days. There was a significant reduction in transfusion requirement and only one major complication. An elderly man with severe steroid dependent chronic obstructive lung disease developed a caecal perforation 7 days after argon laser treatment of a large caecal ectasia; a successful segmental colectomy was performed without sequelae. Right colonic lesions were less likely to rebleed than lesions located elsewhere in the digestive tract.

Lanthier *et al.* reported a similarly successful experience with argon laser photocoagulation in 13 patients with bleeding colonic angiodysplasia as part of a series of 26 patients: the other 13 were treated with electrocoagulation.[58] During a mean follow up of 29 months, 21 patients remained symptom free after a single therapeutic procedure.

The results of neodymium:yttrium-aluminium-garnet (Nd:YAG) laser photocoagulation in the treatment of 33 patients with bleeding colonic angiodysplasia have been reported.[59] A total of 224 lesions were treated using a flexible fibre with coaxial carbon dioxide, a power setting of 65–80 W and short pulse durations of 0·5 s. The fibre tip was placed 1·5–2 cm from the tissue. The endoscopic treatment goal was complete disappearance of the vascular tissue, each pulse causing blanching of a defined area. These patients had a mean number of six lesions and 1·5 treatment sessions. During a mean follow up of 11·5 months, bleeding episodes remained significantly reduced when compared to pretreatment data. Considering the entire group of 57 evaluable patients, including 25 patients with upper tract lesions, transfusion requirement remained significantly reduced during follow up at 1, 6 and 12 months. Endoscopic follow up at 1 week revealed ulceration surrounded by a slightly raised hyperaemic zone that had healed in more than 60% at 2 weeks. Histologically, biopsies from photocoagulated colonic angiodysplasia revealed coagulation necrosis of the mucosa and part of the submucosa, with destruction of the vessels in this region.[59]

Six percent of patients suffered a colonic perforation, and the authors recommend limiting the total energy applied to each lesion to less than 200 J. It was noted that with multiple lesions, some were more likely to be missed at initial colonoscopy and hence the chance of rebleeding was increased.[59]

Electrocoagulation

Monopolar electrocoagulation using the Williams coagulation forceps[65] ("hot biopsy") has been reported in two series each involving more than 25 patients with gastrointestinal blood loss caused by colonic angiodysplasia.[61 63] The lesion may be grasped directly and pulled away from the bowel wall,[61] or it may be gripped at its margin, lifted and angled over itself before coagulation is applied.[63] Rogers used 10 W of current for 1–2 s.[61 66] Neither group reported any serious complications. Monopolar coagulation using the ball tip electrode has also been reported.[64]

Excellent results devoid of any serious complications have been presented in an abstract reporting the treatment of 20 patients who had bleeding colonic "angioma" treated with multipolar electrocoagulation using the BICAP probe[56] (Microinvasive/Boston Scientific). There was a significant reduction in bleeding episodes and a significant increase in mean haematocrit. Bipolar/multipolar electrocoagulation would appear to be safer than heater probe in the treatment of colonic angiodysplasia.[67] Unfortunately there are few clinical papers that discuss the use of bipolar/multipolar electrocoagulation in the treatment of colonic angiodysplasia; most of the work has focused on haemostatic intervention within the upper digestive tract.[68] Endoscopic band ligation of angiodysplasia has recently been reported in the upper gastrointestinal tract but no such experience has been reported for lesions in the lower tract.[69]

A review of the published experience reveals that rebleeding is most likely to occur in those patients with large (greater than 1·5 cm) or multiple lesions, and in those with a defined syndrome such as the Osler–Rendu–Weber syndrome or von Willebrand's disease.[50 54] In the latter two groups, inaccessible untreated lesions in the small bowel may account for continuing blood loss.

Therapeutic efficacy has been established for most photo- and electrocoagulation techniques,[56–59 61 63] but safety is an important consideration. Clinical data suggest that the monopolar coagulation forceps are associated with a small but significant incidence of serious complications, including bleeding and perforation.[70] This has been corroborated by canine experimental data indicating a greater frequency of transmural colonic injury and a significantly greater incidence of colonic perforations for this device when compared with bipolar/multipolar electrocoagulation or the heater probe.[71] In separate experiments, involving the same canine colon model, Nd:YAG laser treatment has been shown to result in a high incidence of transmural injury and perforation similar to that seen with the monopolar coagulation forceps.[72] In contrast, argon laser and bipolar electrocoagulation have been shown to have a safe and comparable low frequency of transmural injury when treating normal canine colonic mucosa and to be 100% effective in controlling haemorrhage from standard canine colonic ulcers.[73] Transmural histological injury and high serosal temperatures are less frequent when bipolar electrocoagulation is compared with the heater probe.[74]

Bipolar electrocoagulation has theoretical safety advantages over monopolar electrocoagulation.[68] The maximum temperature that can be generated with bipolar electrocoagulation is 100°C. As tissue temperature approaches 100°C, tissue water evaporates and tissue resistance is profoundly increased. The comparatively low output of the bipolar generator, unlike that of the monopolar device is unable to drive electrons across the desiccated tissue, effectively shutting off the bipolar probe at 100°C, and thus preventing severe transmural tissue injury.[68]

Argon plasma coagulation

A new technique that holds great promise for the provision of relatively superficial coagulation without tissue vaporisation is argon plasma coagulation.[75] High frequency electrical current is applied to the target tissue via ionised, electrically conductive argon gas. Applicators for argon plasma coagulation consist of a nozzle, through which the argon gas is applied to the tissue, and a monopolar electrode that is positioned to allow ionization of the gas between the electrode and the target tissue. The maximum depth of tissue coagulation is 2–3 mm.[76] Further evaluation of this technique in the treatment of angiodysplasia and radiation induced telangiectasia is awaited.

Doppler ultrasound

Transendoscopic Doppler ultrasound in the diagnosis and treatment of angiodysplasia was first reported by Rutgeerts et al.[77] Thirty-six lesions in the colon and 28 in the upper tract, in 10 patients, were studied using a 2·5 mm probe emitting at 7 MHz. A Doppler signal was detected in more than 75% of lesions and 100% of those larger than 5 mm. Forty-five lesions in 13 patients were then studied before and after YAG laser treatment. Three out of five patients, in whom Doppler positive lesions persisted despite laser treatment, rebled, compared with two out of eight of those in whom lesions were Doppler negative. Disappearance of the Doppler signal from a lesion was not always indicative of successful therapy, and might result from transient laser-induced oedema.[77] The Doppler device may also aid in the differentiation of angiodysplasia from traumatic lesions. Jaspersen et al., have reported success using transendoscopic Doppler (Figure 19.2) in the diagnosis and treatment (by injection of adrenalin/polidocanol) of colorectal angiodysplasia in 15 patients.[78] Good results have also been reported using endoscopic Doppler to guide endoscopic injection therapy in Forrest grade II and III peptic ulcers.[79] Transendoscopic Doppler would seem to be a useful adjunct in the diagnosis and treatment of colonic angiodysplasia, although its exact role still awaits clarification. It may prove to have an important role in determining the correct amount of energy for individual lesions (that is, the dose that obliterates the Doppler signal) and thus potentially limit complications such as perforation or the postcoagulation syndrome (serosal burn).

There are no prospective clinical trials demonstrating a clear therapeutic and safety advantage for any one endoscopic treatment of colonic angiodysplasia. However, from the experimental and theoretical information available, bipolar/multipolar electrocoagulation would appear to be the

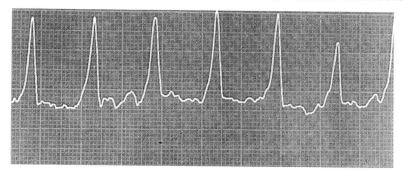

FIGURE 19.2—*Doppler-positive vascular signals from an angiodysplasia of the right colon. Reproduced with permission.*[78]

logical first choice. Its safety profile is superior to that of other modalities, and it is more economical than the argon laser (with which it shares comparable safety). It is the standard therapy for the endoscopic treatment of colonic angiodysplasia at our institution (Figure 19.3). Analogous to the recent experience with saline assisted polypectomy in the removal of sessile right colonic polyps,[80 81] the use of saline or adrenalin assisted coagulation in large (more than 15 mm) right colonic angiodysplastic lesions requires evaluation. Preinjection of such lesions with adrenalin or saline may provide a submucosal fluid cushion or heat sink, and hence limit the possibility of severe transmural injury or perforation.

Postpolypectomy haemorrhage

The incidence of postpolypectomy haemorrhage is 0·5 to 2·2%.[82–86] Haemorrhage may be immediate or delayed, even beyond 2 weeks. Delayed haemorrhage accounts for nearly two-thirds of the total.[84] The use of coagulation current at low settings has been advocated to reduce the risk of postsnare polypectomy haemorrhage,[82 83 87] but there are no clear data to support this assertion.[88] A retrospective analysis of 1485 colonic snare polypectomies revealed that blended current led to eight immediate major haemorrhages (at polypectomy or up to 12 h later) and coagulation current to six delayed bleeds (at 2–7 days).[88] Delayed haemorrhage did not occur with blended current and major immediate bleeding was not observed with coagulation current. Major delayed haemorrhage has also been reported following electrocoagulating ("hot") biopsy of diminutive colonic polyps.[89 90] Preinjection of large polyp stalks with adrenalin has been advocated to decrease the risk of postpolypectomy bleeding.[91] A detachable nylon snare (Olympus Optical, Tokyo, Japan) has also been used to prevent bleeding after the removal of large, stalked polyps.[92] The snare is placed around the base or stalk of the lesion before it is removed, and can also be used in an emergency to control unexpected bleeding from a transected stalk.

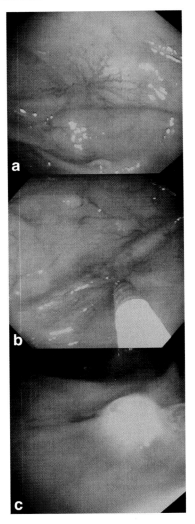

FIGURE 19.3—*Ascending colon angiodysplastic lesion (a) before (b) during and (c) after treatment with bipolar electrocoagulation.*

The control of immediate bleeding complicating polypectomy essentially involves ensnaring the residual pedicle for a further 5–10 min.[82 87 93 94] Further application of current carries the risk of shortening the residual stalk to a point at which it can no longer be grasped and should be avoided.[95] Injection of adrenalin or thermal devices may also be used.

Few studies are reported of endoscopic therapy for delayed postpolypectomy bleeding. Most such bleeding episodes are minor and self-limiting and can be managed expectantly.[83 85 94 95] Rex and colleagues have reported their experience of 29 delayed postpolypectomy bleeds.[94]

Eighteen of these patients were managed by observation alone with or without blood transfusion. One patient underwent angiography, and bleeding was successfully controlled using pitressin infusion. One patient was found to have a malignant polyp in the right colon; when the patient returned with bleeding, a right hemicolectomy was undertaken. The remaining nine patients underwent endoscopic therapy for active postpolypectomy bleeding. All but one had had sessile polyps (6 mm to 3 cm) removed, and presented with bleeding 12 hours to 12 days later. No patient received oral bowel preparation and only two received enemas; nevertheless, the bleeding site (a cautery ulcer) was identified in all cases (Figure 19.4). Six had active oozing and two active arterial haemorrhage. Endoscopic haemostasis was carried out by injection of adrenalin followed by heater probe or bipolar/multipolar electrocoagulation. The authors recommended moderate amounts of energy and only modest appositional force when using these devices in this setting.

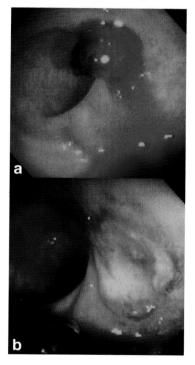

FIGURE 19.4—*(a) Active postpolypectomy bleeding from a site in the sigmoid colon; (b) after removal of the clot and injection with adrenalin 1 in 10 000, a non-bleeding cautery ulcer remains.*

Experimental work discussed earlier has indicated that there is a substantial incidence of transmural injury and, in the case of the hot biopsy forceps, perforation, when standard canine colonic ulcers are treated with bipolar/multipolar electrocoagulation or the heater probe.[72 73] A preliminary adrenalin injection may provide a heat sink or submucosal fluid cushion to prevent severe transmural injury.

Successful endoscopic haemostasis has also been reported using the endoscopic haemoclip in 24 spurting and 18 oozing colonic postpolypectomy bleeds.[44] The stainless steel clips are 6 mm long and 1·2mm wide. Reloading of the clipping device is slow, and the authors recommend having two devices on hand to avoid delay in the application of a second clip. In a series of 88 patients with bleeding from a wide range of sources, the mean number of clips applied per patient was 2·9. The distance between the clip prongs when fully open is 7 mm; it may therefore be difficult to apply a clip to a thick pedicle that is bleeding.

Successful use of suction band ligation has been reported in one patient with three bleeding polyp stalks that adrenalin injection and electrocautery had failed to control.[96] A standard polypectomy snare was used as an alternative to the shorter monofilament trip wire, which cannot transverse the full length of a colonoscope. Clip and ligation techniques are appealing, because they do not involve thermal tissue destruction. However, the application of band ligation is likely to be limited by the pliability of the cautery ulcer and surrounding tissue, as the latter must be sufficiently flexible to be aspirated into the friction fit adaptor. The need to reload the endoscope outside the patient and poor visibility add to the complexity of this technique.

Endoscopic haemostasis of postpolypectomy haemorrhage is effective and safe.[94 95] The bipolar/multipolar probe has a better safety profile than other devices and in combination with injection of adrenalin is the preferred agent. Further studies in this area are required.

Subacute and Chronic Lower Gastrointestinal Bleeding

Inoperable colorectal carcinoma, radiation proctitis, haemorrhoids and colonic angiodysplasia are the most frequent causes of subacute and chronic lower gastrointestinal bleeding that require endoscopic intervention. Angiodysplasia has been discussed earlier.

Colorectal cancer

The most appropriate treatment for colorectal cancer is segmental resection of the primary tumour. However, as many as 30% of rectosigmoid cancers are incurable at presentation because of local extension or distant metastasis.[97 98] The optimal palliative approach to these patients has yet to be defined.[98 99]

The use of laser in the palliation of rectosigmoid cancer has been widely reported.[98–108] We shall focus on the results of this treatment in the control of bleeding.

Brunetaud et al. have reported their results in the palliation of 95 patients with rectosigmoid carcinoma and abnormal rectal discharge (blood, mucus or diarrhoea).[102] A Nd:YAG laser was used at a setting of 70 W in continuous mode with 0·7 s applications at 0·3 s intervals. Exophytic portions of tumour were coagulated, not vaporised. Patients were treated twice weekly until their symptoms resolved. In 10 patients, complete destruction of an exophytic tumour smaller than 3 cm (and with a biopsy negative scar) was accomplished during a mean of 4·8 treatment sessions. These patients suffered no further bleeding. Symptomatic relief in the remaining 85 patients (with tumours larger than 3 cm) depended on the circumference of the tumour. No failures occurred in 11 patients in whom circumferential involvement by tumour was less than one-third, while 12 failures occurred in a group of 36 patients with circumferential involvement in excess of two-thirds. The mean time until improvement was 18 days, with a mean number of 2·5 treatments. Overall, 85% of patients were considered to be improved. Obstructive symptoms responded less well to laser than did other symptoms. Complications were few: one fatal colonic perforation and one perirectal abscess that resolved with medical management. No major laser induced bleeding was recorded. Brunetaud *et al.* contend that the lower complication rate in their series compared with that in others[100 109] is explained by their preference for coagulation of the tumour rather than vaporisation.

Using a vaporisation technique, Loizou *et al.* have reported similarly successful results with Nd:YAG laser in the palliation of 49 patients with rectosigmoid cancer.[105] Initial success was attained in 81% and maintained in 74% over a mean follow up of 4·8 months. A mean of 1·6 treatments over an interval of 9 days was necessary to sustain initial improvement. Median survival was only 4 months, with a 15% 1 year survival. This group also found circumferential tumour extent to be the most valuable indicator of response to laser; patients with greater than two-thirds circumferential involvement did poorly when compared with those having tumours of lesser extent. Two perforations (5%) occurred in this series; both patients had impassable carcinomas at the rectosigmoid junction and both were managed by defunctioning colostomy without sequelae. One patient developed localised peritonism with fever; no leak was detected on gastrograffin enema and the patient settled with conservative management. No other complications were reported. There was no mortality attributable to laser coagulation.

Laser coagulation compares favourably with other palliative modalities. It can be performed on an outpatient basis under minimal sedation after enema bowel preparation. Treatment significantly improves quality of life[103] and is superior to palliative resection in terms of total cost and length of inpatient stay.[104] Other non-operative palliative therapies include electrocoagulation,[110–112] external radiotherapy with or without intracavitary or interstitial irradiation,[113 114] and cryotherapy.[115] Cryotherapy is not suitable for use above the peritoneal reflection because of the risk of perforation. It is not especially effective for bleeding, with response rates of 20–50%.[115–116] Traditional surgical electrocoagulation, using a rigid sigmoidoscope, requires general anaesthesia and cannot easily be used above the peritoneal reflection; it also carries a substantial complication rate of up to 28% including a significant risk of haemorrhage.[110-112] In one study, 9% of patients required operative haemostasis for bleeding induced by electrocoagulation.[110] Radiotherapy is attended by complications in up to 20% of cases.[113] Soft tissue necrosis necessitating colostomy, fistulation and delayed haemorrhage may all occur. Radiotherapy at reduced doses may serve as a useful adjunct to laser therapy[105] but this has not been prospectively evaluated.

In general, these techniques lack the targeted specificity and predictability of endoscopically controlled laser treatment. This lack of precision results in injury to normal tissue both around and beneath the tumour.

Endoscopic bipolar/multipolar electrocoagulation and injection sclerotherapy using absolute alcohol are in clinical use for the palliation of haematochezia in inoperable rectal cancer. Their safety and efficacy have not been prospectively evaluated, and endoscopic laser therapy remains the preferred method for palliation of these patients.

Radiation proctitis

Radiation injury to the rectum and sigmoid, with recurrent bleeding and transfusion dependence, is a difficult clinical problem. The latent period from between the radiotherapy (usually for pelvic malignancy) and the onset of bleeding is often of the order of 6 to 18 months, but intervals of several decades have been reported.[117-120] Surgical management of radiation proctitis is technically difficult, and associated with considerable morbidity and substantial mortality.[121-125] Medical treatment has not been proven to be effective in controlling severe rectal bleeding.[126 127]

Successful endoscopic therapy for bleeding radiation proctitis has been reported with both Nd:YAG[128-130] and argon[131-133] laser therapy. The largest experience is that of Viggiano *et al.*, they assessed the response to Nd:YAG laser therapy in 47 patients with medically refractory haematochezia caused by radiation proctopathy, over a median follow up of 14 months.[130] These workers advocate use of the term "proctopathy" in preference to proctitis, as this lesion is associated with minimal inflammatory changes.[130] A laser setting of 40 W and maximum pulse duration of 0·5 s was used, with the aim of achieving a white coagulum with a single pulse on each individual telangiectatic lesion. Cavitation and charring were avoided. After treatment (median of two sessions, average 7950 J per session) the number of patients with daily haematochezia decreased significantly from 40 (85%) to five (11%). Twenty-three of 27 patients were no longer transfusion dependent. The median haemoglobin level improved from 97 gm/l to 117 gm/l, 3 to 6 months after treatment. Endoscopically, most telangiectasias were noted to have resolved with treatment. Three complications occurred (6%), only one of which was directly attributable to laser. This was a rectovaginal fistula which was managed with rectosigmoid resection and end sigmoid colostomy. No mortality was reported. Six patients, all of whom were transfusion dependent, were regarded as treatment failures, and tended to be women with poorly accessible sigmoid lesions.

Taylor et al. have reported experience with the argon laser in the treatment of 14 patients with daily bleeding from radiation proctitis.[133] All patients experienced improvement or cessation of haematochezia within 5 days of treatment. Ten patients required maintenance therapy for recurrent bleeding, with an average interval of 7 months between treatments. No complications were recorded during a mean follow up of 35 months. Successful control of haematochezia caused by radiation proctitis using bipolar electrocoagulation[134 135] or heater probe[134] has also been reported. During a followup period of 4 months, eight patients have had rectal bleeding caused by radiation proctitis abolished with topical formalin therapy.[136] The technique involves rigid sigmoidoscopy under caudal anaesthesia, and the topical application of gauze soaked in 4% formalin.

Laser is the most comprehensively studied of all endoscopic treatment modalities for bleeding radiation proctitis. It has proved to be highly effective and is associated with minimal morbidity.[129 130 133] Its non-contact nature allowing large areas of proctitis to be treated in a short time.[130] Argon laser has the theoretical advantage over the Nd:YAG of a smaller depth of penetration within the gut wall,[72 73] but the techniques are probably of comparably low risk in experienced hands. No prospective trials comparing the safety and efficacy of the various techniques have been conducted, but experimental data indicate that bipolar electrocoagulation and heater probe are likely to be as safe and effective as laser.[72 73] Both are more economical than laser, but the contact nature of the technique makes treatment slower and more likely to induce bleeding.[130] Despite these drawbacks, the bipolar probe is the preferred technique in our unit. Topical formalin therapy requires further evaluation.

Haemorrhoids

Haemorrhoids are the most common source of lower gastrointestinal bleeding seen in clinical gastroenterological practice. In patients over 40 years of age, other more proximal causes of bleeding should be excluded by colonoscopy before haematochezia can be safely attributed to haemorrhoids.[137] Until recently their treatment has been seen as the preserve of the surgeon, but there are several non-operative therapeutic modalities for the treatment of symptomatic internal haemorrhoids. These include cyrotherapy,[138] injection therapy (via a proctoscope[137] or flexible scope with retroflexion in the rectum[139]), infrared photocoagulation[140] laser[141] rubber band ligation,[142 143] direct current electrocoagulation[144 145] heater probe,[145] and bipolar electrocoagulation.[146]

Cryotherapy is technically cumbersome and associated with a substantial incidence of side effects, including rectal discharge and pain, that necessitate time off work.[137 138] Laser has not been widely studied, but requires local anaesthesia and is expensive in comparison with other highly effective therapies in regular use. Band ligation and injection therapy are effective and economical and widely used in clinical practice. Ligation has the advantage of removing redundant tissue; the resulting ulceration and healing attaches the remaining mucosa to the rectal wall. All but large grade 4 or very small haemorrhoids are amenable to ligation treatment. Serious pelvic and perineal sepsis in a few patients has been reported after both injection and ligation.[147 148] Despite these reports, ligation has achieved excellent results with minimal side effects in large series of patients.[140 143 149] Bat et al. have reported 512 patients who were prospectively evaluated for complications after haemorrhoidal band ligation.[149] Thirteen patients (2·5%) were admitted to hospital, half with delayed massive rectal bleeding and half with pain caused by prolapsed thrombosed haemorrhoids or urinary retention. Only one patient developed a perianal abscess (at 2 months after ligation), which was managed by surgical drainage without sequelae. Five per cent of patients suffered minor complications that did not require hospital admission; half of them had painful thrombosed haemorrhoids. The authors concluded that ligation remains a safe therapeutic approach in the treatment of symptomatic internal haemorrhoids.[149] Bleeding complicating haemorrhoid ligation can be managed endoscopically with bipolar electrocoagulation, injection of adrenalin or further band ligation.

Recent work has demonstrated the efficacy and safety of direct current and bipolar electrocoagulation.[150] Both techniques were around 90% successful in obliteration of haemorrhoids and control of bleeding, but direct current electrocoagulation was associated with greater pain and took significantly longer to perform. These newer techniques have not yet been shown to be superior to the older established therapies such as band ligation. Prospective studies comparing safety, efficacy and efficiency are required. In the meantime, suction band ligation is the non-surgical treatment of choice for symptomatic bleeding internal haemorrhoids.

Uncommon causes of lower gastrointestinal bleeding

Colonic varices are an uncommon cause of lower gastrointestinal bleeding.[151 152] They are most often located in the rectum and most episodes of bleeding arise from this area.[151 153] Definitive therapy to control bleeding has usually involved surgery,[151 154] but long term administration of octreotide has been reported.[155] The use of endoscopic therapy to control bleeding has been reported in only one instance.[156] Five percent sodium morrhuate was successfully used to arrest massive bleeding from a rectal varix. Follow up endoscopy revealed a large rectal ulcer at the site of injection, which eventually healed. The authors recommend caution when using sclerotherapy above the peritoneal reflection, because of the risk of ulceration and perforation. Although not yet reported, endoscopic variceal ligation would probably be a safer alternative.

Successful endoscopic therapy to control bleeding has been reported in one patient with haemorrhagic herpes simplex colitis, using injection of adrenalin and monopolar electrocoagulation,[157] in one patient with a Dieulafoy's lesion of the colon, using monopolar electrocoagulation,[158] and in two patients with visible vessels within solitary rectal ulcers, using the endoscopic hemoclip.[44] These are uncommon indications for endoscopic intervention.

Conclusion

In the early 1980s, studies suggested that routine early endoscopy was of no benefit in the management of patients with upper gastrointestinal tract bleeding.[159 160] However, it is clearly established that early intervention with endoscopic haemostasis in endoscopically defined high risk groups significantly reduces rates of further bleeding, surgery and mortality.[161 162] This disparity can be resolved when one considers that upper gastrointestinal haemorrhage ceases spontaneously in 80% of patients, most of whom have an uneventful recovery without specific intervention.[163] The majority with a good outcome obscured the subgroup of patients who were likely to benefit from early endoscopic intervention—those patients at high risk for rebleeding and death.

Early endoscopy in upper gastrointestinal bleeding has established endoscopic predictors of rebleeding, and in conjunction with clinical parameters, these stigmata can be used to identify high risk patients and direct endoscopic therapy.

Similarly, lower gastrointestinal bleeding ceases spontaneously in 80% of patients. Recurrent or continued bleeding is here too associated with a poor prognosis, and these patients account for most of the deaths. Traditionally, management of acute lower gastrointestinal bleeding has been by angiography and surgery with a limited role for the gastroenterologist/endoscopist. This convention, along with the relative infrequency of the condition and the technical difficulties of endoscopy within an unprepared, blood filled colon, has discouraged physicians from an aggressive endoscopic approach. Recent work suggests that emergency colonoscopy after purge is safe and highly accurate in localising the source of bleeding.[6 10 11 32] In addition, endoscopic haemostasis is highly effective at arresting non-diverticular bleeding.[6 10] Several case reports have shown that endoscopic haemostasis in diverticular bleeding is feasible.[37 39 40 42 43] Randomised prospective trials comparing emergency colonoscopy after purge with the traditional approach of angiography and surgery are required to determine which strategy is superior. Endoscopic stigmata predictive of recurrent or continued bleeding in diverticular haemorrhage (sentinel clot, active bleeding) require elucidation, so that in combination with clinical criteria, they can be used to direct endoscopic therapy towards those at high risk.

269

The past decade has seen a revolution in the approach to upper gastrointestinal bleeding; endoscopic haemostasis is established as the first line therapy and widely practised. Is a similar approach applicable in acute lower gastrointestinal bleeding? This is the question that must be answered by physicians who deal with this condition.

Key points

- New diagnostic techniques—angiography, radionuclide scanning and endoscopy—have improved the mortality rate for lower gastrointestinal bleeding (LGIB) by removing the need for poorly targeted empirical surgical treatment

- After resuscitation, sigmoidoscopy should be a routine part of the primary assessment in severe LGIB

- Emergency colonoscopy after purge is safe and accurate in localising the source of bleeding, and allows the use of endoscopic haemostasis techniques. Prospective trials are needed to compare this approach with angiography plus surgery

- Early endoscopic haemostasis in high risk groups significantly reduces rates of rebleeding, surgery and mortality. It is effective for non-diverticular bleeding, and feasible for diverticular bleeding

---

References

1 Wright HK. Massive colonic haemorrhage. *Surg Clin North Am* 1980;**60**:1297–304.
2 NIH Concensus Conference (Office of Medical Application of Research) Therapeutic endoscopy and bleeding ulcers. *JAMA* 1989;**262**:1369–72.
3 Gilbert DA. Epidemiology of upper gastrointestinal bleeding. *Gastrointest Edosc* 1990;**36**: 5 S8–S3.
4 Kang JY, Piper DW. Improvement in mortality rates in bleeding peptic ulcer disease. *Med J Aust* 1980;**1**:213–5.
5 Hunt RH. Rectal bleeding. *Clin Gastroenterol* 1978;**7**:719–40.
6 Caos AM, Benner KG, Manier J, *et al*. Colonoscopy after Golytely preparation in acute rectal bleeding. *J Clin Gastroenterol* 1986;**8**:46–9.
7 McGuire HH, Haynes BW. Massive haemorrhage from diverticulosis of the colon. *Ann Surg* 1972;**175**:847–53.
8 Casarella WJ, Kanter IE, Seaman WB. Right-sided colonic diverticula as a cause of acute rectal haemorrhage. *N Engl J Med* 1972;**286**:450–3.
9 Drapanas T, Pennington DG, Kappelman M, Lindsey ES. Emergency subtotal colectomy—preferred approach to the management of massively bleeding diverticular disease. *Ann Surg* 1973;**177**:519–26.
10 Jensen DM, Machicado GA. Diagnosis and treatment of severe hematochezia: The role of urgent colonoscopy after purge. *Gastroenterology* 1988;**95**:1569–74.
11 Des Marez B, Adler M, Buset M, *et al*. The value of colonoscopy in the diagnosis and management of severe hematochezia. *Mt Sinai J Med* 1986;**53**:478–81.
12 Elta GH. Approach to the patient with gross gastrointestinal bleeding. In: Yamada T, Alpers DH, Owyang C, eds. *Textbook of gastroenterology*. Philadelphia: JB Lippincott, 1991;591–616.
13 Mant A, Bakey EL, Chapius PH. Rectal bleeding: do other symptoms aid in diagnosis? *Dis Colon Rectum* 1989;**32**:191–6.

14 Church JM. Analysis of the colonoscopic findings in patients with rectal bleeding according to the pattern of their presenting symptoms. *Dis Colon Rectum* 1991;**34**:391–5.

15 Peterson WL, Laine L. Gastrointestinal bleeding. In: Sleisenger MH and Fordham JS, eds. *Gastrointestinal disease. Pathophysiology/diagnosis/management.* Philadelphia: WB Saunders, 1993;162–92.

16 Potter GD, Sellin JH. Lower gastrointestinal bleeding. *Gasteroenterol Clin North Am* 1988; **17**:341–56.

17 Schrock TR. Colonoscopic diagnosis and treatment of lower gastrointestinal bleeding. *Surg Clin North Am* 1989;**69**:1309–25.

18 Waye JD. Diagnostic endoscopy in lower intestinal bleeding. In: Sugawa C, Schuman BM, Lucas CE, eds. *Gastrointestinal bleeding.* New York: Igaku-Shoin, 1992;230–41.

19 Leitman IM, Paull DE, Shires GT III. Evaluation and management of massive lower gastrointestinal haemorrhage. *Ann Surg* 1989;**209**:175–80.

20 Parkes BM, Obeid FN, Sorensen VJ, Horst HM, Fath JJ. The management of massive lower gastrointestinal bleeding. *Am Surg* 1993;**59**:676–8.

21 Berry AR, Campbell WB, Kettlewell MGW. Management of major colonic haemorrhage. *Br J Surg* 1988;**75**:637–40.

22 Baum S, Rösch J, Dotter CT, *et al.* Selective mesenteric arterial infusions in the management of massive diverticular haemorrhage. *N Engl J Med* 1973;**288**:1269–72.

23 Browder W, Cerise EJ, Litwin MS. Impact of emergency angiography in massive lower gastrointestinal bleeding. *Ann Surg* 1986;**204**:530–6.

24 Fiorito JJ, Brandt LJ, Kozicky O, Grosman I, Sprayragen S. The diagnostic yield of superior mesenteric angiography: correlation with the pattern of gastrointestinal bleeding. *Am J Gastroenterol* 1989;**84**:878–81.

25 Wright HK, Pellicia O, Higgins EF, Sreenivas V, Gupta A. Controlled semi-elective, segmental resection for massive colonic haemorrhage. *Am J Surg* 1980;**139**:535–8.

26 Nath RL, Sequeira JC, Weitzman AF, Birkett DH, Williams LF. Lower gastrointestinal bleeding: diagnostic approach and management conclusions. *Am J Surg* 1981;**141**: 478–81.

27 Forde KA. Colonoscopy in acute rectal bleeding. *Gastrointest Endosc* 1981;**27**:219–20.

28 Colacchio TA, Forde KA, Patsos TJ, Nunez D. Impact of modern diagnostic methods on the management of active rectal bleeding. *Am J Surg* 1982;**143**:607–10.

29 Farivar M, Perrotto J. The efficacy of colonoscopy in acute rectal bleeding [Abstract]. *Gastrointest Edosc* 1982;**28**:130.

30 Fabry TL, Waye JD. Emergency colonoscopy in lower gastrointestinal bleeding [Abstract]. *Gastrointest Endosc* 1982;**28**:149.

31 Vellacoff KD. Early endoscopy for lower gastrointestinal haemorrhage. *Ann R Coll Surg Engl* 1986;**68**:243–4.

32 Rossini FP, Ferrari A, Spandre M, *et al.* Emergency colonoscopy. *World J Surg* 1989;**13**: 190–2.

33 Cussons PD, Berry AR. Comparison of the value of emergency angiography and intraoperative colonoscopy with antegrade colonic irrigation in massive rectal haemorrhage. *J R Coll Surg Edinb* 1989;**24**:91–3.

34 Reuter SR. Embolization of gastrointestinal haemorrhage. *Am J Radiol* 1979;**133**:557–8.

35 Forde KA. Lower gastrointestinal bleeding: the magnitude of the problem. In: Sugawa C, Schuman BM, Lucas CE, eds. *Gastrointestinal bleeding.* New York: Igaku-Shoin, 1992; 13–25.

36 Mauldin JL. Therapeutic use of colonoscopy in active diverticular bleeding. *Gastrointest Endosc* 1985;**31**:290–1.

37 Bertoni G, Conigliaro R, Ricci E, Mortilla MG, Bedogni G, Fornaciari G. Endoscopic injection hemostasis of colinic diverticular bleeding: a case report. *Endoscopy* 1990;**22**: 154–5.

38 Andress HJ, Newes A, Lange V. Endoscopic haemostasis of a bleeding diverticulum of the sigma with fibrin sealant. *Endoscopy* 1993;**25**:193.

39 Savides TJ, Jensen DM. Colonoscopic haemostasis for recurrent diverticular haemorrhage associated with a visible vessel: a report of 3 cases. *Gastrointest Endosc* 1994;**40**:70–3.

40 Johnston J, Sones J. Endoscopic heater probe coagulation of the bleeding colonic diverticulum [Abstract]. *Gastrointest Endosc* 1986;**32**:160.

41 Farrands PA, Taylor I. Management of acute lower gastrointestinal haemorrhage in a surgical unit over a 4 year period. *J R Soc Med* 1987;**80**:79–82.

42 Pardoll PM, Neubrand S. Injection control of colonic haemorrhage with hypertonic saline-epinephrine solution [Abstract]. *Am J Gastroenterol* 1989;**84**:1193.

43 Kim Y, Marcon NE. Injection therapy for colonic diverticular bleeding. A case study. *J Clin Gastroenterol* 1993;**17**:46–8.

44 Binmoeller KF, Thonke F, Soehendra N. Endoscopic hemoclip treatment for gastrointestinal bleeding. *Endoscopy* 1993;**25**:167–70.

45 Letourneau JG. Percutaneous biopsy techniques: Radiologic Biopsy of Abdominal Masses. In: Castañeda-Zúñiga WR, Tadavarthy S, eds. *Interventional radiology*. Baltimore: Williams and Wilkins 1992;1255–85.

46 Sugawa C, Schuman BM. Endoscopic injection therapy. In: Sugawa C, Schuman BM, Lucas LE, eds. *Gastrointestinal bleeding*. New York: Igaku-Shoin, 1992;347–57.

47 Margulis AR, Heinbecker P, Bernard HR. Operative mesenteric arteriography in the search for the site in unexplained gastrointestinal haemorrhage. *Surgery* 1960;**48**:534–9.

48 Athanasoulis CA, Galdabini JJ, Waltman AC, Novelline AJ, Greenfield AJ, Ezpeleta ML. Angiodysplasia of the colon: a cause of rectal bleeding. *Cardiovasc Radiol* 1978;**1**:3–13.

49 Boley SJ, DiBiase A, Brandt LJ, Sammartano RJ. Lower interstitial bleeding in the elderly. *Am J Surg* 1979;**137**:57–63.

50 Boley SJ, Brandt LJ. Vascular ectasias of the colon. *Dig Dis Sci* 1986;**31**:(**suppl 9**):26–42.

51 Tedesco FJ, Waye JD, Raskin JB, Morris SJ, Greenwald RA. Colonoscopic evaluation of rectal bleeding. A study of 304 patients. *Ann Intern Med* 1978;**89**:907–9.

52 Reinus JF, Brandt LJ. Vascular ectasias and diverticulosis. Common causes of lower intestinal bleeding. *Gastroenterol Clin North Am* 1994;**23**:1–20.

53 Santos JC, Aprilli F, Guimarães AS, Rocha JJ. Angiodysplasia of the colon: endoscopic diagnosis and treatment. *Br J Surg* 1988;**75**:256–8.

54 Bowers JH, Dixon JA. Argon laser photocoagulation of vascular malformations in the GI tract: short-term results [Abstract]. *Gastrointest Endosc* 1982;**28**:126.

55 Jensen DM, Machicado GA, Tapia JI, Beilin DB. Endoscopic treatment of haemangiomata with argon laser in patients with gastrointestinal bleeding [Abstract]. *Gastroenterology* 1982;**82**:1093.

56 Jensen DM, Machicado GA. Bleeding colonic angioma: Endoscopic coagulation and followup [Abstract]. *Gastroenterol* 1985;**88**:1433.

57 Cello JP, Grendell JH. Endoscopic laser treatment for gastrointestinal vascular ectasias. *Ann Intern Med* 1986;**104**:352–4.

58 Lanthier PH, D'Harveng B, Van Heuverzwyn R, *et al*. Colonic angiodysplasia. Followup of patients after endoscopic treatment for bleeding lesions. *Dis Colon Rectum* 1989;**32**:296–8.

59 Rutgeerts P, Van Gompel F, Geboes K, Vantrappen G, Broeckaert L, Coremans G. Long-term results of treatment of vascular malformations of the gastrointestinal tract by Neodymium Yag laser photocoagulation. *Gut* 1985;**26**:586–93.

60 Rogers BHG, Adler F. Hemangiomas of the caecum: colonoscopic diagnosis and therapy. *Gastroenterology* 1976;**71**:1079–82.

61 Rogers BHG. Endoscopic diagnosis and therapy of mucosal vascular abnormalities of the gastrointestinal tract occurring in elderly patients and associated with cardiac, vascular and pulmonary disease. *Gastrointest Endosc* 1980;**26**:134–8.

62 Rogers BHG. Endoscopic electrocoagulation of vascular abnormalities of the gastrointestinal tract in 51 patients [Abstract]. *Gastrointest Endosc* 1982;**28**:142–3.

63 Howard OM, Buchanan JD, Hunt RH. Angiodysplasia of the colon: experience of 26 cases. *Lancet* 1982;**2**:16–9.

64 Roberts PL, Schoetz DJ, Coller JA. Vascular ectasia. Diagnosis and treatment by colonoscopy. *Am Surg* 1988;**54**:56–9.

65 Williams CB. Diathermy-biopsy: a technique of endoscopic management of small polyps. *Endoscopy* 1973;**5**:215–8.

66 Rogers BHG. The electrocoagulation forceps is ideal for the diagnosis and management of small vascular abnormalities of the caecal area. *Gastrointest Endosc* 1985;**31**:222–4.

67 Jensen DM, Machicado GA. Endoscopic diagnosis and treatment of bleeding colonic angiomas and radiation telangiectasia. *Perspect Colon Rectal Surg* 1989;**2**:99–113.

68 Laine LA. Bipolar/multipolar electrocoagulation. In: Sugawa C, Schuman BM, Lucas CE, eds. *Gastrointestinal bleeding*. New York: Igaku-Shoin, 1992;314–23.

69 Jones WF, Khandelwal M, Akerman P, *et al*. Endoscopic band ligation (EBL) for acute non-variceal/non-ulcer upper gastrointestinal haemorrhage [Abstract]. *Gastrointest Ednosc* 1994;**40**:25.

70 Wadas DD, Sanowski RA. Complications of the hot biopsy forceps technique. *Gastrointest Endosc* 1988;**34**:32–7.
71 Jensen DM, Tapia JI, Machicado GA, Beilin DB, Silpa M. Comparison of electrocoagulation and heater probe for hemostasis in the canine colon [Abstract]. *Gastrointest Endosc* 1982;**28**:151–2.
72 Jensen DM, Tapia JI, Machicado GA, Beilin DB. Hydrothermal probe, hot biopsy forceps and YAG laser for hemostasis in the canine colon [Abstract]. *Gastrointest Endosc* 1983;**29**:189.
73 Jensen DM, Machicado GA, Tapia J, Mautner W. Comparison of argon laser photocoagulation and bipolar electrocoagulation for endoscopic hemostasis in the canine colon. *Gastroenterology* 1982;**83**:830–5.
74 Jensen DM, Shindel N, Brunetaud JM, Hirabayshi K, Harris L. Temperature profiles and transmural injury from heater probe vs BICAP® in the canine colon [Abstract]. *Gastrointest Endosc* 1986;**32**:140–1.
75 Farin G, Grund KE. Technology of argon plasma coagulation with particular regard to endoscopic applications. *Endosc Surg* 1994;**2**:71–7.
76 Grund KE, Storek D, Farin G. Endoscopic argon plasma coagulation. First clinical experiences in flexible endoscopy. *Endosc Surg* 1994;**2**:42–6.
77 Rutgeerts P, Vantrappen G, D'Heygere F, Broeckaert L. Transendoscopic Doppler ultrasound: usefulness for diagnosis and treatment of vascular malformations. *Endoscopy* 1988;**30**:99–101.
78 Jaspersen D, Körner T, Schorr W, Hammar C. Diagnosis and treatment control of bleeding colorectal angiodysplasias by endoscopic Doppler sonography: A preliminary study. *Gastrointest Endosc* 1994;**40**:40–4.
79 Kohler B, Riemann. Endoscopic injection therapy of Forrest II and III gastroduodenal ulcers guided by endoscopic Doppler ultrasound. *Endoscopy* 1993;**25**:219–23.
80 Karita M, Masashiro T, Okita K, Kodama T. Endoscopic therapy for early colon cancer: the strip biopsy resection technique. *Gastrointest Endosc* 1991;**37**:128–32.
81 Karita M, Cantero D, Okita K. Endoscopic diagnosis and resection treatment for flat adenoma with severe dysplasia. *Am J Gastroenterol* 1993;**88**:1421–3.
82 Macrae RA, Tan KG, Williams CB. Towards safer colonoscopy: a report on the complications of 5000 diagnostic or therapeutic colonoscopies. *Gut* 1983;**24**:376–83.
83 Fruhmorgen P, Matek W. Significance of polypectomy in large bowel endoscopy. *Endoscopy* 1983;**15**:155–7.
84 Gilbert DA, Hallstrom AP, Shaneyfelt SL, Mahler AK, Silverstein FE. The national ASGE colonoscopy survey–complications of colonoscopy [Abstract] *Gastrointest Endosc* 1984;**30**:156.
85 Webb WA, McDaniel L, Jones L. Experience with 1000 colonoscopic polypectomies. *Ann Surg* 1985;**201**:626–32.
86 Nivatvongs S. Complications in colonoscopic polypectomy: an experience with 1555 polypectomies. *Dis Colon Rectum* 1986;**29**:825–30.
87 Waye JD. Techniques of polypectomy: Hot biopsy forceps and snare polypectomy. *Am J Gastroenterol* 1987;**82**:615–8.
88 Van Gossum A, Cozzoli A, Adler M, Taton G, Cremer M. Colonoscopic snare polypectomy: analysis of 1485 resections comparing two types of current. *Gastrointest Endosc* 1992;**38**:472–5.
89 Quigley EM, Donovan JP, Linder J, Thompson JS, Straub PF, Paustian FF. Delayed massive haemorrhage following electrocoagulating biopsy ("hot biopsy") of a diminutive colonic polyp. *Gastrointest Endosc* 1989;**35**:559–63.
90 Dyer WS, Quigley EM, Noel SM, Camacho KE, Manela F, Zetterman RK. Major colonic haemorrhage following electrocoagulating (hot) biopsy of diminutive colonic polyps: relationship to colonic location and low dose aspirin therapy. *Gastrointest Endosc* 1991;**37**:361–4.
91. Williams CB. Colonoscopy: general aspects, polyps and cancer. In: Cotton PB, Tytgat GNJ, Williams CB, eds. *Annual of Gastrointestinal Endoscopy*. Current Science, London, 1992;133–46.
92 Hachisu T. A new detachable snare for hemostasis in the removal of large polyps or other elevated lesions. *Surg Endosc* 1991;**5**:70–4.
93 Hunt RH. Toward safer colonoscopy. *Gut* 1983;**24**:371–5.
94 Rex DK, Lewis BS, Waye JD. Colonoscopy and endoscopic therapy for delayed postpolypectomy haemorrhage. *Gastrointest Endosc* 1992;**38**:127–9.

273

95 Rosen L, Bub DS, Reed JF III, Mastasee SA. Haemorrhage following colonoscopic polypectomy. *Dis Colon Rectum* 1993;**36**:1126–31.

96 Slivka A, Parsons WG, Carr-Locke DL. Endoscopic band ligation for treatment of postpolypectomy haemorrhage. *Gastrointest Endosc* 1994;**40**:230–2.

97 Johnson WR, McDermott FT, Pihl E, Milne BJ, Price AB, Hughes ESR. Palliative operative management in rectal carcinoma. *Dis Colon Rectum* 1981;**24**:606–9.

98 Longo WE, Ballantyne GH, Bilchik AJ, Modlin IM. Advanced rectal cancer—what is the best palliation? *Dis Colon Rectum* 1988;**31**:842–7.

99 Moran MR, Rottenberger DA, Lahr CJ, Buls JG, Goldberg SM. Palliation for rectal cancer. *Arch Surg* 1987;**122**:640–3.

100 Mathus-Vliegen EMH, Tytgat GNJ. Laser photocoagulation in the palliation of colorectal malignancies. *Cancer* 1986;**57**:2212–6.

101 Bown SG, Barr H, Matthewson K, *et al.* Endoscopic treatment of inoperable colorectal cancers with the Nd YAG laser. *Br J Surg* 1986;**73**:949–52.

102 Brunetaud JM, Manoury V, Ducrotte P, Cochelard D, Cortot A, Paris JC. Palliative treatment of rectosigmoid carcinoma by laser endoscopic photoablation. *Gasteroenterology* 1987;**92**:663–8.

103 McGowan I, Barr H, Krasner N. Palliative laser therapy for inoperable rectal cancer—does it work? *Cancer* 1989;**63**:967–9.

104 Mellow MH. Endoscopic laser therapy as an alternative to palliative surgery for adenocarcinoma of the rectum—comparison of costs and complications. *Gastrointest Endosc* 1989;**35**:283–7.

105 Loizou LA, Grigg D, Boulos PB, Bown SG. Endoscopic Nd:YAG laser treatment of rectosigmoid cancer. *Gut* 1990;**31**:812–6.

106 Chia YW, Goiss N, Goh PM. Endoscopic Nd:YAG laser in the palliative treatment of advanced low rectal carcinoma in Singapore. *Dis Colon Rectum* 1991;**34**:1093–6.

107 Eckhauser ML, Mansour EG. Endoscopic laser therapy for obstructing and/or bleeding colorectal carcinoma. *Am Surg* 1992;**58**:358–63.

108 Tacke W, Paech S, Kruis W, Stuetzer H, Mueller JM, Ziegenhagen DJ. Comparison between endoscopic laser and different surgical treatments for palliation of advanced rectal cancer. *Dis Colon Rectum* 1993;**36**:377–82.

109 Mathus-Vliegen EM, Tytgat GN. Nd:YAG laser photocoagulation in gastroenterology: its role in palliation of colorectal cancer. *Laser Med Sci* 1986;**1**:75–80.

110 Madden JL, Kandalaft S. Clinical evaluation of electrocoagulation in the treatment of cancer of the rectum. *Am J Surg* 1971;**122**:347–52.

111 Hughes EP, Veidenheimer MC, Corman ML, Coller JA. Electrocoagulation of rectal cancer. *Dis Colon Rectum* 1982;**25**:215–8.

112 Hoekstra HJ, Verschueren RCJ, Oldhoff J, van der Ploeg E. Palliative and curative electrocoagulation for rectal cancer. *Cancer* 1985;**55**:210–3.

113 Puthawala AA, Nisarsyed AM, Gates TC, McNamara C. Definitive treatment of extensive anorectal carcinoma by external and interstitial irradiation. *Cancer* 1982;**50**:1746–50.

114 Papillon J. New prospects in the conservative treatment of rectal cancer. *Dis Colon Rectum* 1984;**27**:695–700.

115 Heberer G, Denecke H, Demmel N, Wirsching R. Local procedures in the management of rectal cancer. *World J Surg* 1987;**11**:499–503.

116 Meijer S, de Rooij PD, Derksen EJ, Boutkan H, Cuesta MA. Cryosurgery for locally recurrent rectal cancer. *Eur J Surg Oncol* 1992;**18**:255–7.

117 Novak J, Collins JT, Donowitz M. Effects of radiation on the human gastrointestinal tract. *J Clin Gastroenterol* 1979;**1**:9–39.

118 DeCosse JJ, Rhodes RS, Wentz WB, Reagan JW, Dworken HJ, Holden WD. The natural history and management of radiation induced injury of the gastrointestinal tract. *Ann Surg* 1969;**170**:369–84.

119 Gilinsky NH, Burns DG, Barbezat GO, Levin W, Myers HS, Marks IN. The natural history of radiation—induced proctosigmoiditis: an analysis of 88 patients. *Q J Med* 1983;**205**:40–53.

120 Galland RB, Spencer J. The natural history of clinically established radiation eneritis. *Lancet* 1985;**1**:1257–8.

121 Cochrane JPS, Yarnold JR, Slack WW. The surgical treatment of radiation injuries after radiotherapy for uterine carcinoma. *Br J Surg* 1981;**68**:25–8.

122 Cooke SAR, DeMoor NG. The surgical treatment of the radiation-damaged rectum. *Br J Surg* 1981;**68**:488–92.

123 Gazet JC. Park's colonal pull—through anastamosis for severe, complicated radiation proctitis. *Dis Colon Rectum* 1985;**28**:110–4.

124 Jao SW, Beart RW, Gunderson LL. Surgical treatment of radiation injuries of the colon and rectum. *Am J Surg* 1986;**151**:272–7.

125 Lucarotti ME, Mountford RA, Bartolo DCC. Surgical management of intestinal radiation injury. *Dis Colon Rectum* 1991;**34**:865–9.

126 Baum CA, Biddle WL, Miner PB Jr. Failure of 5-aminosalicylic acid enemas to improve chronic radiation proctitis. *Dig Dis Sci* 1989;**34**:758–60.

127 Kochhar R, Patel F, Dhar A, *et al.* Radiation-induced proctosigmoiditis:prospective, randomized, double-blind controlled trial of oral sulfasalazine plus rectal steroids versus rectal sucralfate. *Dig Dis Sci* 1991;**36**:103–7.

128 Leuchter RS, Petrilli ES, Dwyer RM, Hacker NF, Castaldo TW, LaGasse LD. Nd:YAG laser therapy of rectosigmoid bleeding due to radiation injury. *Obstet Gynecol* 1982; **59(suppl 6)**:65–7.

129 Alexander TJ, Dwyer RM. Endoscopic Nd:YAG laser treatment of severe radiation injury of the lower gastrointestinal tract: longterm followup. *Gastrointest Endosc* 1988; **34**:407–11.

130 Viggiano TR, Zighelboim J, Ahlquist DA, Gostout CJ, Wang KK, Larson MV. Endoscopic Nd:YAG laser coagulation of bleeding from radiation proctopathy. *Gastrointest Endosc* 1993;**39**:513–7.

131 Buchi KN, Dixon JA. Argon laser treatment of haemorrhagic radiation proctitis. *Gastrointest Endosc* 1987;**33**:27–30.

132 O'Connor JJ. Argon laser treatment of radiation proctitis. *Arch Surg* 1989;**124**:749.

133 Taylor JG, DiSario JA, Buchi KN. Argon laser therapy for haemorrhagic radiation proctitis: longterm results. *Gastrointest Endosc* 1993;**39**:641–4.

134 Jensen DM, Jutabha R, Machiacado GA, Cheng S, Core Hemostasis Group. Prospective study of patients with severe rectal bleeding from radiation telangiectasia [Abstract]. *Gastrointest Endosc* 1994;**40**:94.

135 Maunoury V, Brunetaud JM, Cortot A. Bipolar electrocoagulation treatment for haemorrhage radiation injury of the lower digestive tract. *Gastrointest Endosc* 1991;**37**: 492–3.

136 Seow-Choen F, Goh HS, Eu KW, Ho YH, Tay SK. A simple and effective treatment for haemorrhagic radiation proctitis using formalin. *Dis Colon Rectum* 1993;**36**:135–8.

137 Dennison AR, Whiston RJ, Rooney S, Morris DL. The management of haemorrhoids. *Am J Gastroenterol* 1989;**84**:475–81.

138 Goligher JL. Cryosurgery for haemorrhoids. *Dis Colon Rectum* 1976;**19**:213–8.

139 Ponsky JL, Mellinger JD, Simon IB. Endoscopic retrograde haemorrhoidal sclerotherapy using 23·4% saline: a preliminary report. *Gastrointest Endosc* 1991;**37**:155–8.

140 Ambrose NS, Hares MM, Alexander-Williams J, Keighley MRB. Prospective randomized comparison of photocoagulation and rubber band ligation in treatment of haemorrhoids. *Br Med J* 1983;**286**:1389–91.

141 Wang JY, Chang-Chien CR, Chen JS, Lai CR, Tang R. The role of lasers in haemorrhoidectomy. *Dis Colon Rectum* 1991;**34**:78–82.

142 Weinstein SJ, Rypins EB, Houck J, Thrower S. Single session treatment for bleeding haemorrhoids. *Surg Gynecol Obstet* 1987;**165**:479–82.

143 Marshman D, Huber PJ, Timmerman W, Simonton CT, Odom FC, Kaplan ER. Haemorrhoidal ligation: a review of efficacy. *Dis Colon Rectum* 1989;**32**:369–71.

144 Norman DA, Neuton R, Nicholas GV. Direct current electrotherapy of internal haemorrhoids: an effective, safe, and painless outpatient approach. *Am J Gastroenterol* 1989;**84**:482–7.

145 Zinberg SS, Stern DH, Furman DS, Wittles JM. A personal experience in comparing three non-operative techniques for treating internal haemorrhoids. *Am J Gastroenterol* 1989;**84**:488–92.

146 Griffith CDM, Morris DL, Ellis I, Wherry DC, Hardcastle JD. Outpatient treatment of haemorrhoids with bipolar diathermy coagulation. *Br J Surg* 1987;**74**:827.

147 Ribbans WJ, Radcliffe AG. Retroperitoneal abscess following sclerotherapy for haemorrhoids. *Dis Colon Rectum* 1985;**28**:188–9.

148 Quevedo-Bonilla G, Farkas AM, Abcarian H, Hambrick E, Orsay CP. Septic complications of haemorrhoidal banding. *Arch Surg* 1988;**123**:650–1.

149 Bat L, Melzer E, Koler M, Dreznick Z, Shemesh E. Complications of rubber band ligation of symptomatic internal haemorrhoids. *Dis Colon Rectum* 1993;**36**:287–90.

150 Yang R, Migikovsky B, Peicher J, Laine L. Randomised prospective trial of direct current versus bipolar electrocoagulation for bleeding internal haemorrhoids. *Gastrointest Endosc* 1993;**39**:766–9.

151 Miller LS, Barbareusch C, Friedman LS. Less frequent causes of lower gastrointestinal bleeding. *Gastroenter Clin North Am* 1994;**23**:21–51.

152 Gudjonsson H, Zeiler O, Gamelli RL, Kaye MD. Colonic varices: report of an unusual case diagnosed by radionuclide scanning, with review of the literature. *Gastroenterology* 1986;**91**:1543–7.

153 Goenka MK, Kochhar R, Nagi B, Mehta SK. Rectosigmoid varices and other mucosal changes in patients with portal hypertension. *Am J Gastroenterol* 1991;**86**:1185–9.

154 Orozco H, Takahashi T, Mercado MA, *et al*. Colorectal variceal bleeding in patients with extrahepatic portal vein thrombosis and idiopathic portal hypertension. *J Clin Gastroenterol* 1992;**14**:139–43.

155 Walters AM, Larvin M, Sadek SA. Control of colonic variceal haemorrhage by long term octreotide administration. *Br J Surg* 1994;**81**:289–90.

156 Weiserbs DB, Zfass AM, Menmer J. Control of massive haemorrhage from rectal varices with sclerotherapy. *Gastrointest Endosc* 1986;**32**:419–21.

157 Rothgaber SW, Rex DK. Colonoscopy and endoscopic therapy of haemorrhage from viral colitis. *Gastrointest Endosc* 1993;**39**:737–8.

158 Schmid KW, Pointner R, Feichtinger J, Schmid KW. Exulceratio simplex Dieulafoy of the colon—a case report. *Endoscopy* 1988;**20**:88–9.

159 Petersen WL, Barnett CC, Smith HJ, Allen MH, Corbett DB. Routine early endoscopy in upper gastrointestinal tract bleeding: a randomized controlled trial. *N Engl J Med* 1981;**304**:925–9.

160 Conn HO. To scope or not to scope. *N Engl J Med* 1981;**304**:967–9.

161 Sacks HS, Chalmers TC, Blum AL, Berrier J, Pagano D. Endoscopic haemostasis: an effective therapy for bleeding peptic ulcers. *JAMA* 1990;**264**:494–9.

162 Cook DJ, Guyatt GH, Salena BJ, Laine LA. Endoscopic therapy for acute non-variceal upper gastrointestinal haemorrhage: A meta-analysis. *Gastroenterology* 1992;**102**:139–48.

163 Laine L, Peterson WL. Bleeding peptic ulcer. *N Engl J Med* 1994;**331**:717–27.

20: Surgical management of lower gastrointestinal bleeding

JOHN D CUNNINGHAM AND
ADRIAN J GREENSTEIN

Recent advances in upper endoscopy, both diagnostic and therapeutic, have improved the management of upper gastrointestinal haemorrhage. Advances have also been made in the management of lower gastrointestinal bleeding, but the overall diagnosis and management of this problem remains quite complex. The purpose of this chapter is to determine the indications for, and the optimal timing of, surgical intervention for lower gastrointestinal bleeding.

Patient Evaluation

A history and physical examination are essential components in the evaluation of the patient with a lower gastrointestinal bleed. The physical examination should include a thorough abdominal examination, examination of the perineum and a digital rectal examination. To determine whether the bleeding is from an upper source, proximal to the ligament of Treitz, a nasogastric tube should be passed. One of every 100 patients who has rectal bleeding and a nasogastric aspirate that is free of blood will be found to be bleeding from a duodenal ulcer. Rigid proctoscopy, which can be performed quickly and easily, is an essential initial diagnostic procedure to determine whether an anorectal source is the cause of bleeding. The initial diagnostic test to be performed will depend on the facilities and experience available. The severity of the bleeding needs to be quantified before sending patients for diagnostic tests. Patients who present in shock or require multiple units of blood within hours of admission, or both, are considered to have massive bleeding and are not candidates for time consuming procedures during which patient monitoring is difficult. Patients who stop bleeding shortly after admission are able to undergo an urgent workup rather than an emergency one.

The Role of Surgery

I shall discuss in turn the place of surgery in the management of diverticular disease, vascular ectasias, ischaemic bowel, colonic polyps and carcinoma, inflammatory bowel disease, occult bleeding, and bleeding from the small intestine.

Diverticular disease

Diverticular disease occurs in the elderly and it is estimated that 50% of people over the age of 70 have diverticula. The number of diverticula varies between individuals, but most are found in the left colon. About 20% of people with diverticula will bleed at some time.[12] Bleeding from diverticula is usually sudden and often massive, but in most patients will stop spontaneously. The diagnosis of diverticular disease can be made by most of the diagnostic tests used for lower gastrointestinal bleeding. Conservative management is successful in up to 90% of patients.[23] The rate of rebleeding is 15–40% at 1 year[24] and those who rebleed should be operated upon.

Most bleeding that does not stop spontaneously responds to vasopressin, which is effective in 66–100% of cases.[5-7] However, the control is usually temporary and most patients eventually need surgery.[56]

The decision to resect the colon for diverticular disease is made easier if the diverticula are located on one side of the colon or if the bleeding is localised by the diagnostic workup. These patients should undergo segmental resection. In one study,[8] nine patients had segmental resection for diverticular disease localised by angiography and all patients had residual diverticula after resection. None of these patients rebled. However, if the diagnostic workup reveals diverticula on both sides of the colon and the bleeding cannot be localised, yet bleeding continues, a subtotal colectomy should be performed. Any left sided diverticula encountered at the time of colon resection for bleeding from vascular ectasia should not be resected,[9] as the risk of bleeding from these lesions is small.

Vascular ectasias

There have been numerous reports of bleeding from vascular ectasia of the cecum since the initial observations of Margulis.[10 11] Bleeding from ectasias, which are capillary or venular in origin, is most often recurrent and low grade. Approximately 15% of patients, some of whom are in shock, present with acute massive haemorrhage.[12] In more than 90% of patients, the bleeding stops spontaneously.[11]

The management of patients with vascular ectasias is controversial. For patients with active bleeding or extravasation on angiography, surgical resection was formerly the mainstay of therapy. Now, in institutions where physicians experienced in endoscopic surgery are available, endoscopic ablation is the primary mode of therapy. In cases of moderate bleeding, or following cessation of bleeding, endoscopic coagulation of the vascular ectasias can often be accomplished by using a heater probe. In these cases, especially if the bleeding has ceased completely, the entire right colon should be carefully examined for telangiectasia, and coagulation of all significant ectasias carried out. However, it is not necessary to obliterate all visible vascular ectasias to stop bleeding in the acute situation, if the precise bleeding point can be identified.

Right hemicolectomy is now reserved for the patient in whom the bleeding cannot be stopped—if an endoscopist experienced in transcolonoscopic ablation is not available—or in cases when endoscopic ablation has been unsuccessful or is not feasible.[12] When surgery is performed, the resection should not be influenced by the presence or absence of diverticulosis in the left colon, as the risk of bleeding from these lesions is small.[13 14] Trudel[15] treated 28/57 patients with vascular ectasias with colonoscopic ablation. The rebleeding rate was 14/28 (50%) and five of these patients were controlled with repeat endoscopy and coagulation, to give an overall success rate of 68%. Seven of the rebleeders were treated surgically and one of these rebled. Of the 17 patients treated primarily with surgery in this study, four patients rebled and bleeding was controlled in two of these patients with endoscopic treatment. The overall surgical success rate was 77%. Rogers[16] controlled bleeding by endoscopic coagulation in all but one of 44 patients with vascular ectasias. These excellent results, combined with the minimal morbidity, make colonoscopic ablation the therapy of choice for patients with colonic vascular ectasias.

Ischaemic bowel

Patients with ischaemic bowel are usually older and are known to have atherosclerotic disease. The usual presentation is left lower quadrant abdominal pain and bloody diarrhoea. Endoscopy is the best diagnostic test and generally reveals sparing of the rectal mucosa with involvement of the sigmoid or descending colon, or splenic flexure. Laparoscopy is of value in diagnosing ischaemic bowel, either small or large, and assessing the depth of the ischaemic process. The recognition of transmural disease at laparoscopy, especially in less commonly involved segmental areas of small bowel, the ileocaecal region, and the right or transverse colon, is an indication for early surgery. Early exploration should prevent progression to perforation or septic shock. Once the diagnosis of gangrenous bowel is made, the patient should be explored and the involved segment resected with the creation of an end colostomy and mucous fistula.

Colonic polyps and carcinoma

These lesions rarely cause massive lower gastrointestinal haemorrhage. The classical presentation is occult bleeding discovered by guaiac testing, or anaemia. The work-up for these patients should include colonoscopy, which allows for the visualisation and biopsy of any lesions present.

Colonoscopy can also be used to remove polyps. Surgery is recommended for polyps that cannot be removed endoscopically, those that are found to contain malignancy, and for all carcinomas.

Inflammatory bowel disease

Gastrointestinal haemorrhage is a major clinical feature of inflammatory bowel disease. It may be acute or chronic; occult, overt, or massive.[17] Chronic haemorrhage is common, especially in disease involving the most distal bowel, colon and rectum (Figure 20.1). Almost all patients with ulcerative colitis have overt bleeding, and about one-third of those with Crohn's disease. Although haemorrhage is uncommon in regional enteritis confined to the small bowel, in a few cases persistent, recurrent haemorrhage can be a major diagnostic problem, causing great difficulty in localising the site of the bleeding.

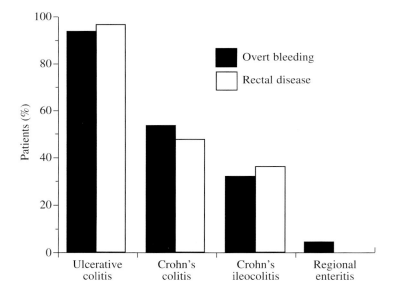

FIGURE 20.1—*The relationship between gastrointestinal bleeding and distal colonic disease in Crohn's disease and ulcerative colitis. The incidence of haemorrhage correlates with that of distal disease, and bleeding is present in almost all cases of ulcerative colitis. Adapted with permission from Greenstein AJ et al*. Crohn's disease of the colon. II. Controversial aspects of hemorrhage, anemia, and rectal involvement in granulomatous disease involving the colon. *Am J Gastroenterol* 1975;**63**:40–8.[17]

Severe bleeding is occasionally (0–6%) encountered in patients with Crohn's disease,[17-20] and is rarely the first manifestation of disease. In a comprehensive review of patients with Crohn's disease,[20] only 21 of 1526 (1·4%) patients were found to have severe bleeding from the lower intestinal tract. (Severe haemorrhage was defined as a transfusion requirement of at least four units of blood during an interval not exceeding 2 weeks.) Patients were more likely to have bled if the colon was involved (1·9% v 0·7%, p<0·001) rather than the small bowel (see Figures 20.1–20.3). The diagnosis of Crohn's disease was made with the usual clinical, radiographic, and endoscopic criteria. Only five patients had angiography and the bleeding site was identified in two of these patients. Surgery was performed in 11 patients for the first bleed and only one of these patients rebled. Of the 10 patients treated medically, three rebled massively. One patient was operated upon and two patients died. These results suggest that, in patients with severe haemorrhage from Crohn's disease, the primary treatment should be surgical resection.

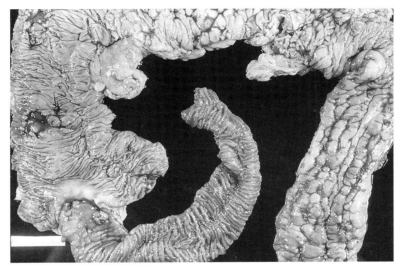

FIGURE 20.2—*Subtotal colectomy specimen from a 41 year old woman who presented with massive haemorrhage from a deep geographic ulcer of the mid ascending colon during an episode of active Crohn's ileocolitis. The distal ileum also shows ulcerating disease. The transverse and distal colon show "cobblestoning" and the descending colon longitudinal ulceration. Reproduced with permission from Greenstein AJ. Surgical management [of Crohn's disease]. In: Berk JE, ed. Bockus Gastroenterology. Philadelphia: WB Saunders 1985; 2331 Figure 127–74.*

Severe haemorrhage in ulcerative colitis is also rare[21–23]; from 1959 to 1986, 25 patients with ulcerative colitis who had bled massively were identified.[23] Surgery was performed in 22 of 25 patients, urgently in 11 and semi-electively in 11. Subtotal colectomy was performed in 10 of 11 emergency procedures and in 7 of 11 semi-elective procedures. Rebleeding was noted in 2 of 11 emergency procedures. Six patients who received a subtotal colectomy subsequently required abdominal resection of the rectum, because of persistent mucous and bloody discharge. Subtotal colectomy in this situation allows one to perform a second-stage procedure—construction of a pelvic pouch, with ileoanal pull-through, and reconstruction of intestinal continuity with continence. The latter may be

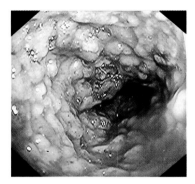

FIGURE 20.3—*An area of cobblestoning in the colon of a 34 year old woman, associated with a stricture of the descending colon. The lesions were associated with prolonged chronic and acute gastrointestinal blood loss and anaemia requiring multiple transfusions. Ultimately segmental left colectomy was carried out (courtesy of Dr Paul Basuk).*

done with or without a temporary proximal diverting loop ileostomy. Subtotal colectomy can, therefore, be undertaken in patients with massive bleeding from ulcerative colitis, provided one is prepared for a 12% risk of persistent or recurrent rectal haemorrhage. Total protocolectomy is the procedure of choice if it is determined by sigmoidoscopy that the major haemorrhage originates in the rectum. A pelvic pouch may still be created at a later date if the anal sphincter muscles are preserved at the primary procedure, either by simultaneous stripping, or by transection of the low rectum at or just above the anal sphincters.

After construction of a pelvic pouch, "pouchitis" with bleeding and anaemia may develop in a few cases. These patients usually respond to metronidazole or ciprofloxacin. We have seen a single case of severe recurrent haemorrhage in a J pelvic pouch, associated with a solitary circumscribed ulcer adjacent to the inflow tract (Figure 20.4).

Occult bleeding

The most difficult problem in managing patients with lower intestinal bleeding is the patient who continues to bleed despite an exhaustive diagnostic work-up. Szold[24] developed a treatment algorithm for patients with obscure gastrointestinal bleeding, which included preoperative endoscopy and small bowel enteroscopy (Figure 20.5). Between 1985 and 1990, 71 patients, all of whom were exhaustively evaluated before entering the study, were managed according to this algorithm. The average duration of bleeding was 26 months. Ninety percent of the patients had been transfused, with an average transfusion requirement of 20 units (range 1–100 units). The source of bleeding was identified by preoperative endoscopy in three (4%) and preoperative small bowel enteroscopy in 50 (70%), and not identified in 17 (24%). In one patient with metastatic colon cancer the procedure failed. Of the 50 presumed localised lesions inferred by small bowel enteroscopy only 26 (52%) were identified by laparotomy alone; 24 patients (48%) still required intraoperative enteroscopy. In all 71 patients a pathological lesion was identified that

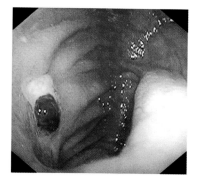

FIGURE 20.4—*Endoscopic view of a visible vessel. This 50 year old woman had a total proctocolectomy and J pelvic pouch in 1984 for ulcerative colitis. She did well, with occasional episodes of pouchitis responding to metronidazole, until 1991, when she suffered an episode of pouchitis associated with a severe gastrointestinal haemorrhage. Endoscopy revealed a solitary ulcer with a visible vessel at the upper end of the pouch, adjacent to the inflow tract, which required injection. She has since had three further bleeding episodes requiring transfusion of as much as four units of blood. These episodes have ceased spontaneously or responded to repeat endoscopic coagulation or injection (courtesy of Dr Blair Lewis).*

could explain the bleeding, and in all except one the segment of the bowel responsible was resected. The exception had diffuse arteriovenous malformations and a resection was not feasible. The source of bleeding was vascular ectasias in 28 (40%) cases, a tumour of the small bowel in 19 (27%) cases, and a host of other causes in the remaining 24 (33%) cases. The overall rebleeding rate was 21%, which is similar to that reported after initial bleeds. No one under the age of 50 years had a lesion that was not obvious at the time of laparotomy. Therefore, this algorithm should be followed in patients presenting with occult bleeding. In younger patients, the workup can be brief and proceed quickly to laparotomy.

Small intestinal bleeding

The history and physical examination of the patient with gastrointestinal bleeding may suggest the small intestine as the site of bleeding. However, it is difficult to diagnose the source and nature of small bowel haemorrhage (Figure 20.5), as most of the small bowel is out of range of the endoscope, although the push-type enteroscope has provided an added diagnostic dimension.[24–26]

If surgery is required, intraoperative arteriographic localisation of the bleeding site may be determined by leaving the catheter in place for intraoperative contrast infusion or the injection of dye to visualise the site of bleeding.[27–29] Vasopressin and gel embolisation are less successful in the control of haemorrhage from the small bowel than in that of colonic

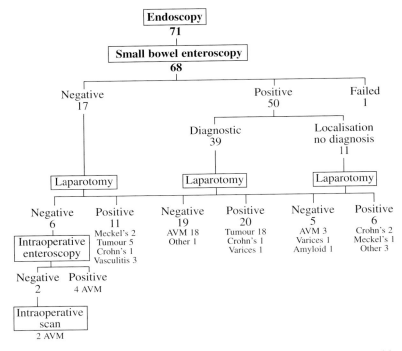

FIGURE 20.5—*A diagnostic-therapeutic algorithm used to evaluate 71 patients with small bowel haemorrhage of obscure cause. Preoperative enteroscopy revealed a precise diagnosis in 50 of 71 patients (70%). All patients were operated upon and a bleeding lesion found in all. Six patients died of recurrent bleeding and six cancer. AVM, arteriovenous malformation; Meckel's, Meckel's diverticulum; Crohn's, Crohn's disease. Adapted with permission from Szold et al.*[24]

bleeding. Small bowel lesions that cause bleeding should be resected whenever possible. Intraoperative endoscopy can enhance and refine information previously obtained, as well as discover new lesions.[24]

Rebleeding

For patients who present with lower gastrointestinal bleeding the overall rate of rebleeding depends on the initial method of management. Orecchia[30] evaluated patients with lower intestinal bleeding using labelled red blood cell scans. Of the 26 patients with a positive scan, 15 had emergency surgery and 11 stopped bleeding. No patients in either group rebled during a mean follow up of 20 months. No bleeding was detected in the 38 patients with negative scans during a mean follow up of 21 months. However, further evaluation of these 38 patients with negative scans revealed eight patients who required surgery for lesions found with other diagnostic tests. These results illustrate the importance of fully evaluating the gastrointestinal tract in a patient who stops bleeding, to prevent progression of a treatable lesion or rebleeding at a later date.

Morbidity and Mortality

The overall mortality for patients who present with lower intestinal bleeding is 0–24%.[8 27 31 32] Prognostic factors predicting death in one series[27] included shock upon admission and steroid use but outcome was not affected by age, sex, associated medical conditions or transfusion requirements. Leitman[27] showed that the mortality rate is lower when the bleeding site is localised than when it is not (17% v 27%), and when a segmental resection is performed rather than blind subtotal colectomy (13% v 40%). Most other studies agree with this finding.[38 32] The questions that remain unanswered are the increased mortality attributable to the operation itself, and to the delay in operating on patients in whom a bleeding source cannot be localised.

Morbidity rates after surgery vary from 9% to 37%.[8 27] Several series have shown no complication following colonoscopy or barium enema.[15 33] No reports give the morbidity following angiography. Patients undergoing transcolonic ablation of bleeding vascular ectasias have a higher complication rate than patients having colonoscopy only.[34 35]

Indications for Surgery

The optimum timing of surgical intervention is not clear, but most clinicians would consider the six unit transfusion requirement established in the management of upper gastrointestinal bleeding as a reasonable guide to the need for urgent surgery. Segmental resection is indicated when diagnostic studies localise the bleeding to a specific site.[5 31 36] When the bleeding cannot be localised, the decision to perform subtotal resection becomes more reasonable. Subtotal colectomy should be used for patients in whom active colonic bleeding persists, the angiogram is normal, and the colonoscopy is either negative or not helpful. Because it is associated with a higher mortality and morbidity rate, this operation should be used with discretion.

Conclusions

Lower intestinal haemorrhage remains a diagnostic dilemma for the physician, who must use the resources available at his or her institution to determine the site of bleeding as expeditiously as possible.

Diverticular disease, vascular ectasias, and ischaemic and inflammatory bowel diseases remain the primary causes of lower intestinal bleeding. Management depends on the diagnosis, the location of the lesion, and the severity of the bleeding. In severe acute haemorrhage a bleeding scan followed by angiography will localise the bleeding site in approximately half the patients and even allow for therapy by using vasopressin (generally a temporising measure) or transcatheter embolisation. Patients who stop bleeding still require a complete diagnostic evaluation to determine the cause of bleeding. Colonoscopy has the highest diagnostic yield, and will generally give a precise pathological diagnosis. Surgery can be performed with acceptable morbidity and mortality. Rebleeding can occur in up to 25% of patients evaluated. Segmental resection should be performed for all localised bleeding. Subtotal colectomy should be performed only for patients in whom bleeding persists and a probable cause cannot be identified.

The source and nature of haemorrhage originating in the small bowel is more difficult to ascertain. Bleeding scan and angiography are seldom of value and enteroscopy is difficult and limited. CT scanning, the recent use of longer enteroscopes, push enteroscopy, formal enteroscopy (a 6 h procedure available at only a few institutions), and intraoperative enteroscopy have improved our diagnostic ability, but the small bowel remains the area with the highest incidence of obscure bleeding and a diagnostic challenge to the most astute physician.

Key points

- Patients with diverticular disease who rebleed require surgery—either segmental resection or subtotal colectomy, according to the redistribution of the diverticula

- First line treatment for bleeding vascular ectasias is endoscopic coagulation. Where this fails or is unavailable, right hemicolectomy is performed

- Early surgery is indicated in ischaemic bowel disease if laparoscopy reveals transmural disease. Gangrenous bowel requires resection with creation of an end colostomy and mucous fistula

- For severe haemorrhage from Crohn's disease, surgical resection should be the primary treatment

- For massive bleeding in ulcerative colitis, subtotal colectomy can be followed by creation of a pelvic pouch, which maintains continence

- Bleeding lesions of the small bowel should be resected where possible

- Full diagnostic evaluation of the patient who has stopped bleeding is essential, to prevent later rebleeding or progression of a treatable lesion

---

References

1 Alexander J, Karl RC, Skinner DB. Results of changing trends in the surgical management of complications of diverticular disease. *Surgery* 1983;**94**:683–90.
2 Ulin AW, Peare AF. Diverticular disease of the colon: surgical perspectives in the last decade. *Dis Colon Rectum* 1981;**14**:176–281.

3 Boley SJ, DiBiase A, Brandt LJ, Sammartano RJ. Lower intestinal bleeding in the elderly. *Am J Surg* 1979;**137**:57–64.
4 Quinn WC. Gross hemorrhage from presumed diverticular disease of the colon: results of treatment in 103 patients. *Ann Surg* 1961;**153**:851–60.
5 Athanasoulis CA, Baum SAR, Rosch J, *et al*. Mesenteric arterial infusions of vasopressin for hemorrhage from colonic diverticulosis. *Am J Surg* 1975;**129**:212–6.
6 Robinette C, Gerlock AJ. Intra-arterial vasopressin infusion in treating acute gastrointestinal bleeding. *South Med J* 1980;**73**:209–13.
7 Eisenberg H, Laufler I, Skillman JJ. Arteriographic diagnosis and management of suspected colonic diverticular hemorrhage. *Gastroenterology* 1973;**64**:1091–1100.
8 Browder W, Cerise EJ, Litwin MS. Impact of emergency angiography in massive lower gastrointestinal bleeding. *Ann Surg* 1986;**204**:530–6.
9 Talman EA, Dixon DS, Gutierrez FE. Role of arteriography in rectal hemorrhage due to arteriovenous malformations and diverticulosis. *Ann Surg* 1979;**190**:203–12.
10 Margulis AR, Heinbecker P, Bernard HR. Operative mesenteric arteriography in the search for the site of bleeding in unexplained gastrointestinal hemorrhage. *Surgery* 1960; **48**:534–9.
11 Boley SJ, Brandt LJ. Vascular ectasias of the colon. *Dig Dis Sci* 1986;**31**:26–42.
12 Richter JM, Christensen MR, Colditz GAI, Nishoika NS. Angiodysplasia: natural history and efficacy of therapeutic interventions. *Dig Dis Sci* 1984;**34**:1542–6.
13 Baum S, Athanasoulis CA, Waltman AC, *et al*. Angiodysplasia of the right colon; a cause of gastrointestinal bleeding. *Am J Roentgenol* 1977;**129**:789–94.
14 Boley SJ, Sammartano R, Brandt LJ, Sprayregen S. Vascular ectasias of the colon. *Surg Gynecol Obstet* 1979;**149**:353–9.
15 Trudel JL, Fazio VW, Sivak MV. Colonoscopic diagnosis and treatment of arteriovenous malformation in chronic lower gastrointestinal bleeding. *Dis Colon Rectum* 1988;**31**:107–10.
16 Rogers BHG. Endoscopic electrocoagulation of vascular abnormalities of the GI tract in 51 patients. *Gastrointest Endosc* 1982;**28**:142–3.
17 Greenstein AJ, Kark AE, Dreiling DA. Crohn's disease of the colon. II. Controversial aspects of hemorrhage, anemia and rectal involvement in granulomatous disease involving the colon. *Am J Gastroenterol* 1975;**63**:40–8.
18 Yuan JG, Sachar DB, Koganei K, Greenstein AJ. Refractory anemia, enterolithiasis, and stricturing Crohn's disease. *J Clin Gastroenterol* 1994;**18**:105–8.
19 Farmer RG, Hawk WA, Turnbull RB. Indication for surgery in Crohn's disease. Analysis of 500 cases. *Gastroenterology* 1976;**71**:245–50.
20 Robert JR, Sachar DB, Greenstein AJ. Severe gastrointestinal hemorrhage in Crohn's disease. *Ann Surg* 1991;**213**:207–11.
21 Edwards FC, Truelove SC. The course and prognosis of ulcerative colitis. *Gut* 1964;**5**: 1–26.
22 Farmer RG. Clinical features and natural history of inflammatory bowel disease. *Med Clin North Am* 1980;**64**:1161–71.
23 Robert JH, Sachar DB, Aufses AH, Greenstein AJ. Management of severe hemorrhage in ulcerative colitis. *Am J Surg* 1990;**159**:550–5.
24 Szold A, Katz LB, Lewis BS. Surgical approach to occult gastrointestinal bleeding. *Am J Surg* 1992;**163**:90–3.
25 Bowden TA. Endoscopy of the small intestine. *Surg Clin North Am* 1989;**69**:1237–47.
26 Lewis BS, Waye JD. Total small bowel enteroscopy. *Gastroint Endosc* 1987;**33**:435–8.
27 Leitman IM, Paul DE, Shires GT. Evaluation and management of massive lower gastrointestinal hemorrhage. *Ann Surg* 1989;**209**:175–80.
28 Beaton H. Small intestinal bleeding: method for intraoperative localisation. *NY State J Med* 1982;**82**:171–4.
29 Athanasoulis CA, Moncure AC, Greenfield AJ, Ryan JA, Dodsen TF. Intraoperative localisation of small bowel bleeding sites with combined use of angiographic methods and methylene blue injection. *Surgery* 1980;**87**:77–84.
30 Orecchia PM, Hensley EK, McDonald PT, Lull RJ. Localization of lower gastrointestinal hemorrhage: experience with red blood cells labeled in vitro with technetium Tc 99m. *Arch Surg* 1985;**120**:621–4.
31 Nath RL, Sequeira JC, Weitzman AF, Birkett DH, Williams LF. Lower gastrointestinal bleeding. Diagnostic approach and management conclusions. *Am J Surg* 1981;**141**:478–81.
32 Colacchio TA, Forde KA, Patsos TJ, Nunez D. Impact of modern diagnostic methods on the management of active rectal bleeding: a ten year experience. *Am J Surg* 1982;**143**: 607–10.

33 Tedesco FS, Gottfried EB, Corless JK, Brownstein RE. Prospective evaluation of hospitalized patients with non-active lower intestinal bleeding: timing and role of barium enema and colonoscopy. *Gastrointest Endosc* 1984;**30**:281–3.

34 Cello JP, Grendell JH. Endoscopic laser treatment for gastrointestinal vascular ectasias. *Ann Intern Med* 1986;**104**:352–4.

35 Howard OM, Buchanan JD, Hunt RH. Angiodysplasias of the colon: experience of 26 cases. *Lancet* 1982;**2**:16–20.

36 Boley SJ, Brandt L, Frank M. Severe lower intestinal bleeding: diagnosis and treatment. *Clin Gastroenterol* 1981;**10**:65–91.

Part VII
Paediatric gastrointestinal bleeding

21: Gastrointestinal bleeding in infants and children

M STEPHEN MURPHY AND IAN W BOOTH

The differential diagnosis for gastrointestinal haemorrhage in early life differs significantly from that in adult patients.[1] To adopt a sensible investigative strategy in young patients, it is essential to be aware of the possible causes of bleeding throughout infancy and childhood (Box 21.1).

Box 21.1   Significant causes of gastrointestinal bleeding in infancy and childhood

Neonate
- Swallowed blood (maternal)
- Vitamin K deficiency
- Necrotising enterocolitis

Infancy/early childhood
- Peptic oesophagitis
- Portal hypertension
- Allergic enterocolitis
- Meckel's diverticulum
- Intestinal duplication

The older child
- Peptic oesophagitis
- Portal hypertension
- Gastric/duodenal ulcers
- Eosinophilic gastroenteropathy
- Crohn's disease

- Allergic proctocolitis
- Congenital anomalies
- Intussusception
- Bacterial gastroenteritis
- Amoebic colitis
- Juvenile polyp
- Anal fissure
- Ulcerative colitis
- Peutz–Jeghers syndrome
- Haemorrhoids

The quantity of blood loss may be trivial, but if the source is in the distal bowel blood is readily seen in the stool and this usually evokes great anxiety. Whatever the severity, bleeding may indicate a significant underlying disorder. As in adults, chronic blood loss, particularly from the upper gastrointestinal tract, may not be clinically apparent and may present as unexplained iron deficiency anaemia. Occasionally bleeding in children is sudden and severe, and this may be particularly hazardous in very young patients in whom haemodynamic homeostatic mechanisms are relatively immature.[1]

This chapter focuses mainly on disorders that may cause gastrointestinal bleeding in infancy and childhood. The principles underlying investigation and treatment are generally comparable with those that apply in adult patients. General approaches to management are outlined, with an emphasis on those aspects that are particularly important in the young. In many cases the facilities and expertise of a tertiary referral are necessary for the optimal management of these children.

Aetiology

It may be advisable to confirm the history of gastrointestinal bleeding, if possible, before undertaking complex investigations. If blood is swallowed, haematemesis or melaena may result. Newborn infants often swallow maternal blood during delivery and older children may do so during episodes of epistaxis. Various medicines and dietary constituents may alter the appearance of the vomitus or faeces leading to unnecessary concern. For example, haematemesis may be suspected in children who vomit after drinking tomato juice; iron supplements, bismuth, spinach, and even dog biscuit, may each darken the stool and suggest melaena. An unexplained anaemia may suggest occult gastrointestinal bleeding. Pulmonary haemosiderosis, a rare disorder associated with chronic intrapulmonary haemorrhage, may present with unexplained anaemia, and if the respiratory symptoms are subtle occult gastrointestinal bleeding may be falsely suspected.

Occasionly Munchausen's syndrome by proxy presents as real or apparent gastrointestinal bleeding.[2] Failure to consider this entity in appropriate circumstances may result in extensive and unnecessary investigations and in a delay in diagnosis.

In the discussion that follows it is not possible to consider the many relevant disorders in a sequence that is particularly helpful from a diagnostic standpoint. The individual diseases may present in many ways, depending on site and severity, and there is considerable overlap in the ages of presentation. The various entities are therefore grouped under general headings relating to their pathology.

Mucosal injury and ulceration in the foregut

Reflux oesophagitis

Gastro-oesophageal reflux is common in infancy. Occasionally it causes an erosive oesophagitis, which may be painless in spite of being responsible for a severe iron deficiency anaemia. In some cases coffee-ground vomiting, haematemesis or even melaena may occur. Severe oesophagitis is particularly frequent in children with cerebral palsy or other major neurological disorders.[3] It is also common in children who have undergone surgery for oesophageal atresia.[4]

Mallory–Weiss syndrome

Severe vomiting may cause haemorrhage because of a traumatic mucosal tear at the gastro-oesophageal junction—the Mallory–Weiss syndrome.[5] This disorder should be suspected if there is a history of forceful or persistent vomiting followed by haematemesis. The amount of blood loss is often small, and in children usually resolves spontaneously.

Gastritis and ulceration

Gastric and duodenal erosions often occur in seriously ill children receiving intensive care.[6] Bleeding is usually slight but occasionally there is life threatening haemorrhage.[7] Gastric bleeding also occurs in ill premature infants and this also may be from stress induced ulceration. Severe bleeding has been described in apparently healthy newborn infants in the first 48 h of life, and in several such cases haemorrhagic gastritis or duodenal ulceration have been documented.[8]

An unexplained haemorrhagic gastritis is occasionally reported in older children.[9] This has been described in association with a lymphocytic gastritis similar to that seen in some adults with gastric bleeding. Severe haemorrhagic gastritis was reported in several Australian children during an epidemic of influenza A.[10]

Although chronic peptic ulcer disease is predominantly a disease of adult life, its occurrence is well documented even in young children.[11] A significant minority first present with haematemesis or melaena. Gastric and duodenal ulcers occur in association with *Helicobacter pylori* colonisation in about 50% of children. Non-steroidal anti-inflammatory agents are widely used in the treatment of juvenile chronic arthritis, and may cause gastric and duodenal ulceration with bleeding in children.[12]

Children with short bowel syndrome may develop hypergastrinaemia with acid hypersecretion, peptic ulceration and bleeding.[13] The Zollinger–Ellison syndrome has occasionally been reported in children[14]; it may be suspected in those with an unusual distribution or severity of ulceration, or if there is associated steatorrhoea or diarrhoea.

Disorders associated with an enteropathy or colitis

Necrotising enterocolitis

Necrotising enterocolitis occurs chiefly in premature infants in the neonatal intensive care unit. Term infants are occasionally affected, particularly in association with perinatal asphyxia, intrauterine growth retardation, polycythaemia or cyanotic heart disease or after exchange transfusions.[15 16] Its aetiology is unknown, but immaturity of the mucosal barrier is probably a significant factor. The characteristic pathological findings include mucosal ulceration, necrosis and the presence of intramural gas collections. It most frequently affects the ileum and the proximal colon but intestinal involvement may be extensive. Infants with necrotising enterocolitis often present with non-specific signs suggestive of sepsis. In some cases there is abdominal distension and vomiting. Blood is often present in the stool. A plain abdominal radiograph may be diagnostic, the classic sign being pneumatosis intestinalis (Figure 21.1).

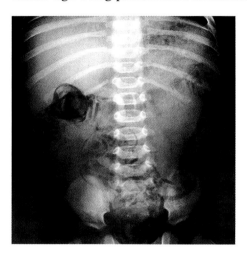

FIGURE 21.1—*Necrotising enterocolitis with radiological signs of extensive pneumatosis.*

Allergic enterocolitis

A syndrome is described in breast fed infants that is characterised by the passage of loose blood-streaked stools.[17-19] This usually presents in the first 3 months of life, and has been termed "benign infantile proctitis". These infants appear well, they are not anaemic or hypoalbuminaemic, and peripheral eosinophilia is not usually noted. Sigmoidoscopy reveals inflammation, occasionally with aphthoid ulcers, in the distal colon and rectum. A patchy focal mixed inflammatory infiltrate is present in which eosinophils may predominate.[19 20] Occasionally crypt abscesses are seen. These infants respond to feeding with a casein hydrolysate formula in place of breast milk, and relapse on reintroduction of breast milk. Small but immunologically significant quantities of maternal dietary proteins are normally present in human milk, and it is assumed that these may provoke this allergic disorder in susceptible infants.

A potentially more severe enterocolitis may occur in infants receiving cow's milk protein either in formula or whole milk.[21-25] These infants usually present in the early months of life with vomiting, failure to thrive or bloody diarrhoea. They may be anaemic or hypoalbuminaemic and there is often a marked peripheral eosinophilia. Occasionally the onset is delayed, with presentation in later infancy, and it has been suggested that in such cases it may be provoked by the change from formula to whole milk.[19] It has been said that whole milk induces gastrointestinal bleeding in many infants, but not all studies support this contention.[26] In some infants biopsy of the small bowel may reveal patchy partial villous atrophy, while in others sigmoidoscopy may demonstrate colitis with an associated patchy focal eosinophilic infiltrate.[20] Although occasional crypt abscesses may be seen, the crypt architecture is preserved.

Cow's milk enterocolitis responds rapidly to the use of a protein hydrolysate formula in place of cow's milk. Soy formula is not generally recommended because it is alleged that a substantial proportion of these infants are also intolerant to soy protein. In most cases cow's milk can be tolerated by 18 to 24 months of age. It has been reported that infants with cow's milk intolerance may rarely exhibit intolerance to various other dietary constituents including beef, pork, fish and wheat.[25] Confirmation of such sensitivity states by double blind placebo controlled testing has not always been possible.

Eosinophilic gastroenteropathy

Eosinophilic gastroenteropathy is an uncommon disorder characterised by the presence of an intense eosinophilic infiltrate in the gut, usually associated with a pronounced peripheral eosinophilia.[27] This disorder may occur at any age, although the peak incidence is in the second and third decades of life. It often follows a chronic relapsing course. Some have reported an increased prevalence of atopy in these patients. Eosinophilic gastroenteropathy, especially in infancy, may represent a sensitivity to dietary constituents, but in most cases no precipitating factors can be identified. The commonest sites of involvement are the gastric antrum and the small intestine, but any region in the gut may be affected. The eosinophilic infiltrate is often associated with mucosal erythema, friability and ulceration. Symptoms may include abdominal pain, vomiting and diarrhoea, and failure to thrive. In children with proximal disease anaemia may occur as a result of chronic blood loss, while in those with colonic disease blood may be observed in the stool.

Crohn's disease and ulcerative colitis

In older children classical inflammatory bowel disease becomes more important as a cause of intestinal inflammation. In about 25% of patients with Crohn's disease or ulcerative colitis the first symptoms occur in childhood or adolescence.[28] In these disorders inflammation and ulceration often cause gastrointestinal haemorrhage. In small bowel Crohn's disease anaemia may occur because of chronic blood loss, and rarely this may be the sole manifestation of the disease (Figure 21.2). Occasionally Crohn's disease may cause severe gastrointestinal bleeding.[29] Both ulcerative colitis and Crohn's colitis may cause bloody mucoid diarrhoea and severe colitis can quickly lead to anaemia.[30]

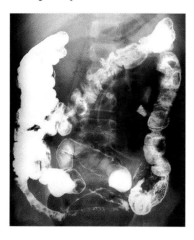

FIGURE 21.2—*Radiological signs of ileal Crohn's disease, including stricture formation, in a child presenting with iron deficiency anaemia.*

Intestinal ischaemia and vascular disorders

Ischaemia

Intussusception is an important cause of acute intestinal obstruction in childhood (Figure 21.3).[31] It usually causes severe episodic colic with vomiting, and an abdominal mass may be palpable. In young infants the initial presentation may be subtle and intestinal infarction may be more likely to occur. Intestinal ischaemia causes loss of epithelial and vascular integrity and consequently may be associated with bleeding. Intussusception is often associated with the passage of blood and mucus per rectum—the "redcurrant jelly" stool. Most patients present during the first year of life, although intussusception does occur in older children and in these a "lead point" such as a Meckel's diverticulum, duplication, polyp, haemangioma or neoplasm is more often present.[32] There is an increased frequency of intussusception in children with cystic fibrosis and in those with Henoch Schoenlein purpura.

Vasculitis

Henoch Schoenlein purpura is a vasculitic disorder that occurs quite often in infants and children.[33] It is characterised by a vasculitic skin rash,

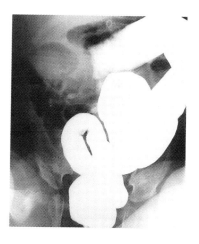

FIGURE 21.3—*Barium enema demonstrating an intussusception in a child presenting with episodic abdominal pain and "redcurrant jelly" stools (that is, blood and mucus).*

arthritis and abdominal pain. The rash is initially urticarial with subsequent development of non-blanching purpuric lesions. In older children it chiefly affects the extensor surface of the limbs (Figure 21.4). In infants, however, the scalp and face are often involved and subcutaneous oedema may also be prominent. Gross or microscopic haematuria is often present. Overt gastrointestinal bleeding is common; this may present with haematemesis and melaena or unaltered blood may be present in the stool. Rarely other vasculitic disorders such as lupus erythematosus, polyarteritis nodosa or Behçet's disease may be responsible for gastrointestinal bleeding in childhood.

Focal gastrointestinal lesions

Congenital anomalies

Meckel's diverticulum, a remnant of the vitellointestinal duct, is present in about 2% of the population (Figure 21.5). It is found on the antimesenteric border of the intestine about 50–75 cm from the ileocaecal junction. Ectopic gastric tissue is present in 30% of cases and may lead to ulceration in the diverticulum or in the adjacent ileum. These children typically present in the first two years of life with passage of maroon or bright red blood per rectum.[34] The episode is usually painless apart from mild intestinal cramping secondary to the intraluminal blood.

Gastrointestinal duplications may occur at any level throughout the gut. These are cystic or tubular structures located on the mesenteric aspect of the gut. They possess a smooth muscle coat and a mucosal lining and they share their blood supply with the adjacent intestine. Tubular duplications frequently communicate with the gut lumen. They often contain ectopic gastric mucosa and so may ulcerate and bleed.[35]

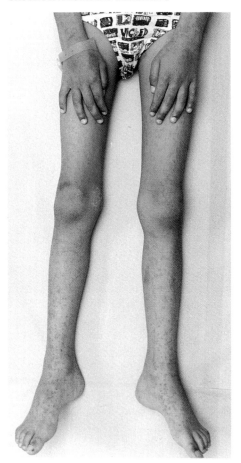

FIGURE 21.4—*Extensive vasculitic rash associated with arthralgia, abdominal pain, bloody stools, and haematuria in a child with severe Henoch Schoenlein purpura.*

Gastrointestinal haemorrhage has occasionally been described in association with a wide range of other anomalies including intestinal webs, atresias and pancreatic rests. Colonic leiomyomas have been reported as a rare cause of severe bleeding in infancy and childhood.[36]

Vascular anomalies

A variety of vascular anomalies may be responsible for gastrointestinal bleeding in childhood. These lesions may be solitary or multiple or they may affect the gut diffusely. They can cause sudden severe haemorrhage or chronic blood loss with anaemia. They may occur in isolation or as a part of a recognised syndrome with extraintestinal manifestations. They encompass a variety of lesions including malformations and neoplasia. Their classification in the literature is confusing because specimens have

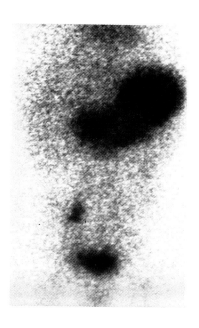

FIGURE 21.5—*$^{99}Tc^m$-pertechnetate scan revealing ectopic gastric mucosa associated with a Meckel's diverticulum in a child presenting with sudden painless passage of blood per rectum. The isotope is simultaneously taken up by the gastric mucosa and excreted in the urine, so that the stomach and bladder are outlined.*

often been inadequate, histological interpretation may be difficult and an agreed terminology has been lacking.

Haemangiomas consist of discrete foci of vascular proliferation. They are classified as capillary or cavernous on the basis of the histological appearance. Cavernous haemangiomas are larger and may cause repeated or severe bleeding.[37] Gastrointestinal haemangiomas may be numerous and are sometimes accompanied by cutaneous, hepatic and pancreatic lesions.[37] Children with Turner's syndrome may suffer from persistent gastrointestinal bleeding from diffuse intestinal haemangiomatosis.[38] Gastrointestinal haemorrhage may also occur in Klippel–Trénaunay syndrome, which is characterised by the presence of cutaneous and visceral haemangiomas and varicosities associated with secondary soft tissue and bony hypertrophy.[39–41] In the blue rubber bleb naevus syndrome cutaneous and intestinal cavernous haemangiomas are present, and these patients may present with massive gastrointestinal bleeding.[42] Large haemangiomas may be responsible for platelet sequestration and fibrinogen consumption—the Kasabach–Merritt syndrome.

A form of congenital intestinal vascular ectasia has been described that is macroscopically similar to the well recognised degenerative ectasia (angiodysplasia) seen in the elderly.[43] The excised lesions are distinguishable histologically from the adult disorder, however. Secondary vascular ectatic lesions also occur in children with various disorders including portal hypertension, congenital aortic valve disease, von Willebrand's disease, graft-versus-host disease and renal failure.[44–46]

Hereditary haemorrhagic telangiectasia is an autosomal dominant disorder in which characteristic red vascular lesions are seen in the mouth and on the face and fingers. These are composed of ectatic veins, venules and capillaries. These patients often present in adolescence with recurrent epistaxis. Gastrointestinal haemorrhage may be the only manifestation, however, and it may occur in children before the first of the tell-tale external lesions appear.[47] Telangiectasia may occur throughout the gastrointestinal tract and in the liver, and they may be seen on the intestinal serosa at laparotomy.[48]

The term arteriovenous malformation is properly applied to a particular form of hamartoma that contains large arterial and venous structures and occupies the full thickness of the bowel wall.[49] Spontaneous or iatrogenic arteriovenous fistulae may also develop between mesenteric arterial vessels and the portal venous system.

Ehlers–Danlos syndrome (cutis elastica) encompasses several related hereditary disorders that are characterised by fragile, hyperelastic skin and subcutaneous tissue, hypermobile joints and a tendency to easy bruising. Ehlers–Danlos syndrome type IV in particular is associated with a propensity to rupture of major blood vessels, and both gastrointestinal perforation and haemorrhage have been reported in affected patients.[50 51] Pseudoxanthoma elasticum is another inherited connective tissue disorder associated with a risk of bleeding, particularly from the upper gastrointestinal tract.[52]

Gastrointestinal polyps

Several forms of gastrointestinal polyp may occur in infants and children, and these lesions may bleed because of necrosis, trauma or avulsion. Juvenile polyps, acquired lesions of unknown aetiology, are by far the most frequent (Figure 21.6).[53] They are an important cause of painless colorectal haemorrhage in childhood, and although blood loss is often slight it may be sudden and severe.[54 55] In the past it was assumed that these polyps were solitary, but colonoscopy has now shown that several are often present and may be located in the proximal colon.[56] Juvenile polyposis is a rare disorder with numerous polyps in the colon and sometimes throughout the gastrointestinal tract.[57]

Peutz–Jeghers syndrome is an uncommon autosomal dominant disorder associated with gastrointestinal hamartomatous polyps throughout the gastrointestinal tract but especially in the small intestine. Most affected children have freckle-like pigmented lesions in and around the mouth and at other cutaneous sites (Figure 21.7). The cutaneous freckles tend to fade with age. Patients may present with intussusception or mechanical obstruction by a large polyp. Occasionally these polyps bleed resulting in chronic iron deficiency or overt haemorrhage.

Familial adenomatous polyposis is an autosomal dominant disorder characterised by the presence of numerous adenomas throughout the colon. It occurs as a sporadic mutation in 20% of cases. In some patients adenomas

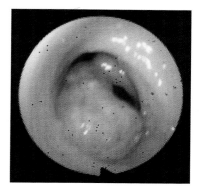

FIGURE 21.6—*Juvenile polyp in the sigmoid colon in a child with a history of recurrent passage of bright red blood per rectum.*

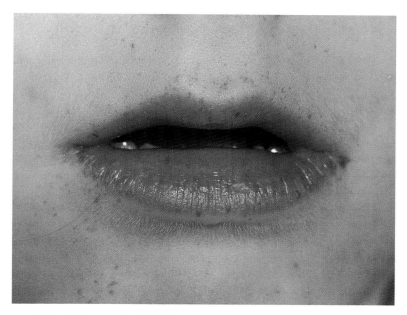

FIGURE 21.7—*Faint perioral freckling in a child with anaemia and evidence of gastrointestinal blood loss. This child had Peutz–Jeghers syndrome with hamartomatous polyps in the small intestine.*

are also found in the stomach and small intestine. Gardner's syndrome is a closely related condition with extracolonic features including osteomas and epidermoid cysts. Polyps appear in early adult life in most patients, but there is considerable variation in this regard and they have been detected as early as 4 years of age. Without surgical treatment patients with familial adenomatous polyposis almost invariably develop adenocarcinoma but obviously this is a greater concern later in adult life. Extensive polyposis often causes diarrhoea but bleeding may also occur.

Several rare polyposis syndromes exist that might potentially cause bleeding. Cowden's disease is an autosomal dominant disorder associated with both gastrointestinal and orocutaneous hamartomas. Turcot's syndrome is an autosomal recessive condition with colonic adenomas and central nervous tumours.

Gastrointestinal neoplasia

Gastrointestinal malignant tumours are uncommon in children, and are rarely suspected in young patients with bleeding. Lymphomas account for 10% of malignancies in children, and occasionally present as primary gastrointestinal tumours.[58] There is an increased incidence of lymphoma in patients with various immunodeficiency states. Overall the stomach is more often involved, while in the small intestine the terminal ileum is the commonest site. These tumours may ulcerate, leading to acute or chronic blood loss (Figure 21.8).

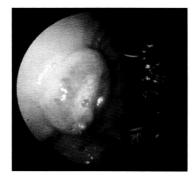

FIGURE 21.8—*Ulcerating lymphoma in the gastric antrum in a boy presenting with abdominal pain and haematemesis.*

Colonic carcinoma is rare in childhood but it does exist and has even been reported in infants.[59 60] The incidence is higher in patients with familial adenomatous polyposis, ulcerative colitis and following ureterosigmoidostomy. In such cases the risk may not be increased in the first 10 years. Children with colonic carcinoma may present with rectal bleeding, although this has usually been accompanied by other symptoms.[61] Adenocarcinoma accounts for 50% of small intestinal malignancies in childhood but it is nevertheless very rare.

Miscellaneous anorectal disorders

A variety of disorders affecting the anorectum and the perianal region can be responsible for the actual or apparent passage of bright red blood. Anal fissures are common in infants and young children, and may be caused by trauma from the passage of hard stool. Typically these fissures are superficial splits usually located in the midline, either anteriorly or posteriorly. In many cases they are associated with painful defaecation and blood is present on the surface of the stool or on the toilet paper. Rectal prolapse is a relatively common disorder in young children and may lead to mucosal trauma and bleeding. The mucosal prolapse syndrome is a different disorder that includes both the "solitary rectal ulcer syndrome" and the "inflammatory cloacogenic polyp"; it is believed to represent a response to mucosal ischaemic injury secondary to mucosal prolapse and stretching. It is well recognised in adults but it may also occur in older children.[62] It presents with tenesmus and persistent rectal bleeding. Haemorrhoids can cause bleeding even in young children. In children with severe irritation and excoriation because of chronic diarrhoea or threadworm infestation, bleeding may occur from the perianal region.

Gastrointestinal infection

Various bacteria including *Campylobacter*, *Salmonella*, and *Shigella* species and enteroinvasive *Escherichia coli* (EIEC) may cause gastroenteritis with bloody diarrhoea. *Campylobacter* and *Salmonella* species are frequent causes of gastroenteritis in childhood in western countries, while EIEC appears to be more important in the developing world.

Enterohaemorrhagic *E. coli* (EHEC) may cause severe bloody diarrhoea in children and this can be followed by development of the haemolytic uraemic syndrome.[63] Various strains of EHEC, particularly *E. coli* O157: H7, have been responsible for local epidemics.[64 65] The mucosal injury in this disorder is caused by a shiga-like toxin known as verotoxin.[66]

Clostridium difficile may be responsible for an antibiotic associated colitis. The illness may vary from mild diarrhoea to severe haemorrhagic colitis with pseudomembrane formation. The organism may play a significant role in the enterocolitis that occurs in infants with Hirschsprung's disease.[67] Curiously, *C. difficile* and its toxin can be detected in the stool of many neonates, and asymptomatic colonisation remains common during the first year of life. Detection of this organism is therefore more likely to be of significance in older children.

Acute amoebic dysentery or chronic amoebic colitis with bloody diarrhoea may be caused by infection with virulent strains of *Entamoeba histolytica*. This is rare in infants and children in western countries.

Although viral gastroenteritis is not usually associated with gastrointestinal bleeding, cytomegalovirus may cause a severe enterocolitis with bloody diarrhoea.[68] Associated mucosal ulceration occasionally causes massive gastrointestinal haemorrhage. This is most commonly seen in patients with immune deficiency states.

Immune deficiency states

Opportunistic gastrointestinal infections are common in the immunodeficient child and can cause bleeding. Children may suffer from a wide range of primary and secondary immune deficiency states. Susceptibility to infection varies depending on the severity of the disorder and on the specific components of immunity affected. Children with severe combined immunodeficiency disorders and some with "common variable immunodeficiency" states (acquired immunodeficiency states affecting both humoral and cellular immunity) have persistent diarrhoea and malabsorption associated with enterocolitis. In many of these cases specific gastrointestinal pathogens can be identified. Some patients develop severe oral, oesophageal or perianal candidiasis. Herpes simplex and cytomegalovirus infections are common. Chronic salmonella and EPEC infections may occur. All of these may be responsible for gastrointestinal bleeding. A similar pattern of infection is seen in acquired immunodeficiency syndrome.[69-71] Administration of chemotherapeutic or immunosuppressive agents may also lead to severe or persistent gastrointestinal infections.

Primary or secondary disorders of phagocytic function may cause gastrointestinal disease associated with bleeding. In chronic granulomatous disease, for example, there is an inherited defect of neutrophil function with impaired intracellular killing of micro-organisms. Patients with this disorder may present with enterocolitis and bloody diarrhoea.[72] Children with marrow suppression caused by cytotoxic agents may develop a neutropenic enterocolitis (typhilitis). In this disorder the ileocaecal region becomes inflamed, ulcerated and focally necrotic. These children are profoundly ill and may develop bloody diarrhoea.

Chemotherapy, radiotherapy and bone marrow transplantation

Many cytotoxic agents used in the treatment of malignant disorders can cause a form of mucosal injury known as mucositis by their action in arresting crypt cell mitotic activity. Methotrexate, doxorubicin, cytosine arabinoside, actinomycin D, 5-fluorouracil and bleomycin are especially potent in this respect.[73] Abdominal radiation therapy may compound the effects of these agents, increasing the incidence and severity of the enteropathy. Mucositis is often a patchy focal disorder associated with erosions and ulceration. Small bowel mucosal biopsy may reveal patchy villous atrophy.[73] These changes are occasionally associated with significant bleeding, especially if there is accompanying marrow suppression and thrombocytopenia.

Almost 50% of bone marrow recipients develop clinical evidence of intestinal graft-versus-host disease. In the most severe cases this leads to extensive mucosal sloughing with severe watery diarrhoea. Faecal occult blood tests are often positive, but overt and even severe bleeding may occur.

Portal hypertension

Portal hypertension can cause severe and often life threatening upper gastrointestinal haemorrhage, even in young children.[74] Bleeding may arise from a ruptured varix or, in those with portal hypertensive gastropathy, it may be from the mucosal surface.

In infants and children, portal hypertension is often associated with hepatic cirrhosis. In these cases bleeding usually occurs in the setting of known hepatic dysfunction and clinical manifestations of liver disease are usually present. Extrahepatic biliary atresia is the commonest cause of cirrhosis in infancy and childhood; here, portal hypertension often develops rapidly unless biliary drainage has been achieved with a successful portoenterostomy procedure. Evidence of portal hypertension, including splenomegaly and varices, may develop within months. Many other congenital and acquired liver disorders can also cause cirrhosis and portal hypertension in infancy or in later childhood (Box 21.2).

Box 21.2   Disorders causing portal hypertension in infancy and childhood

Hepatic disorders

- Extrahepatic biliary atresia
- Alagille's syndrome (syndromic bile duct paucity)
- Non-syndromic bile duct paucity
- Caroli's disease
- Neonatal hepatitis (idiopathic)
- Congenital viral hepatitis (for example, cytomegalovirus)
- Acquired viral hepatitis (for example hepatitis B and C)

- Metabolic disorders (for example, alpha-1-antitrypsin deficiency, tryosinaemia type 1, Wilson's disease)
- Autoimmune chronic active hepatitis
- Parenteral nutrition
- Cystic fibrosis
- Congenital hepatic fibrosis

Vascular disorders

- Congenital and acquired obstruction of the hepatic vein or the internal vena cava (Budd–Chiari syndrome)
- Portal vein or splenic vein thrombosis

Portal vein thrombosis is an important extrahepatic cause of portal hypertension in childhood. In many cases the first presentation is with severe haematemesis and melaena. On examination splenomegaly is usually noted. Sometimes a history of umbilical vein catheterisation or omphalitis in the neonatal period may be elicited as a possible cause. Alternatively congenital anomalies affecting the portal vein may be responsible.

Disorders of haemostasis and coagulation

Patients with bleeding disorders are at increased risk of severe bleeding if there is an underlying gastrointestinal disorder predisposing to haemorrhage. Infants and children may suffer from a wide spectrum of congenital and acquired disorders of haemostasis and coagulation. There is an increased incidence of gastrointestinal bleeding in children with moderate or severe factor VIII or IX deficiencies.[75] Vitamin K deficiency can occur in breast fed infants and in children with cholestasis and fat malabsorption, and this may cause a severe coagulopathy. Advanced liver disease may be associated with impaired synthesis of clotting factors. Treatment with agents such as warfarin is associated with an increased risk of gastrointestinal haemorrhage, particularly if the level of anticoagulation is excessive.[76]

Investigation

Clinical assessment

The approach to the investigation of gastrointestinal haemorrhage is governed by the specific clinical features in individual cases (Box 21.3). In those with overt bleeding it is often possible to determine the approximate region in which the blood loss is likely to have occurred. The clinical history and physical examination may limit the differential diagnosis or may even point to a specific diagnosis. Finally, as previously discussed, the age of the child is a key element in the differential diagnosis, and is crucial in determining investigative priorities.

Box 21.3   Potentially useful investigations in gastrointestinal haemorrhage in infants and children

Suspected site

- Oesophagus/stomach/duodenum

- Small intestine

- Terminal ileum/colon/rectum

Investigations

- Apt test (neonates)
- Upper gastrointestinal endoscopy
- $^{99}Tc^{m}$-pertechnetate scan
- $^{99}Tc^{m}$-red cell scan
- Angiography
- Enteroscopy
- Laparotomy
- Stool microscopy and culture
- *Clostridium difficile* toxin
- Flexibile sigmoidoscopy or colonoscopy

continued

- Occult bleeding

- Upper gastrointestinal endoscopy
- Colonoscopy
- $^{99}Tc^m$-red cell scan
- Angiography
- Small bowel contrast radiology

Haematemesis indicates blood loss from above the ligament of Treitz. Melaena or the passage of maroon stools indicate a moderate to large haemorrhage usually proximal to the hepatic flexure of the colon. Severe bleeding from any site may result in the passage of a large quantity of red blood. Smaller quantities of blood mixed with the stool usually indicate colonic bleeding. Blood streaked on the surface of the stool suggests an anorectal source.

A history of persistent vomiting, retrosternal pain or dysphagia may point to an underlying oesophageal disorder. Epigastric pain with nocturnal wakening may suggest peptic ulcer disease, particularly if there is a family history of this disorder. A history of mucoid diarrhoea would suggest the presence of chronic inflammation. A careful physical examination is essential to identify potentially important extraintestinal signs, such as cutaneous vascular anomalies. Nutritional assessment is important, because in disorders such as Crohn's disease growth failure may be the only obvious manifestation. An abdominal mass may be palpable in children with an intussusception or in Crohn's disease. In those with portal hypertension prominent venous collaterals may be visible on the abdominal wall and there may be significant splenomegaly. Inspection of the perianal region may reveal the presence of haemorrhoids or excoriation, while other lesions such as skin tags, fissures, sinuses and fistulae may suggest Crohn's disease. Digital rectal examination may reveal the presence of a polyp.

In all cases of unexplained gastrointestinal bleeding a coagulation screen should be performed. In the newborn infant, swallowed maternal blood can be identified using the Apt test, in which adult and fetal haemoglobin are differentiated on the basis of the different colour changes induced by alkaline denaturation.

When a child presents with unexplained melaena or with the passage of copious blood, a nasogastric tube should be passed to determine whether there is blood in the stomach, and hence whether the source of bleeding is proximal to the ligament of Treitz. If no blood is aspirated from the stomach the source must be presumed to be distal to the pylorus.

Endoscopy

In children with a history suggestive of upper gastrointestinal bleeding, early endoscopy should be considered. Small fibreoptic endoscopes are available that are suitable for use even in young infants. Early endoscopy after an acute haemorrhage may increase the diagnostic yield. Endoscopy permits direct inspection of the mucosa, thus revealing superficial lesions that may be missed with contrast radiology.[77] Oesophagitis, Mallory–Weiss tears, varices and portal hypertensive gastropathy, peptic ulcers and a variety of other less common lesions may be identified. Mucosal biopsies can be obtained and may be essential to establishing a specific diagnosis; for example, histological evidence of *Helicobacter pylori* colonisation, Crohn's disease or malignant lesions may be found. Finally, as discussed later, endoscopy may permit the performance of various therapeutic procedures designed to control or prevent bleeding.

Colonoscopy may be indicated in children who pass blood rectally. The extent of the endoscopic examination is influenced by the history and by the findings in the distal bowel. Flexible sigmoidoscopy is nowadays preferred to the rigid sigmoidoscope for limited examinations. Endoscopic examination and biopsy may be helpful in identifying a wide range of disorders, including various forms of colonic inflammation and localised lesions such as polyps or vascular anomalies. A variety of therapeutic procedures are possible during colonoscopy.

Highly specialised enteroscopes suitable for examination of the entire small bowel are being developed and may facilitate the investigation of obscure intestinal bleeding. These long, flexible endoscopes are introduced into the upper intestine and are drawn by peristalsis to the distal ileum. The endoscopist then examines the mucosa while slowly withdrawing the instrument. There are still considerable technical difficulties with these instruments.[1]

Radiology

Radionuclide scintigraphy using red blood cells labelled with $^{99}Tc^m$ locate a bleeding site, provided that the rate of blood loss at the time of examination is in the order of 0·1 ml per min.[78 79] After intravenous administration of radio labelled red cells, scintigraphic images are obtained at intervals over many hours, thus increasing the chance of demonstrating extravasation of blood (Figure 21.9). This is a moderately sensitive technique that may be particularly helpful in the investigation of those in whom the source of blood loss is beyond reach of the endoscope and also in those with intermittent bleeding. Scintigrapic studies require expert interpretation to avoid false positive results. Endoscopy or angiography may confirm a positive scan and identify the source. This may be advisable before proceeding to surgery.

Angiography performed by selective mesenteric artery catheterisation may demonstrate an actively bleeding source. Alternatively a vascular abnormality that is likely to be responsible for bleeding may be identified. Although a positive angiogram may be more informative than $^{99}Tc^m$-red cell scintigraphy, it is somewhat less sensitive, requiring blood loss at a rate of at least 0·5 ml per min during the examination.[80]

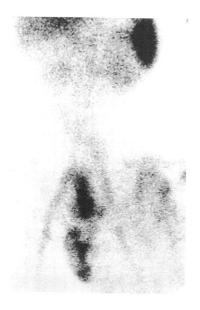

FIGURE 21.9—*Radionuclide scintigraphy with ⁹⁹Tcᵐ-labelled red blood cells revealing the presence of haemangiomas in the distal colon and rectum.*

Ectopic gastric tissue in a Meckel's diverticulum or duplication may be demonstrated with a $^{99}Tc^m$-pertechnetate scan (Figure 21.5). Intravenously administered $^{99}Tc^m$-pertechnetate is selectively taken up by gastric parietal cells. This is an appropriate investigation in children who present with episodes of painless bleeding associated with passage of maroon or red blood.

Laparotomy

In carefully selected cases exploratory laparotomy may be useful in establishing the cause of gastrointestinal haemorrhage. Ill considered surgery is rarely helpful, the source of blood loss often remaining inapparent. In patients in whom investigations, such as angiography, have successfully identified a bleeding site, surgical exploration may be necessary to establish the nature of the lesion. Intra-operative endoscopy may also be helpful. Here the surgeon facilitates the passage of the instrument by sliding the bowel over it, thus allowing the endoscopist to perform a more extensive examination of the mucosa. Endoscopic transillumination of the bowel wall during this process may also prove helpful.

Investigation of occult blood loss

Children may present with iron deficiency anaemia resulting from unrecognised low grade chronic blood loss. In such cases faecal occult blood tests may be positive. $^{99}Tc^m$-red cell scintigraphy is more useful if performed during an episode of bleeding, so repeated testing for faecal occult blood may be valuable. Upper gastrointestinal endoscopy or colonoscopy or both should also be considered in these cases. Small bowel contrast radiology may be indicated in children with unexplained intestinal bleeding, as unsuspected disorders such as Crohn's disease may be present.

Management

Infants and children with acute gastrointestinal bleeding should be assessed without delay to determine their haemodynamic status. Even after a severe haemorrhage, tachycardia may be the only manifestation of instability. Further bleeding is often likely, so hypovolaemia and anaemia should be corrected without delay. Continued observation is of fundamental importance and the vital signs should be closely monitored. Before initiating specific investigations the patient's condition should be stabilised. Subsequently, however, investigation may reveal a disorder for which specific therapy is available either to control bleeding or to reduce the risk of recurrence. Placement of a nasogastric tube is an important aspect of management in those in whom upper gastrointestinal haemorrhage is suspected. Gastric aspiration can provide an early warning of continued or recurrent bleeding. Aspiration of blood from the stomach may alleviate vomiting and in patients with hepatic insufficiency it may reduce the risk of encephalopathy.

Correction of abnormal haemostasis/clotting

In patients with thrombocytopenia platelets should be administered to maintain the serum level above $50 \times 10^9/l$. Children with variceal bleeding associated with end-stage liver disease often have a significant coagulopathy. Vitamin K deficiency may be an important contributor to this, so intravenous vitamin K should be administered empirically. In most cases, however, the coagulopathy reflects a severe defect in hepatic synthetic function and correction therefore requires intravenous administration of clotting factors, usually as fresh frozen plasma.

Variceal haemorrhage

In children with active variceal bleeding pharmacological agents, including vasopressin, glypressin and octreotide, may be effective in controlling haemorrhage.[81] These agents seem to reduce portal blood flow by increasing splanchnic arteriolar tone. Although there is some uncertainty about the efficacy of these drugs, they are widely used in the management of variceal bleeding in adults and children. The largest experience is with vasopressin, which is administered as an intravenous bolus followed by a continuous infusion. Unfortunately it causes several side effects including pallor, hypertension, abdominal pain and arrhythmias. The vasopressin analogue triglycyl-lysine vasopressin (glypressin or terlipressin) may be preferable as it has fewer side effects.[82] Somatostatin and its long acting analogue octreotide appear to be efficacious and are relatively free of side effects.[83] Experience with these newer agents is limited in infants and children.

In a significant proportion of children variceal haemorrhage persists or recurs in spite of such pharmacotherapy. In such cases endoscopic sclerotherapy may prove effective. A sclerosing agent such as ethanolamine or tetradecyl sulphate is injected in small aliquots (for example, 0·5–1 ml) either directly into the varix or immediately adjacent to it. Variceal bleeding may also be controlled by mechanical compression using the Sengstaken–Blakemore tube. Tubes of appropriate size are available even for young children. This technique of balloon tamponade can lead to several complications, including pressure necrosis, pulmonary aspiration and airway obstruction.[81] It is perhaps most useful as a temporising measure and best restricted to children who are intubated and receiving mechanical ventilation. This facilitates close monitoring of the child, and ensures protection of the airway. Ultimately surgical intervention may be required, and in many cases liver transplantation is the definitive procedure.

Bleeding ulcers

In children with bleeding ulcers a variety of endoscopic techniques may be used to control blood loss, including electrocoagulation, heat probe treatment or injection of vasoconstricting or sclerosing agents.[84] There is relatively little experience with endoscopic laser therapy in these circumstances in very young patients.[85] Endoscopic therapy is unnecessary in most cases, however, and should be reserved for those in whom there has been substantial blood loss together with an actively bleeding ulcer or an ulcer with a recognisable blood vessel in its crater.[85] These techniques have occasionally been used in the treatment of bleeding vascular anomalies in children.[41]

Conclusion

Gastrointestinal bleeding is common in children and may be caused by a wide range of disorders. Although it is often quantitatively trivial its presence may indicate a significant underlying abnormality. Occult bleeding may be responsible for iron deficiency and anaemia. Rarely severe life threatening haemorrhage occurs in childhood. The principles of investigation and management are in general similar to those which apply in the adult patient. The differential diagnosis is wide, however, and it differs significantly at each stage throughout infancy and childhood. A tertiary referral centre with appropriate facilities and expertise is the most appropriate setting for the investigation and management of many children presenting with gastrointestinal blood loss.

Key points

- The differential diagnosis for gastrointestinal bleeding in early life differs significantly from that in the adult

- Chronic blood loss may present as unexplained iron deficiency anaemia

- Severe bleeding is particularly hazardous in the very young, in whom haemodynamic homeostatic mechanisms are immature

- Investigation and management is similar to that in adults, but in many cases only a tertiary referral centre can provide optimal care

- Intussusception is an important cause of acute intestinal obstruction in childhood, and often associated with the passage of blood and mucus per rectum—the "redcurrant jelly stool"

- Portal hypertension, usually associated with hepatic cirrhosis, can cause severe, life threatening haemorrhage, even in young children

- Nutritional assessment is important, because growth failure may be the only obvious manifestation of some disorders, such as Crohn's disease

- Small fibreoptic endoscopes are available for use in young infants

References

1 Berry R, Perrault J. Gastrointestinal bleeding. In: Walker WA, Durie PR, Hamilton JR, Walker-Smith JA, Watkins JB, eds. *Pediatric gastrointestinal disease—pathophysiology diagnosis management*. Philadelphia: BC Decker, 1991;111–31.
2 Mills RW, Burke S. Gastrointestinal bleeding in a 15 month old male. A presentation of Munchausen's syndrome by proxy. *Clin Pediatr* 1990;**29**:474–7.
3 Ross MN, Haase GM, Reiley TT. The importance of acid reflux patterns in neurologically damaged children detected by four-channel pH monitoring. *J Pediatr Surg* 1988;**23**:573–6.
4 Orringer MB, Kirsch MM, Sloan H. Long term esophageal function following repair of esophageal atresia. *Ann Surg* 1977;**91**:550–4.
5 Cannon RA, Lee G, Cox R. Gastrointestinal haemorrhage due to Mallory–Weiss syndrome in an infant. *J Pediatr Gastroenterol Nutr* 1985;**4**:323–4.
6 Lopez-Herce J, Dorao P, Elola P, Delgado MA, Ruza F, Madero R. Frequency and prophylaxis of upper gastrointestinal hemorrhage in critically ill children: a prospective study comparing the efficacy of almagate, ranitidine and sucralfate. *Crit Care Med* 1992; **20**:1082–9.
7 Lacroix J, Nadeau D, Laberge S, Gauthier M, Lapierre G, Farrell CA. Frequency of upper gastrointestinal bleeding in a pediatric intensive care unit. *Crit Care Med* 1992;**2**: 35–42.
8 Goyal A, Treem WR, Hyams JS. Severe upper gastrointestinal bleeding in healthy full-term neonates. *Am J Gastroenterol* 1994;**89**:613–6.
9 Caporali R, Luciano S. Diffuse varioliform gastritis. *Arch Dis Child* 1986;**61**:405–7.
10 Armstrong K, Fraser DK, Faoagali JL. Gastrointestinal bleeding with influenza virus. *Med J Austral* 1991;**154**:180–2.
11 Murphy MS, Eastham EJ, Jimenez M, Nelson R, Jackson RH. Duodenal ulceration: review of 110 cases. *Arch Dis Child* 1987;**62**:554–8.
12 Langman MJS, Morgan L, Worrall A. Use of anti-inflammatory drugs by patients admitted with small or large bowel perforations and haemorrhage. *BMJ* 1985;**290**:347–9.
13 Bohane TD, Haka-Ikse K, Biggar WD, Hamilton JR, Gall DG. A clinical study of young infants after small intestinal resection. *J Pediatr* 1979;**94**:552–8.
14 Buchta RM, Kaplan JM. Zollinger-Ellison syndrome in a nine year old child: case report and a review of this entity in childhood. *Pediatrics* 1971;**47**:594–8.

15 Kliegman RM, Hack M, Jones P, Fanaroff AA. Epidemiologic study of necrotizing enterocolitis among low birth weight infants: absence of identifiable risk factors. *J Pediatr* 1982;**100**:440–4.

16 Wiswell TE, Robertson CR, Jones TA, Tuttle DJ. Necrotizing enterocolitis in full term infants: a case-control study. *Am J Dis Child* 1988;**142**:532–5.

17 Lake AM, Whittington PF, Hamilton SR. Dietary protein-induced colitis in breast fed infants. *J Pediatr* 1982;**101**:906–10.

18 Dupont C, Badoual J, LeLuyer B, LeBourgeois C, Barbet J-P, Voyer M. Rectosigmoidoscopic findings during isolated rectal bleeding in the neonate. *J Pediatr Nutr* 1987;**6**:257–64.

19 Lake AM. Food-induced gastroenteropathy in infants and children. In: Metcalfe DD, Sampson HA, Simon RA, eds. *Food allergy. Adverse reactions to foods and food additives.* Boston, Massachusetts: Blackwell Scientific Publications, 1991:173–85.

20 Odze RD, Bines J, Leichtner AM, Goldman H, Antonioli DA. Allergic proctocolitis in infants: a prospective clinicopathologic biopsy study. *Hum Pathol* 1993;**24**:668–74.

21 Gryboski JD, Burkle F, Hillman R. Milk induced colitis in an infant. *Pediatrics* 1966;**38**:299–302.

22 Powell GK. Milk- and soy-induced enterocolitis of infancy. *J Pediatr* 1978;**93**:553–60.

23 Jenkins HR, Pincott JR, Soothill JF, Milla PJ, Harries JT. Food allergy: the major cause of infantile colitis. *Arch Dis Child* 1984;**59**:326–9.

24 Goldman H, Proujanski R. Allergic proctitis and gastroenteritis in children. Clinical and mucosal biopsy features in 53 cases. *Am J Surg Pathol* 1986;**10**:75–86.

25 Hill SM, Milla PJ. Colitis caused by food allergy in infants. *Arch Dis Child* 1990;**65**:132–40.

26 Fuchs G, DeWier M, Hutchinson S, Sundeen M, Schwartz S, Suskind R. Gastrointestinal blood loss in older infants: impact of cows' milk versus formula. *J Pediatr Gastroenterol Nutr* 1993;**16**:4–9.

27 Whitington PF, Whitington GL. Eosinophilic gastroenteropathy in childhood. *J Pediatr Gastroenterol Nutr* 1988;**7**:379–85.

28 Mendeloff AI. The epidemiology of inflammatory bowel disease. *Clin Gastroenterol* 1980;**9**:258–62.

29. Roberts JR, Sachar DB, Greenstein AJ. Severe gastrointestinal hemorrhage in Crohn's disease. *Ann Surg* 1991;**213**:207–11.

30 Robert JH, Sachar DB, Aufses AH, Greenstein AJ. Management of severe hemorrhage in ulcerative colitis. *Am J Surg* 1990;**159**:550–5.

31 Bruce J, Huh YS, Cooney DR. Intussusception: evolution of current management. *J Pediatr Gastroenterol Nutr* 1987;**6**:663–4.

32 Schuh S, Wesson DE. Intussusception in children two years of age and older. *Can Med Assoc J* 1987;**136**:269–72.

33 Rosenblum ND, Winter HS. Steroid effects on the course of abdominal pain in children with Henoch Schoenlein purpura. *Pediatrics* 1987;**79**:1018–21.

34 Seagram CGF, Louch RE, Stephens CA, *et al.* Meckel's diverticulum: a 10 year review of 218 cases. *Can J Surg* 1968;**11**:369–73.

35 Wardell S, Vidican DE. Ileal duplication cyst causing massive bleeding in a child. *J Clin Gastroenterol* 1990;**12**:681–4.

36 Cummings SP, Lally KP, Pineiro-Carrero V, Beck DE. Colonic leiomyoma—an unusual cause of gastrointestinal hemorrhage in childhood. Report of a case. *Dis Col Rectum* 1990;**33**:511–4.

37 Abrahamson J, Schandling B. Intestinal haemangiomata in childhood and a syndrome for diagnosis: a collective review. *J Pediatr Surg* 1973;**8**:487–95.

38 Rosen KM, Sirota DK, Marinoff SC. Gastrointestinal bleeding in Turner's syndrome. *Ann Intern Med* 1967;**67**:145–50.

39 Schmitt B, Posselt HG, Waag KL, *et al.* Severe hemorrhage from intestinal hemangiomatosis in Klippel–Trénaunay syndrome: pitfalls in diagnosis and management. *J Pediatr Gastroenterol Nutr* 1986;**5**:155–8.

40 Azizkhan RG. Life-threatening hematochizia from a rectosigmoid vascular malformation in Klippel–Trénaunay syndrome: long-term palliation using an argon laser. *J Pediatr Surg* 1991;**26**:1125–7.

41 Myers BM. Treatment of colonic bleeding in Klippel–Trénaunay syndrome with combined partial colectomy and endoscopic laser. *Dig Dis Sci* 1993;**38**:1351–3.

42 Wong SH, Lau WY. Blue rubber-bleb nevus syndrome. *Dis Colon Rectum* 1982;**25**:371–4.

43 Sasaki K, Nakagawa H, Takahashi T, Sato E. Bleeding ectatic vascular lesion involving the sigmoid colon endoscopically indistinguishable from angiodysplasia in an 8-year-old boy. *Am J Gastroenterol* 1991;**88**:105–8.

44 Duray PH, Marcal JM, Livolsi VA, Fisher R, Scholhamer C, Brand MH. Gastrointestinal angiodysplasia: a possible component of von Willebrand's disease. *Hum Pathol* 1984;**15**: 539–41.

45 Marcuard SP, Weinstock JV. Gastrointestinal angiodysplasia in renal failure. *J Clin Gastroenterol* 1988;**10**:482–4.

46 Marmaduke DP, Greenson JK, Cunningham I, Herderick EE, Cornhill JF. Gastric vascular ectasia in patients undergoing bone marrow transplantation. *Am J Clin Pathol* 1994;**102**: 194–8.

47 Mestre JR, Andres JM. Hereditary hemorrhagic telangiectasia causing hematemesis in an infant. *J Pediatr* 1982;**101**:577–9.

48 Vase P, Grove O. Gastrointestinal lesions in hereditary hemorrhagic telangiectasia. *Gastroenterology* 1986;**91**:1079–83.

49 Moore JD, Thompson NW, Appleman HD, Foley D. Arteriovenous malformations of the gastrointestinal tract. *Arch Surg* 1976;**111**:381–9.

50 Beighton PH, Murdoch JL, Votteler T. Gastrointestinal complications of Ehlers–Danlos syndrome. *Gut* 1969;**10**:1004–8.

51 Silva R, Cogbill TH, Hansbrough JF, Zapata-Sirvent RL, Harrington DS. Intestinal perforation and vascular rupture in Ehlers–Danlos syndrome. *Int Surg* 1986;**7**:48–50.

52 Kundrotas L, Novak J, Kremzier J, Meenaghan M, Hassett J. Gastric bleeding in pseudoxanthoma elasticum. *Am J Gastroenterol* 1988;**83**:868–72.

53 Latt TT, Nicholl R, Domizio P, Walker-Smith JA, Williams CB. Rectal bleeding and polyps. *Arch Dis Child* 1993;**69**:144–7.

54 Toccalino H, Guastavino E, de Pinni F, O'Donnell JC, Williams CB. Juvenile polyps of the rectum and colon. *Acta Paediatr Scand* 1973;**62**:337–40.

55 Mazier WP, Bowman HE, Sun KM, Muldoon JP. Juvenile polyps of the colon and rectum. *Dis Col Rectum* 1974;**17**:523–8.

56 Douglas JR, Campbell CA, Salisbury DM, Walker-Smith JA, Williams CB. Colonoscopic polypectomy in children. *BMJ* 1980;**281**:1386–7.

57 Veale AMO, McColl I, Bussey HJR, Morson BC. Juvenile polyposis coli. *J Med Genet* 1966;**3**:5–10.

58 Herrman R, Panahon AM, Barcos MP, Walsh D, Stutzman L. Gastrointestinal involvement in non-Hodgkin's lymphoma. *Cancer* 1980;**46**:215–22.

59 Kern WH, White WC. Adenocarcinoma of the colon in a 9-month-old infant: report of a case. *Cancer* 1958;**11**:855–7.

60 Odone V, Chang L, Caces J, George SL, Pratt CB. The natural history of colorectal carcinoma in adolescents. *Cancer* 1982;**49**:1716–20.

61 Middlekamp JN, Haffner H. Carcinoma of the colon in children. *Pediatrics* 1963;**32**: 558–71.

62 Du Boulay CEH, Fairbrother J, Isaacson PG. Mucosal prolapse syndrome—a unifying concept for solitary ulcer syndrome and related disorders. *J Clin Pathol* 1983;**36**:1264–8.

63 Spika JS, Parsons JE, Nordenberg D, Wells JG, Gunn RA, Blake PA. Hemolytic uremic syndrome and diarrhea associated with *Escherichia coli* O157:H7 in a day care center. *J Pediatr* 1986;**109**:287–91.

64 Griffin PM, Tauxe RV. The epidemiology of infections caused by *Escherichia coli* O157: H7, other enterohemorrhagic *E. coli* and the associated haemolytic uremic syndrome. *Epidemiol Rev* 1991;**13**:60–98.

65 Swerdlow DL, Woodruf BA, Brady RC, *et al.* A waterborne outbreak in Missouri of *Escherichia coli* O157:H7 associated with bloody diarrhea and death. *Ann Intern Med* 1992; **117**:812–9.

66 Karmali MA, Petric M, Lim C, Fleming PC, Arbus GS, Lior H. The association between idiopathic haemolytic uremic syndrome and infection by verotoxin-producing *Escherichia coli*. *J Infect Dis* 1985;**151**:775–81.

67 Qualman SJ, Petric M, Karmali MA, Smith CR, Hamilton SR. Clostridium difficile invasion and toxin circulation in fatal pediatric pseudomembranous colitis. *Am J Clin Pathol* 1990;**94**:410–6.

68 Weber JN, Thom S, Barrison I, *et al.* Cytomegalovirus colitis and oesophageal ulceration in the context of AIDS. *Gut* 1987;**28**:482–7.

69 Dolgin SE, Larsen JG, Shah KD, David E. CMV enteritis causing haemorrhage and obstruction in an infant with AIDS. *J Pediatr Surg* 1990;**25**:696–8.
70 Kawimbe B, Bem C, Patil PS, Bharucha H. Cytomegalovirus ileitis presenting as massive rectal bleeding in infancy. *Arch Dis Child* 1991;**66**:883–4.
71 Cappell MS, Gupta A. Gastrointestinal hemorrhage due to gastrointestinal *Mycobacterium avium intracellulare* or oesophageal candidiasis in patients with the acquired immunodeficiency syndrome. *Am J Gastroenterol* 1992;**87**:224–9.
72 Ament ME, Ochs HD. Gastrointestinal manifestation of chronic granulomatous disease. *N Engl J Med* 1983;**288**:382–7.
73 Mitchell EP, Schein PS. Gastrointestinal toxicity of chemotherapeutic agents. *Semin Oncol* 1982;**9**:52–64.
74 Bernard P, Alvarez F, Brunelle F. Portal hypertension in children. *Clin Gastroenterol* 1985;**14**:33–55.
75 Mittal R, Spero JA, Lewis JH, *et al.* Patterns of gastrointestinal haemorrhage in hemophilia. *Gastroenterology* 1985;**88**:515–22.
76 Jick H, Porter J. Drug-induced gastrointestinal bleeding. *Lancet* 1978;2:87–9.
77 Ament ME, Berquist WE, Vargas J, Perisic V. Fibreoptic upper intestinal endoscopy in infants and children. *Pediatr Clin North Am* 1988;**35**:141–55.
78 Datz FL, Thorne DA, Remley K. Determination of bleeding rates necessary for imaging acute gastrointestinal bleeding with Tc-99m labeled red blood cells. *J Nucl Med* 1986;**27**:956.
79 Smith R, Copley DJ, Bolen FH. ^{99m}Tc RBC scintigraphy: correlation of gastrointestinal bleeding rates with scintigraphic findings. *Am J Roentgenol* 1987;**148**:869–74.
80 Afshani E, Berger PE. Gastrointestinal tract angiography in infants and children. *J Pediatr Gastroenterol Nutr* 1986;**5**:173–86.
81 Shneider BL, Groszmann J. Portal hypertension. In: Suchy FJ, ed. *Liver disease in children*. St Louis: Mosby, 1994;249–66.
82 Soderlund C, Magnusson I, Torngren S, Lundell L. Terlipressin (triglycyl-lysine vasopressin) controls acute bleeding oesophageal varices. A double-blind randomised, placebo-controlled trial. *Scand J Gastroenterol* 1990;**25**:622–30.
83 Burroughs AK. Octreotide in variceal bleeding. *Gut* 1994;**35**(**suppl 3**):S23–7.
84 Laine L, Peterson L. Bleeding peptic ulcer. *N Engl J Med* 1994;**331**:717–27.
85 Tedesco FJ. Endoscopic therapy for vascular lesions: new challenges. *J Pediatr Gastroenterol Nutr* 1988;**7**:321–2.

Part VIII
Conclusions

22: Audit of the management of gastrointestinal bleeding

J M T WILLOUGHBY

Any audit of clinical practice, if it is to be done well, must be seen at the outset of planning as a potentially laborious and expensive task. This should ensure that its subject is carefully chosen, not only as representing a real problem in management but also as amenable to this specialised—and to most clinicians still unfamiliar— form of investigation. Audit is not research, but rather an examination of whether, in a particular setting, the fruits of research are being applied as effectively as possible. The very selection of a topic for audit implies that this may well not be the case, and so from the start there must be a strategy for securing the indispensable co-operation of colleagues (often in two or more distinct medical disciplines) who are quite aware that by taking part they may be helping to expose significant defects in their own service. This will be easier if the topic is acknowledged across specialty boundaries to be a weak area in which attention to any one aspect would be unlikely to make sufficient progress. Not only will individual participants then feel less vulnerable, but also there will be a better chance of obtaining from all of them the wholehearted and sustained commitment without which the project cannot be carried through to completion.

Such conditions are well met by gastrointestinal bleeding, in several of its varied manifestations. To date it is acute upper gastrointestinal haemorrhage that has attracted most of the effort devoted to audit in this field. This common emergency challenges the primary care physician, the medical gastroenterologist, and the surgeon, and, as often as not, shows up the frailty of co-operation between the various teams involved in its management. The difficulty is not in knowing what to do, but in how to put into practice the precepts established by a series of important studies, each of which tends to support the conclusions of its predecessors while adding refinements in diagnosis and treatment made possible by the latest technological progress. The lesions liable to bleed at this level are few, and usually easy enough to diagnose with precision; the signs of significant bleeding are clearly characterised; the principles of medical and surgical

319

management are theoretically straightforward; and death is the simplest possible among several measures of failure. Combining as it does so many of the features that favour effective medical audit, acute upper gastrointestinal haemorrhage would be hard to better as a model for study.

Perhaps equally common, but more difficult to tackle because of its chronicity, is the slow, occult bleeding which may arise at almost any level of the alimentary tract and which rivals excess menstrual loss as the most important single cause of iron deficiency in the developed world. This, and other less critical forms of gastrointestinal haemorrhage, remain virtually untouched by the process of audit, but it is not too soon to explore ways in which the knowledge compiled over decades of research may be applied to improving our management of these problems too.

The Development of Audit in Upper Gastrointestinal Bleeding

The first audit, in all but name, was that designed 50 years ago as a prospective study by Avery Jones[12] at the Central Middlesex Hospital, London, to cover all patients bleeding acutely from peptic ulceration and admitted to his own wards. By combining early gastroscopy in selected cases with a barium meal later in most, he achieved a higher rate of precise diagnosis than his predecessors. He appreciated also that much of the mortality in previous studies had stemmed from tentative use of blood transfusion, dehydration from inappropriate prohibition of oral intake (at a time when there was no intravenous alternative), and reluctance to operate on relatively young, healthy patients debilitated solely by loss of blood. Avery Jones was the first investigator to base his practice on the prognostic significance of age over 60 and co-morbidity, as well as to recognise how much outcome could be improved by close co-operation between physician and surgeon. Data he derived from the investigations and from autopsy showed a clear distinction between acute and chronic ulcers as threats to survival, leading him to the conclusion, later confirmed by use of fibrendoscopy, that rebleeding as such mattered less than erosion of a major artery.

Changes early this century in the epidemiology of peptic ulcer, combined with widely differing criteria for case selection in studies from the 1920s and 1930s, render Avery Jones' figure of 7·8% for mortality in acutely bleeding peptic ulcer the first with which those published since may realistically be compared. This was acknowledged by Lewin and Truelove,[3] who attributed their much higher mortality of 18·8% to the fact that there was no special interest in acute upper gastrointestinal haemorrhage at Oxford. Once again, age was identified as the single most important prognostic factor.

The earliest published report on the subject by a hospital's audit committee came from the Maine Medical Centre in 1972.[4] Numbers were small and analysis sketchy, but the role of a non-steroidal anti-inflammatory drug (NSAID), aspirin, was discussed and attention was drawn to how the lethal nature of bleeding from oesophageal varices could affect the overall mortality rate.

It is apparent that if the specialists of a single unit wish to investigate their own management of upper gastrointestinal haemorrhage, they may succeed not only in this but also in conveying to others how useful the small internal audit can be when well conducted. In what has become the model study from a British district general hospital, Madden and Griffiths[5] examined retrospectively the records of all emergency admissions for upper gastrointestinal bleeding at Newport, Wales, in the years 1980 and 1981. The particular relevance of their findings, judged by the frequency with which subsequent authors have cited them in some detail, derives from three central factors. Their hospital, in size, catchment population, and medical staffing, is so nearly typical of its kind as to reflect accurately the conditions in most of its counterparts elsewhere. A good choice was made of the data to extract, and—perhaps most important of all—details of the clinical histories, examination, investigation, and treatment of the 330 patients included were unusually complete. Few units could boast either note keeping or record retrieval of so high a standard; but it could also be argued that, after this study, there would be no further need for a description of practice untouched by the recognition that guidelines based on a few simple points made repeatedly over the years might enhance the efficiency of management and reduce mortality within the constraints of existing resources.

Where management has already changed—for reasons that may not be explicit—there has been a place for the relatively simple retrospective form of audit in which the outcome of treatment in two or more successive periods may be compared, and conclusions drawn as to which policy best suits that institution.[67] The special circumstances obtaining in Nottingham, England, during the 1970s allowed a comparison of outcome in two hospitals that simultaneously admitted patients from the same population but differed in their views on the value of surgery as a treatment for the bleeding peptic ulcer.[8] The findings of this study gave rise to a suspicion that, for some patients, surgery was reducing the chances of survival, whereas review of a change towards early surgery in Stockholm, Sweden, had suggested that this more aggressive policy was saving lives.[7] Such a discrepancy illustrates well how the handicap of small numbers, compounded in this instance by differences in case-mix and almost certainly too by variables relating to the concept of "early surgery", can limit the general applicability of conclusions that may be valid enough in the local context.

Despite their limitations, however, local audits and allied studies have encouraged clinicians in comparable units elsewhere to examine their own practice more closely and have served in a cumulative fashion to focus attention on certain clinical features that may generally be taken as indicators of high risk (see Chapter 6) and thus also on those aspects of management that merit special consideration. Perhaps the most important result of this process is a nascent consensus on certain key points, such as the importance of medicosurgical co-operation,[1 2 5 6 8 9 11–14] the role of dedicated units,[1 9–13 15–19] the status of early endoscopy,[13–15 20–28] and the quantitative use of blood transfusion requirements in deciding the best timing for surgery,[14 16 18 19 28–30] that is now clearly detectable in the similar starting protocols of most recent studies.

One form of audit long practised in surgical units, the death review, was applied to good effect in the context of upper gastrointestinal haemorrhage by Devitt *et al.*[9] They studied the course of treatment in 50 consecutive fatal cases that had been managed by 85 clinicians at Ottowa Civic Hospital, Canada, over a period of 9 years. An experience so dilute could have taught each individual doctor very little at the time, yet when thus concentrated and analysed it showed at once that most avoidable deaths could be ascribed to inadequate blood transfusion and delayed surgery. This finding inspired a simple protocol, derived from the patient's age, the chronicity of the bleeding lesion, and the surprisingly constant pattern of rebleeding first described by Avery Jones, which enabled the quantity and rapidity of transfusion to be tailored to each individual case (with the help of central venous monitoring if necessary), and in which surgery was recommended after one or two recurrent bleeds according to the calculated level of risk.

The Prospective Study and Its Role in Audit

Obvious advantages of the prospective trial design include the opportunity to ensure that all the most relevant data are recorded and to avoid the loss of cases and possible bias, through failure to recover patient files, that may handicap the retrospective study.[10 31 32] It does in itself, however, constitute an incentive to improve performance, and so tends to mask those very faults in current management that the audit was intended to expose. This is a defect that, once acknowledged, must nevertheless be accepted as unavoidable and is more than compensated by its positive features. The modern concept of medical audit incorporates an intention to change the protocol of management evaluated wherever any weakness has been identified, and finally to close the loop by similarly testing the revised scheme. Unless it uses a survey of past practice to influence the design of the initial protocol it is wholly prospective. In so far as adherence to this pattern is a necessary part of the definition of audit, many studies that have contributed over the years to our current understanding of what constitutes good practice in the management of acute upper gastrointestinal haemorrhage cannot be so designated.

However, it is possible to trace in single or successive reports the sustained operation of audit by certain individual units. At the Central Middlesex Hospital, Avery Jones and his surgical colleagues deliberately increased the operation rate in selected cases and thereby improved the prognosis of patients otherwise similarly treated in the same unit for many years.[2] Hunt et al.[11] and Duggan[17] were able to demonstrate how mortality in two Australian centres was lower for patients admitted to a special unit than for those treated in general wards, whether in the recent past or studied concurrently. When the comparative study at Nottingham[8] found evidence to suggest that an aggressive surgical policy might be increasing mortality, a more conservative protocol was adopted and was shown to be no less effective.[33]

Out of a detailed prospective enquiry at Birmingham, UK, published in 1976[10] came a further study[16] and a policy of constant review in regular surgical audit meetings. By 1990 this had so improved the local management of bleeding ulcers as to allow the implementation there of a firm protocol[30] that closely resembled those of other units appearing in print at this time. In Glasgow, a dramatic reduction of deaths from ulcer haemorrhage had been achieved by assigning patients to a team of interested physicians and surgeons.[13]

Away from the principal teaching centres, it was not until 1986 that poor mortality figures were first used to advocate the establishment of special units in district general hospitals,[5] but already some such hospitals with relatively generous staffing for their gastrointestinal services had recognised that need and were finding that specialist care could deliver the benefits predicted.[14 18 19]

Multicentre Audit

The first of two projects designed to audit the management of upper gastrointestinal haemorrhage over a wide range of institutions was undertaken for the American Society of Gastrointestinal Endoscopy (ASGE) and published in 1981.[25 26 34] A standardised form was issued to 269 ASGE members throughout the United States for recording the main clinical features and details of treatment in cases handled between May 1978 and October 1979. Of these, 2225 were included in an analysis that enabled the authors to examine minutely the effect of all possible risk factors considered in the literature to date (eight different general medical historical categories could be separately analysed), and also to relate the use of endoscopy, blood transfusion, and surgery to outcome. Their figure of 10·8% for overall mortality (8·7% in patients under 60 years of age, 13·4% in those over 60) confirmed the apparent failure of early endoscopic diagnosis and safer surgery to improve survival: a point on which most investigators in non-specialised units, before and since, have been agreed. Little that was new came out of the ASGE survey, but this in itself was an encouragement to all whose studies had been, or could only hope to be, on a much smaller scale. Its principal recommendation was a plea for the development of endoscopic haemostasis, which only now is coming into use widely enough to be considered suitable for inclusion in a general audit.[35] Above all, the survey showed that the formidable task of organising an audit on this scale was feasible, and it would be only a matter of time before the data from a variety of units came to be harnessed to the next stage: that of determining whether lessons learned from such an initial survey could be used to raise the general standard of management in cases of acute haemorrhage.

The necessary foundation for a complete process of audit in this field was laid in 1991 by a working party on which the British Society of Gastroenterology, the Royal College of Physicians of London and the Royal College of Surgeons of England were represented. This group published a comprehensive set of "National Guidelines"[35]; these distilled from the literature all those pointers to good practice that had received most frequent emphasis and that accorded with the experience of its members. The guidelines have formed the basis for an audit that is being carried out in a large group of English hospitals and is designed to establish whether a second phase, conducted in the full knowledge of those defects in management that were exposed by the first, can in fact demonstrate an improvement in practice and, if so, whether this has affected mortality.[36 37]

Acute Lower Gastrointestinal Bleeding

Acute haemorrhage from the lower gastrointestinal tract is uncommon except in the context of ulcerative, infective, or ischaemic colitis, when it is most usefully considered under the relevant diagnostic heading. As such it makes an unsuitable subject for audit at any but the largest of centres, and is unlikely to inspire even a multicentre study until more is known about the pathogenesis and distribution of the small vascular lesions from which it usually arises. Both this and the setting of worthwhile standards for management will require much higher sensitivity than has yet been attained in techniques for establishing the site(s) of haemorrhage.

Chronic Bleeding from the Gastrointestinal Tract

If colitis is excluded, overt bleeding into the faeces for periods exceeding a few days is seldom other than intermittent. Its origins are diverse; from the haemorrhoids most often incriminated (and posing no major problem in either diagnosis or treatment), through the adenomas, benign or malignant, of the large bowel, to the same range of vascular pathologies with which acute haemorrhage is chiefly associated. Such bleeding has acquired the epithet "obscure" whenever routine tests fail to identify its source. Thorough reviews of practice in the investigation of obscure gastrointestinal bleeding at tertiary referral centres have been published,[38-43] but formal prospective audit in this field is still lacking.

Apart from the special place for angiography and scanning methods when bleeding is overt, much of the material in these studies has an obvious and particular relevance to the far more common occult form of obscure bleeding that presents as iron deficiency anaemia, often requiring multiple admissions to hospital for blood transfusion, and always potentially a marker of intestinal cancer.

Anaemia was the sole criterion for entry to a prospective study in Australia,[44] though careful note was taken of any gastrointestinal symptoms and whether these suggested proximal or distal pathology, as well as of NSAID intake. Of 100 patients, all underwent upper gastrointestinal endoscopy. The colon was examined in 90, of whom 67 had colonoscopy and 53 the combination of flexible sigmoidoscopy with barium enema, so that in 30 the colon was surveyed twice. The protocol had demanded coverage of the colon for all patients in whom this was not positively contraindicated, and the finding of three colorectal cancers and four large polyps in seven out of 54 patients whose benign upper gastrointestinal lesions could have explained their anaemia led the authors to advocate study of the large bowel as an essential part of the diagnostic process. However, such a conclusion seems less well supported by their data when it is noted that three of these patients had bled per rectum and none had an upper gastrointestinal lesion commonly associated with anaemia. In two subsequent prospective studies of patients referred with iron deficiency only one out of 100[45] and two out of 93[46] patients subjected to both upper gastrointestinal endoscopy and colonic investigation were found to have a potential cause at both sites. For one group, the patients' symptoms offered a fairly accurate guide to the site of the putative bleeding lesion, enabling the authors to conclude that most patients need undergo no more than one examination,[45] but unfortunately this has not been the experience elsewhere.[44 46 47] Nevertheless, at Nottingham no patient under 60 had even benign adenomas of the colon, prompting the recommendation that if upper gastrointestinal endoscopy (with routine duodenal biopsy for coeliac disease) is always performed first and happens to yield a plausible explanation for the anaemia, there should be no need for barium enema (or, presumably, colonoscopy) below this age.[46]

It would seem that, for a variable proportion of patients with gastrointestinal symptoms and for all those without (together perhaps encompassing most cases of iron deficiency), the most efficient sequence of investigations will be arrived at only by deploying the diagnostic facilities available at each individual centre in accordance with the differing patterns of pathology characteristic of different age groups. Whether or not that sequence should ever exclude colonoscopy for the "younger" patient and, if so, what upper age limit should be taken as defining that group, would be appropriate subjects for an audit that should also help decide when investigation may be abandoned after a series of negative results. Two follow up studies of patients in whom multiple tests had failed to make a diagnosis found that such failure is almost always indicative of a benign aetiology,[48 49] so attention to this aspect might be expected to identify the potential for appreciable savings in financial and other resources as well as sparing patients much of the anxiety and discomfort that at present is regarded as inevitable.

Themes for Development in the Audit of Gastrointestinal Haemorrhage

The character of acute upper gastrointestinal bleeding as an instantly recognisable and potentially lethal event has led to a maturity in the study of its management that sets it apart from all other forms of bleeding into the alimentary tract.

Concern during the 1970s that no consistent fall in mortality was being recorded despite the revolution in speed and accuracy of diagnosis that came with fibrendoscopy, and the concomitant progress made in techniques for monitoring a patient's haemodynamic state, was in time dispelled by closer scrutiny of changes in the population treated. It is agreed now that a real improvement in care had been masked by increases in the mean age at admission and therefore also in the proportion of patients with serious co-morbidity. Moreover two particular measures, one long established but still surprisingly neglected, the other relatively new, have each been shown capable of over-riding this effect and actually reducing mortality in the relevant group by as much as 50%. Although a diversity of variables from one series to another allows few direct comparisons, there has emerged over the years an impressive trend to higher survival when patients receive the co-ordinated care of medical and surgical teams in special units.[1 11 15–19] More recently three meta-analyses have demonstrated a significant reduction in mortality, as well as in quantity of blood transfused and the need for surgery, in patients whose ulcers were recognised at endoscopy to be still bleeding or at high risk of rebleeding and were then submitted to local haemostatic procedures.[50–52] It is probable that an overall mortality in the region of 5% is approaching the lowest that will ever be obtained in an unselected series of patients with acute upper gastrointestinal haemorrhage, and certain that it will never be bettered across the whole range of institutions receiving such cases unless both key measures are adopted generally. Guidelines incorporating these measures would set a standard for audit without which no hospital could either realise its potential or maintain that level of performance in the management of the acute bleed.

The dramatic contribution made by endoscopic haemostasis to the treatment of bleeding in those ulcers with the worst prognosis will require some refinement of the criteria for surgical intervention.[53–57] Much more of a challenge is posed by that still relatively small proportion of patients, nearly always having other severe, pre-existing disease, in whom peptic ulceration with bleeding first develops during their treatment in hospital.[2 34 58] The average mortality in this group stands at more than 30%, and will never be made to approach that for patients in whom ulcer haemorrhage is the primary event; nevertheless, audit tailored to the patient in intensive care, high dependency units or elderly care should enable some impression to be made on this alarming figure.

As yet the element of audit in studies of bleeding that is chronic or originates exclusively in the lower gastrointestinal tract is hard to discern, save when occult haemorrhage has led to anaemia. However, current obstacles to its development—chiefly the poor sensitivity of diagnostic tests and the inadequacy of patient numbers at any one centre—will in time be overcome by a combination of technological advance and co-operative ventures of the sophistication already shown in the case of upper gastrointestinal haemorrhage to be perfectly feasible, when the will and the resources come together.

Key points

- Local audits and allied studies of the management of upper gastrointestinal haemorrhage have focused attention on indicators of high risk and related aspects of management. Protocols in use now reflect a consensus on certain points:
    —the importance of medicosurgical co-operation
    —the role of dedicated units
    —the status of early endoscopy
    —the quantitative use of blood transfusion requirements in deciding the timing of surgical intervention

- Audit of the management of bleeding that is chronic or originates exclusively from the lower gastrointestinal tract is made difficult by the poor sensitivity of diagnostic tests and the small patient numbers at individual centres

---

References

1 Avery Jones F. Haematemasis and melaena: with special reference to bleeding peptic ulcer. *BMJ* 1947;**ii**:441–6,477–86.
2 Avery Jones F. Hematemesis and melena: with special reference to causation and to the factors influencing the mortality from bleeding peptic ulcers. *Gastroenterology* 1956;**30**:166–90.
3 Lewin DC, Truelove S. Haematemesis: with special reference to chronic peptic ulcer. *BMJ* 1949;**i**:383–6.
4 Augur NA. Medical audit committee report on gastrointestinal bleeding. *J Maine Med Ass* 1972;**63**:237–8,259.
5 Madden MV, Griffith GH. Management of upper gastrointestinal bleeding in a district general hospital. *J R Coll Physicians Lond* 1986;**20**:212–5.
6 Schiller KFR, Truelove SC, Gwyn Williams D. Haematemesis and melaena: with special reference to factors influencing the outcome. *BMJ* 1970;**i**:7–14.
7 Hellers G, Ihre T. Impact of change to early diagnosis and surgery in major upper gastrointestinal bleeding. *Lancet* 1975;**ii**:1250–1.
8 Dronfield MW, Atkinson M, Langman MJS. Effect of different operation policies on mortality from bleeding peptic ulcer. *Lancet* 1979;**i**:1126–8.
9 Devitt JE, Brown FN, Beattie WG. Fatal bleeding ulcer. *Ann Surg* 1966;**164**:840–4.

10 Allan R, Dykes P. A study of the factors influencing mortality rates from gastrointestinal haemorrhage. *Q J Med* 1976;**45**:533–50.

11 Hunt PS, Hansky J, Korman MG. Mortality in patients with haematemesis and melaena: a prospective study. *BMJ* 1979;**1**:1238–40.

12 Rofe SB, Duggan JM, Smith ER, Thursby CJ. Conservative treatment of gastrointestinal haemorrhage. *Gut* 1985;**26**:481–4.

13 Murray WR, Birnie GG. Special units for acute upper gastrointestinal bleeding. *BMJ* 1987;**295**:51–2.

14 Clements D, Aslan S, Foster D, Stamatakis J, Wilkins WE, Morris JS. Acute upper gastrointestinal haemorrhage in a district general hospital: audit of an agreed management policy. *J R Coll Physicians Lond* 1991;**25**:27–30.

15 Dronfield MW. Special units for acute upper gastrointestinal bleeding. *BMJ* 1987;**294**: 1308–9.

16 Morris DL, Hawker PC, Brearley S, Simms M, Dykes PW, Keighley MRB. Optimal timing of operation for bleeding peptic ulcer; prospective randomised trial. *BMJ* 1984; **288**:1277–80.

17 Duggan JM. Haematemesis patients should be managed in special units. *Med J Aust* 1986; **144**:247–50.

18 Holman RAE, Davis M, Gough KR, Gartell P, Britton DC, Smith RB. Value of a centralised approach in the management of haematemesis and melaena: experience in a district general hospital. *Gut* 1990;**31**:504–8.

19 Sanderson JD, Taylor RFH, Pugh S, Vicary FR. Specialized gastrointestinal units for the management of upper gastrointestinal haemorrhage. *Postgrad Med J* 1990;**66**:654–6.

20 Walls WD, Glanville JN, Chandler GN. Early investigation of haematemesis and melaena. *Lancet* 1971;**ii**:387–90.

21 Cotton PB, Rosenberg MT, Waldram RPL, Axon ATR. Early endoscopy of oesophagus, stomach and duodenal bulb in patients with haematemesis and melaena. *BMJ* 1973;**2**: 505–9.

22 Morgan AG, McAdam WAF, Walmsley GL, Jessop A, Horrocks JC, de Dombal FT. Clinical findings, early endoscopy and multivariate analysis in patients bleeding from the upper gastrointestinal tract. *BMJ* 1977;**2**:237–40.

23 Foster DN, Miloszewski KJA, Losowsky MS. Stigmata of recent haemorrhage in diagnosis and prognosis of upper gastrointestinal bleeding. *BMJ* 1978;**1**:1173–7.

24 Griffiths WJ, Neumann DA, Welsh JD. The visible vessel as an indicator of uncontrolled or recurrent gastrointestinal hemorrhage. *N Engl J Med* 1979;**300**:1411–13.

25 Silverstein FE, Gilbert DA, Tedesco FJ, *et al.* The national ASGE survey on upper gastrointestinal bleeding. I. Study design and baseline data. *Gastrointest Endosc* 1981;**27**: 73–9.

26 Gilbert DA, Silverstein FE, Tedesco FJ, *et al.* The national ASGE survey on upper gastrointestinal bleeding. III. Endoscopy in upper gastrointestinal bleeding. *Gastrointest Endosc* 1981;**27**:94–102.

27 Storey DW, Bown SG, Swain CP, Salmon PR, Kirkham JS, Northfield TC. Endoscopic prediction of recurrent bleeding in peptic ulcers. *N Engl J Med* 1981;**305**:915–6.

28 Berry AR, Collin J, Frostick SP, Dudley N, Morris PJ. Upper gastrointestinal haemorrhage in Oxford. A prospective study. *J R Coll Surg Edin* 1984;**29**:134–8.

29 Himal HS, Watson WW, Jones CW, Miller L, Maclean LD. The management of upper gastrointestinal hemorrhage: a multiparametric computer analysis. *Ann Surg* 1974;**179**: 489–93.

30 Wheatley KE, Dykes PW. Upper gastrointestinal bleeding—when to operate. *Postgrad Med J* 1990;**66**:926–31.

31 Dunnill MGS, Gould SR. Audit of gastrointestinal bleeding in a district general hospital. *BMJ* 1992;**304**:383–4.

32 Clements D. Audit: the crucial role of medical records. *BMJ* 1992;**304**:643.

33 Vellacott KD, Dronfield MW, Atkinson M, Langman MJS. Comparison of surgical and medical management of bleeding peptic ulcers. *BMJ* 1982;**284**:548–50.

34 Silverstein FE, Gilbert DA, Tedesco FJ, *et al.* The national ASGE survey on upper gastrointestinal bleeding. II. Clinical prognostic factors. *Gastrointest Endosc* 1981;**27**:80–93.

35 Report of a joint working group of the British Society of Gastroenterology, the Research Unit of the Royal College of Physicians of London, and the Audit Unit of the Royal College of Surgeons of England. Guidelines for good practice in and audit of the

management of upper gastrointestinal haemorrhage. *J R Coll Physicians Lond* 1992;**26**: 281–9.

36 Rockall TA, Logan RFA, Devlin HB, Northfield TC on behalf of the steering committee and members of the National Audit of Acute Upper Gastrointestinal Haemorrhage. Incidence of and mortality from acute upper gastrointestinal haemorrhage in the United Kingdom. *BMJ* 1995;**311**:222–6.

37 Rockall TA, Logan RFA, Derin HB, Northfield TC on behalf of the Steering Committee Members of the National Audit of Acute Upper Gastrointestinal Haemorrhage. Influencing practice and outcome in acute upper gastrointestinal haemorrhage (in preparation).

38 Spiller RC, Parkins RA. Recurrent gastrointestinal bleeding of obscure origin: report of 17 cases and a logical guide to management. *Br J Surg* 1983;**70**:489–93.

39 Thompson JN, Salem RR, Hemingway AP, *et al.* Specialist investigation of obscure gastrointestinal bleeding. *Gut* 1987;**28**:47–51.

40 Lau WY, Fan ST, Wong SH, *et al.* Preoperative and intraoperative localisation of gastrointestinal bleeding of obscure origin. *Gut* 1987;**28**:869–77.

41 Lewis BS, Waye JD. Chronic gastrointestinal bleeding of obscure origin: role of small bowel enteroscopy. *Gastroenterology* 1988;**94**:1117–20.

42 Desa LA, Ohri SK, Hutton KAR, Lee H, Spencer J. Role of intraoperative endoscopy in obscure gastrointestinal bleeding of small bowel origin. *Br J Surg* 1991;**78**:192–5.

43 Morris AJ, Wasson LA, MacKenzie JF. Small bowel enteroscopy in undiagnosed gastrointestinal blood loss. *Gut* 1992;**33**:887–9.

44 Cook IJ, Pavli P, Riley JW, Goulson KJ, Dent OF. Gastrointestinal investigation of iron deficiency anaemia. *BMJ* 1986;**292**:1380–2.

45 Rockey DC, Cello JP. Evaluation of the gastrointestinal tract in patients with iron-deficiency anaemia. *N Engl J Med* 1993;**329**:1691–5.

46 McIntyre AS, Long RG. Prospective survey of investigations in outpatients referred with iron deficiency anaemia. *Gut* 1993;**34**:1102–7.

47 Fagan PA. The "red herring" barium meal x-ray examination in carcinoma of the right side of the colon. *Med J Aust* 1969;**i**:276–7.

48 Bannerman RM, Beveridge BR, Witts LJ. Anaemia associated with unexplained occult blood loss. *BMJ* 1964;**i**:1417–9.

49 Sahay R, Scott BB. Iron deficiency anaemia—how far to investigate? *Gut* 1993;**34**:1427–8.

50 Sacks HS, Chalmers TC, Blum AL, Berrier J, Pagano D. Endoscopic hemostasis. An effective therapy for bleeding peptic ulcers. *JAMA* 1990;**264**:494–9.

51 Cook DJ, Guyatt GH, Salena BJ, Laine LA. Endoscopic therapy for acute nonvariceal upper gastrointestinal hemorrhage: a meta-analysis. *Gastroenterology* 1992;**102**:139–48.

52 Lam SK, Lai KC. Endoscopic haemostasis for gastrointestinal bleeding: the dawning of a new era. *J Gastroenterol Hepatol* 1994;**9**:69–74.

53 Watson RGP, Porter KG. An audit of hospital admissions for acute upper gastrointestinal haemorrhage. *Ulster Med J* 1989;**58**:140–4.

54 Villanueva C, Balanzo J, Espinos JC, *et al.* Prediction of therapeutic failure in patients with bleeding peptic ulcer treated with endoscopic injection. *Dig Dis Sci* 1993;**38**:2062–70.

55 Williams RA, Vartany A, Davis IP, Wilson SE. Impact of endoscopic therapy on outcome of operation for bleeding peptic ulcers. *Am J Surg* 1993;**166**:712–5.

56 Qvist P, Arnesen KE, Jacobsen CD, Rosseland AR. Endoscopic treatment and restrictive surgical policy in the management of peptic ulcer bleeding. Five years' experience in a central hospital. *Scand J Gastroenterol* 1994;**29**:569–76.

57 Palmer KR, Choudari CP. Endoscopic intervention in bleeding peptic ulcer. *Gut* 1995;**37**:161–4.

58 Loperfido S, Monica F, Maifreni L, *et al.* Bleeding peptic ulcer occurring in hospitalized patients: analysis of predictive and risk factors and comparison with out-of-hospital onset of hemorrhage. *Dig Dis Sci* 1994;**39**:698–705.

23: Overview and conclusions

NEVILLE KRASNER

Patients admitted to hospital with gastrointestinal haemorrhage account for about 8% of the acute medical intake in the UK. The annual admission rate which has stood at about 50 per 100 000 population for more than 30 years[1-3] is, in the 1990s, 103 per 100 000;[4] around 14% of this figure represents bleeds occurring in established inpatients. The latter is a high risk group with a mortality of 33%; of the acute admissions, 11% succumb, a proportion that might suggest advances in endoscopy and radiology, both in diagnosis and therapy, to have had no significant impact on mortality. However, in the absence of malignancy or organ failure the National Audit of acute gastrointestinal bleeding reports a mortality rate in those aged less than 60 years of only 1·3%. The steep increase in mortality that is associated with advancing age and co-morbidity is compounded by the ingestion of non-steroidal anti-inflammatory drugs (NSAIDs); it is likely that about one-third of all patients over the age of 60 years who are admitted with upper gastrointestinal bleeding will have taken one of these preparations.[5]

Peptic ulceration remains the single most common cause of upper gastrointestinal bleeding on both sides of the Atlantic. There is general acceptance of the causative role of *Helicobacter pylori* infection in the development of peptic ulceration and it is further recognised that the prevalence of *H. pylori* infection increases with age. It might be reasonable to assume, therefore, that the presence of *H. pylori* is a major contributor to NSAID related haemorrhage. Current data, however, suggest that NSAIDs and *H. pylori* are independent risk factors for ulcer bleeding.

Approximately 80% of patients with upper gastrointestinal haemorrhage will stop bleeding spontaneously. The endoscopic identification of those most at risk from continued bleeding has helped concentrate efforts on those most in need of therapeutic endoscopy or treatment via interventional radiology. Conventional wisdom requires an endoscopy to be performed on all "bleeders" within 24 to 48 h of admission and certainly before discharge from hospital; this inevitably places additional strains on already hard pressed endoscopy services. An audit conducted by Whatley and colleagues[6] suggested that haemodynamically stable patients, with "coffee grounds" haematemesis and a haemoglobin concentration of greater than

100 g/l, could be discharged immediately on a proton pump inhibitor and have endoscopy arranged on an outpatient basis. Patients with a haemoglobin of less than 100 g/l and showing clinical evidence of active bleeding require resuscitation and consideration for urgent endoscopy.

While several endoscopic stigmata of recent bleeding have been described, only the visible vessel protruding from the ulcer base carries prognostic significance, with a rebleeding rate of nearly 60%.[7] Presence of a visible vessel or active bleeding, rather than oozing, from an ulcer requires active intervention by endoscopic methods or arterial embolisation; if these methods do not effect rapid haemostasis, timely surgical intervention is required. Therapeutic endoscopy encompasses an ever expanding array of methods to stop ulcer bleeding, some fascinating in their ingenuity and attractive because of their very simplicity. Injection therapy includes the instillation of 1 in 10 000 or 1 in 100 000 adrenaline, with or without a sclerosant, the use of tissue adhesives, and clot promoting agents (fibrin sealants). Thermal methods of inducing haemostasis involve the application of heater probes, mono- or bipolar electrodes and Nd:YAG or more recently Aluminium Gallium Arsenide (AlGaAs) diode lasers. The newest techniques include the application of clips and an endoscopic "sewing machine". In terms of efficacy, there is little to choose between the technologies. However, the considerable expense of lasers limits their widespread availability and injection therapy with adrenaline seems the most cost effective option. Injection of sclerosant and thermal methods can also be used in the management of vascular malformations, in both the upper and lower gastrointestinal tract, from angiomatous lesions to telangiectasia or angiodysplasia; lasers are particularly useful for this indication. More inaccessible lesions such as angiodysplasia in the small bowel have also proved amenable to heater probe therapy, via push enteroscopy.[8]

Traditionally, where the endoscopic service is run primarily by physicians, the latter assume responsibility for the initial management of patients with upper gastrointestinal bleeding. Although H_2 receptor antagonists and the newer, proton pump inhibitors undoubtedly promote and accelerate ulcer healing, they have not been clearly shown to have any direct influence on the bleeding process, whether in peptic ulcer disease, erosions or other causes of upper gastrointestinal haemorrhage. The application of therapeutic endoscopy has allowed physician gastroenterologists a glimpse into the realms of minimal access surgery, and they have been ready to take up the challenge. Nevertheless, a team approach is essential to the management of acute bleeding problems, and early recourse must be made to a surgical opinion. This in no way commits either the surgeon or the patient to an operation, but allows an early assessment of the surgical options if conservative methods of treatment fail. For example, a bleeding site identified endoscopically may prove inaccessible to the therapeutic modality being applied. Embolisation may be life-saving in this situation. Whether patients are best managed in a specialised bleeding unit remains a subject for debate, but the essence of good management is early assessment, the maintenance of vital signs and the rapid institution of supportive measures.

Bleeding from oesophageal varices carries the highest mortality rate of common conditions presenting with acute upper gastrointestinal haemorrhage. Advances have been made in pharmacological treatment with vasopressin analogues with or without nitrates, and with synthetic somatostatin derivatives, but these agents, combined if necessary with mechanical tamponade, serve mainly to buy time that allows the safe endoscopic application of injection sclerotherapy, ligating bands or clips. Beta blockers have not realised their initial promise in the management of varices; although they may reduce somewhat the risk of bleeding or rebleeding, there is no convincing evidence of any reduction in mortality rates.[9] Congestive gastropathy appears to occur more often in patients whose varices have been treated with sclerotherapy.[10] Beta blockers may prove to be more useful in this situation.

It is the onset of hepatic coma that is more often responsible for death from bleeding from oesophageal or gastric varices than the bleeding episode itself, so there is a prime need for early and accurate diagnosis, urgent and active treatment, and vigilant monitoring. In the past, when conservative methods failed to arrest variceal haemorrhage, there was little recourse but to refer the patient for portosystemic shunt surgery, which has a distressingly high mortality rate in all but the elective procedure. However, an ingenious minimal access technique, available as yet in only a few centres, has opened new avenues in the management of uncontrolled variceal bleeding. Insertion of an expanding metal mesh stent to produce a portosystemic shunt by the transjugular intrahepatic route—the TIPS procedure—gains time to allow the patient to be fully resuscitated and prepared for the major surgical undertaking of liver transplantation. It offers also the prospect of helping to establish, in patients who have symptoms relating primarily to portal hypertension, suitability for formal shunt surgery: the circle has turned fully.

Acute lower gastrointestinal bleeding is usually defined as bleeding from lesions distal to the ligament of Treitz. Although much less attention is paid to such bleeding than to its upper counterpart, and best estimates suggest that it represents only about 20% or about 6000 cases annually, the incidence may be substantially higher. The issue is further complicated by the proportion of rectal bleeding episodes that originate from the upper rather than the lower gastrointestinal tract. If rapid, high volume bleeding occurs from an upper lesion, then blood passed per rectum may be unaltered; such patients are likely to present with shock, a scenario uncommon with an acute left sided colonic bleed. Information of the kind we have on upper gastrointestinal bleeding[11] is not available or perhaps in prospect for bleeding problems from the lower gut. It is generally assumed that severe lower gastrointestinal haemorrhage is uncommon and that transfusion is not usually required. Nevertheless, a recent Scandinavian series showed a mortality rate of 4%, and in 17% of the cases included, the cause of the bleeding remained unclear.[12]

Bleeding of rectal origin is more common in patients under 50 years of age, whereas a left colonic site and diverticular disease are more frequent in those over 70 years. While acute massive lower gastrointestinal bleeding is more likely to occur from a benign than a malignant lesion as a potentially life threatening condition it requires a full range of diagnostic and treatment facilities. Carcinoma of the colon, diverticular disease and angiodysplasia account for most cases of bleeding from the lower gut. Colonoscopy and selective angiography have enabled the localisation of angiodysplastic lesions; these are found mainly in elderly subjects in the ascending colon and caecum, and while they are usually responsible for occult bleeding, leading in some cases to profound anaemia, they occasionally present with significant acute bleeding. Angiodysplasia also occurs in younger individuals, where it is most commonly encountered in the stomach and small bowel and is best identified with some form of angiography. Identification by small bowel enteroscopy is effective but this technique is not widely available. The value of radionuclide scanning, using sulphur colloid or red blood cells labelled with $^{99}Tc^m$, is restricted by the requirement for active bleeding at the time of investigation. Many of the causes of gastrointestinal bleeding are common to all age groups, but the conditions and presentations specific to infancy and the neonatal period, and the impracticability of managing young children in adult wards, usually requires referral to tertiary centres. The principles of resuscitation, investigation and management remain universally applicable.

The rate of haemorrhage and the site of the source determine the character of blood loss from the lower gut. Patients with brisk haemorrhage and those with distal lesions tend to pass red blood while more gentle bleeding or that from the proximal colon leads to the passage of dark red blood mixed with faeces. Melaena may result from angiodysplasia in the ascending colon or caecum rather than from, for instance, bleeding peptic ulceration. Colonoscopy offers greater diagnostic accuracy than barium contrast radiology, as well as the therapeutic potential of snare cautery, electrocoagulation, injection or laser therapy. Furthermore, retained barium within bowel loops may interfere at subsequent angiography. Interventional radiology has undoubtedly expanded diagnostic and therapeutic options in the management of gastrointestinal bleeding. The ultimate resort in cases of major bleeding from the lower gastrointestinal tract is on-table lavage of the bowel with intraoperative colonoscopy if the patient can be maintained in a stable condition during the procedure. If bleeding continues and a site can not be identified, subtotal colectomy with ileorectal anastomosis may be the only option.

Haemorrhoids remain the most prominent cause of overt chronic bleeding, and while in most cases the origin is idiopathic and benign, full bowel investigations are necessary to exclude treatable causes. For all the sophistication of modern surgical and endoscopic techniques, band ligation and injection remain the most effective management for all except the largest of haemorrhoids.

Occult blood loss from the lower bowel should be an important indicator of potentially serious pathology and yet we still lack a sensitive, specific test that can be used reliably in colonic cancer screening programmes. Such screening can, and perhaps should, be organised from the primary care setting, where the performance of rigid sigmoidoscopy at least could be more widespread and some practitioners have introduced flexible sigmoidoscopy. Considerable debate surrounds the issue of endoscopy in general practice, but it is clearly not a practical alternative when there is acute bleeding, whether from the upper or lower gastrointestinal tract. Endoscopic screening for colonic polyps or overt tumours remains controversial, and presents major logistic problems. While overt bleeding from the lower gut usually requires endoscopic investigation, unexplained anaemia demands surveillance of all accessible areas within reach of the endoscope; it is not uncommon for dual pathology to exist. Diagnosing a hiatus hernia or mucosal erosions in the stomach or duodenum does not help the patient with occult colonic malignancy. The old adage that "if you don't put your finger in, you will put your foot in it" emphasises the need for rectal examination in the diagnosis of rectal malignancy: it is sound advice for all clinicians, and not just for students.

Why does the mortality from gastrointestinal haemorrhage remain, apparently, at such an unacceptable level? The problems and pitfalls of audit are well illustrated in Chapter 22. The relative reluctance, in the UK and elsewhere, to undertake studies on the prevalence of lower gastrointestinal bleeding accounts for the paucity of reliable information in this area, while a lack of uniform protocols and specific parameters to study confound accurate audit on the management of haemorrhage from the upper gastrointestinal tract. The use of endoscopy has revolutionised the diagnostic and therapeutic opportunities, but there remains much debate about the optimum timing of the procedure. Medical/surgical co-operation is an accepted tenet of the management of gastrointestinal bleeding, but its implementation is at best patchy and sometimes unnecessarily delayed by the enthusiasm of medical gastroenterologists for pursuing endoscopic therapeutic options. Monitoring the volume of blood transfused might be considered a valuable guide to best timing for surgery, but what might reasonably be considered as a "high risk indicator" is far from being universally applied.

The role of dedicated, high dependency units in the management of gastrointestinal bleeding is a further topic of unresolved debate. While in one such unit in Glasgow, a reduced mortality rate from ulcer haemorrhage was demonstrated,[13] a European study proposed that the major efforts of a specialised gastrointestinal team would be best directed at reducing the morbidity associated with acute bleeding and the overall cost of care.[14] We should be aware also that the resources available both with regard to staff and equipment in teaching hospitals and major district general hospitals provides the opportunities for management of patients which may not be available in smaller units. It is probable that an overall mortality in the region of 5% is approaching the lowest that would be obtained in an unselected series of patients with gastrointestinal haemorrhage. Future studies should therefore be directed at the most cost effective and beneficial management strategies for both upper and lower gastrointestinal bleeding, whether acute or chronic, overt or occult, that can be widely applied in any hospital setting.

References

1 Rockall TA, Logan RFA, Devlin HB, Northfield TC. Proceedings of the British Society of Gastroenterology, September 1994, Abstract: GUT Suppl. S47, T188.

2 Allen R, Dykes P. A study of the factors influencing mortality rates from gastrointestinal haemorrhage. *Quart J Med* 1976;**45**:533–50.

3 Dronfield MW, Langman MJS, Atkinson M, *et al*. Outcome for endoscopy and barium radiology for acute upper gastrointestinal bleed; controlled trial in 1037 patients. *BMJ* 1982;**284**:545–8.

4 Madden MV, Griffiths GH. Management of upper gastrointestinal haemorrhage in a district general hospital. *J R Coll Physicians Lond* 1986;**20**:212–5.

5 Dronfield MW. Upper gastrointestinal bleeding. In: *Diseases of the gut and pancreas*. Vol I. Oxford: Blackwell Scientific, 1994;370.

6 Whatley G, Khan A, Loft DE, Nwokolo CU. Does dark-blood (coffee grounds) haematemesis predict a good prognosis in upper gastrointestinal haemorrhage [abstract]. *Gut* 1994; suppl 5,S35,S59,F236.

7 Swain CP, Story DW, Bown SG, *et al*. Nature of the bleeding vessel in recurrently bleeding gastric ulcers. *Gastroenterology* 1986;**90**:595–608.

8 Morris AJ, Mokhasi M, McKenzie JF. Push enteroscopy and heater probe therapy for small bowel bleeding [abstract]. *Gut* 1994;suppl 5,35,S36,T144.

9 Richter GM, Noeldge G, Palmaz JC, *et al*. The transjugular intrahepatic porto-systemic shunt (TIPSS); the results of a pilot study. *Cardiovasc Intervent Radiol* 1990;**13**:200–7.

10 McCormack TT, Simms J, Eyre-Brooke I, *et al*. Gastric lesions in portal hypertension; inflammatory gastritis or congestive gastropathy? *Gut* 1985;**26**:1226–32.

11 Rockall TA, Logan RFA, Devlin HB, Northfield TC. Incidence of and mortality from acute upper gastrointestinal haemorrhage in the United Kingdom. *BMJ* 1995;**311**:222–6.

12 Mäkelä JT, Kiviniemi H, Laitinen F, Kairaluoma MJ. Diagnosis and treatment of acute lower gastrointestinal bleeding. *Scand J Gastroenterol* 1993;**28**:1062–6.

13 Murray WR, Birnie CG. Special units for acute upper gastrointestinal bleeding. *BMJ* 1987;**295**:31–2.

14 Jostout CJ, Wang KK, Ahlquist DA, *et al*. Acute gastrointestinal bleeding. Experiences of a specialised management team. *J Clin Gastroenterol* 1992;**14**:260–7.

Index

Page numbers in **bold type** refer to figures; those in *italic* refer to tables or boxed material.

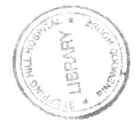
**This book is to be returned on or before
the last date stamped below.**

26 MAR 2012

11 JUL 2003

21 JUL 2003

0 2 OCT 2003

22 AUG 2008

28 JAN 2011